HEARING
AND DEAFNESS

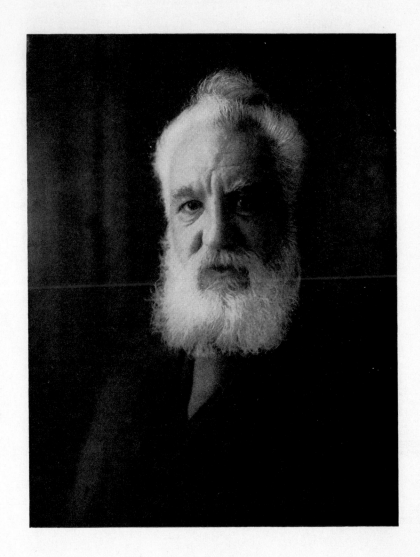

To the memory of

ALEXANDER GRAHAM BELL

A versatile genius, inventor, scientist, teacher of speech, and organizer, he invented the telephone, from which later grew the electric hearing aid. His scientific genius and his humanitarian spirit epitomize the ideals of audiology.

HEARING AND DEAFNESS

EDITED BY *Hallowell Davis, M.D.*

COEDITOR FOR THE REVISED EDITION
S. Richard Silverman, Ph.D.

REVISED EDITION

Holt, Rinehart and Winston, Inc.
NEW YORK

October, 1961

CONTENTS

APPENDIX

THE EDITORS' FOREWORD
TO THE REVISED EDITION

More than eleven years have elapsed since the publication of the first edition of this book. Our friends still seem to find it useful, but they have told us with increasing insistence that several sections of that first edition were out of date and also that the book would be more useful if it contained certain new material or more detail on some of the old. On the other hand, we believe that the main substance of the book is still sound and that the need for a guide to audiology still exists among laymen with impaired hearing themselves or with children, relatives, or friends who are deaf or hard of hearing. Somewhat to our surprise our book has proved most popular and useful as an introductory textbook for students of audiology. When the book was written in 1946 there were almost no such students! Since that time, however, several of the authors have themselves recommended the book to their own students and to teachers in training.

Many of the additions in this second edition have been provided particularly for the benefit of beginning students of audiology. Hence the omission, from this edition, of the original subtitle, "A Guide for Laymen." We have retained, nevertheless, the original organization and, as far as possible, our original statements and language. One important change is the introduction of several rather new terms, such as "hearing level," that we have found useful in our teaching and writing and that we hope will be adopted generally. We hope that with the changes and new additions our book will continue to be helpful to students and laymen alike.

In Chapter 1 is a brief summary of the contents of each of the later chapters. The original statements remain virtually unchanged, but to each we have added new paragraphs that tell what has been added or how the material has been rearranged. Actually, very little that was included in the first edition has been omitted except for some out-of-date details concerning hearing aids and the chapter on military aural rehabilitation.

Our original group of authors remains almost intact. We have lost Dr. Helmer Myklebust, but in his place Mr. Boyce R. Williams, who is Consultant (Deaf and the Hard of Hearing) in the Office of Vocational Rehabilitation of the Department of Health, Education, and Welfare, has written a new chapter on vocational guidance for the deaf. We have omitted the chapter on military aural rehabilitation and thus have lost Drs. Norton Canfield and Leslie Morrissett. In their stead Dr. Bernard M. Anderman, Chief, Audiology and Speech Correction, of the Department of Medicine and Surgery of the Veterans Administration, describes the VA program in audiology. Professors E. P. Fowler, Jr., M. D. Pauls, and T. E. Walsh, and Mr. S. Gordon Taylor have revised their chapters from the first edition. Miss Betty Wright, Dr. Raymond Carhart, and Dr. Donald Ramsdell did not add any new material. The minor changes in their chapters were made by Miss Ada M. Hill, Dr. S. R. Silverman, and Dr. H. Davis respectively. Our new collaborators are Dr. Robert Goldstein, of Washington University, and Dr. Donald G. Doehring, of the research staff at Central Institute for the Deaf.

For criticism of our revisions and additions we thank particularly Drs. Ira J. Hirsh, Jerome R. Cox, Jr., Donald H. Eldredge, Irvin Shore, and Frank R. Kleffner, all of whom are members of the staff of Central Institute for the Deaf. For valuable comments on Chapters 4, 5, and 6 we are indebted to Dr. Ben H. Senturia. Dr. S. Richard Silverman, the coeditor of this revised edition, has taken the primary responsibility for the last three sections, which deal with rehabilitation, education, psychology, and economic and social problems, and has shared the responsibility for the chapters on hearing aids.

For the many new drawings as well as for the revision or modification of several earlier ones we are grateful to Mr. Joseph Odenbach.

HALLOWELL DAVIS
S. RICHARD SILVERMAN

St. Louis, Missouri
January, 1960

FOREWORD TO THE
FIRST EDITION

Granted that the first handicap of deafness lies in communication, it has often seemed to me that a close second might be the attitude of hearing people toward it and that the former would be considerably lessened if we could do something to improve the latter.

Man's need for communication with his fellow man is possibly his greatest need and the fulfillment of his other needs and desires is largely dependent upon, or at the last greatly facilitated by, his ability to satisfy this basic one. The development of language, both spoken and written, as a means of communication is one of mankind's greatest achievements. Yet, because from birth we hearing people effortlessly, almost unconsciously, have *absorbed* this magnificent tool simply because we are lucky enough to hear, we take it very much for granted and tend to belittle, to shun, or to look somewhat askance at anyone who has had to fashion, bit by bit, word by word, sound by sound, a workable, even though imperfect, language tool for himself.

By turns I have been amused, annoyed, angry, and frustrated by this attitude and its various manifestations. However, I have tried to remind myself that people are like this because they don't know any better. Some thought and perhaps a little effort often *are* required to understand the speech and to follow the language of a deaf or severely hard-of-hearing person. It often *does* entail more attention than we usually give to our casual conversations to enable the deaf or hard-of-hearing person, who must depend mainly upon our lip movements, to understand what we are saying. I find very few people who are willing to give this attention or make this effort. Perhaps most people's impatience, even their rudeness, is partly due to this too swiftly paced, this tabloid, he-who-runs-may-read age and partly to a natural laziness of mind. However, I believe a great deal of it is due to almost complete lack of understanding of the problems faced by those with a

xi

hearing loss and to the narrowness and fear and insecurity bred of ignorance.

There is no other subject that vitally affects the lives of so many people on which there is so little positive information and so much fuzzy and widespread misinformation and misunderstanding. I doubt if over five per cent of our population has ever read anything authentic on the deaf or the hard of hearing. And yet the impression that the deaf have no vocal chords and so cannot speak is widespread. It might surprise you to know how many people ask if the deaf learn to read Braille.

A great many of the misconceptions concerning the deaf undoubtedly can be traced to that inaccurate and unfortunate term "deaf and dumb." The implications it has given rise to in the minds of generations of hearing children and the attitudes it has engendered, not to mention the devastation it has caused in the hearts of parents, are incalculable. Fortified with those words alone, many people are almost determined in their belief that the totally deaf cannot possibly speak.

Education for the deaf, speech reading, and speech are not new. Speech has been taught in this country for close to a century. And yet, accurate, not to mention easy-to-read, articles or books for the layman, this fellow whom we must reach, whose attitudes we must change, are so few as to be almost non-existent. I often have said that educators of the deaf talk to other educators of the deaf, write for other educators of the deaf in magazines for educators of the deaf and nothing reaches the layman—the layman who one day may be the totally unprepared mother or father of a little deaf baby, the layman who himself may become deaf or hard of hearing.

So my spirits leapt when I read the title of this book, *Hearing and Deafness: A Guide for Laymen.* Here at last is information, correct, easy to read, covering nearly every phase of the problem in a manner suited to that numerically large and needy group of people—laymen.

Hearing and Deafness should do much to change an attitude and, in consequence, be the means of greatly lessening the handicap of deafness.

I feel very honored and happy to be able to have even such a small finger in this notable work.

LOUISE TRACY

The John Tracy Clinic
Los Angeles, California
August, 1947

INTRODUCTION TO
THE FIRST EDITION

If there is another book which fulfills the aims and purposes of this one, I have not seen it. In my opinion the resolution of the editor

. . . to answer the thousand and one questions that are continually being asked by all sorts of people about the nature of hearing and the problem of deafness, . . .

has been most effectually carried out.

When one desires to read something concerning his own problem, he turns naturally to pertinent articles that are easy to get and simple to understand. A large number of such writings on the treatment of deafness has recently appeared in some of our popular magazines. These commentaries, written ostensibly in an informative vein but produced plainly for "reader appeal," were composed by professional lay writers who have constantly before them two cardinal questions in journalism: (1) Is it new or unusual? and (2) Does it have human or dramatic appeal?

These articles, semi-scientific in character but produced in journalistic style and given extensive circulation, seem to have aroused in an untold number of persons an interest in their deafness that long had remained dormant, and that never would have been so completely stimulated, had it not been for the journalist and his manner of writing.

Similarly, new interests in the problems of deafness, new operations to restore hearing, new electrical apparatus to give more perfect sound reception to improperly functioning ears, new methods of ensuring the preservation of speech, and a new understanding of the mental attributes of the hard of hearing have made almost mandatory the publication of an up-to-date, authoritative, and comprehensible reference work that covers the field of *audiology* both as a textbook and as a guide.

Hearing and Deafness: A Guide for Laymen is just such a text. Not without a dash of the "new and unusual" and not without its human appeal, this "guide" contains factual and instructive discussions of various phases of audiology. In the early pages we are informed that the sequence of chapters is "from inanimate nature to the individual human to complex social problems" and that in spite of this shift "there is one theme that runs evenly throughout the book." That theme, we are told, is *psychology.* Unquestionably, this topic reaches its climax when we are enlightened concerning the importance of "auditory backgrounds" which are responsible for that "comfortable sense-of-being-a-part-of-a-living-active-world," and also when we recognize the significance of the *three psychological levels of hearing.* Furthermore, suspicion, so characteristic a feature of the hard of hearing, is admirably discussed and is a matter that should be thoroughly understood by all deafened persons who retain it.

Every otologist, every teacher of the deaf, every social worker, every chapter of the American Hearing Society, and every other person "concerned with auditory rehabilitation or with the conservation of hearing" should welcome the publication of this book, for in what other compact form can one find reliable answers to such questions as (1) "Why did I lose my hearing?" (2) "Is my deafness bad enough to require the use of a hearing aid?" (3) "Should I buy a bone or air conduction instrument?" and (4) "In which ear should I wear the 'aid'?"

Or if the problem involves a congenitally deaf child, we have replies to such queries as (1) "Why doesn't my child talk?" (2) "Will he be able to talk?" and (3) "What about his education?"

Among the other "thousand and one questions that are continually being asked" and that have received such impressive answers are (1) "Why do I hear a buzzer when I cannot hear a doorbell or telephone?" (2) "Will the fenestration operation cure my deafness?" (3) "Does industry discriminate against the hard of hearing?" (4) "Why do people stop talking when I come into the room?" and (5) "Why does the intense stillness so depress me?"

Further perusing the pages of this work, we become interested in the variations of normal hearing, and in finding out just what Miss Brown, Mr. Jones, and Mrs. Smith can expect from the use of a hearing aid. And while the mechanically minded inquirers are running their fingers up and down the "Cause, Test and Remedy" columns of the "Troubleshooting Chart," and as the speech-reading class is memorizing the twelve suggestions for "ease of communication," the daring among us are venturing to trespass upon that special preserve where the more erudite disquisitions are lurking.

Surely this work, so extensive in scope, so practical in application and so expert in composition will serve a real need. Conceived, as it is, in the spirit of altruism and occupying, as it does, a niche not held by any other work, it deserves highest commendation and should be in the hands of all the thousands upon thousands of those who ask the questions and want to get the correct answers.

C. STEWART NASH, *President*
American Hearing Society

Rochester, New York
September 5, 1947

THE EDITOR'S FOREWORD
TO THE FIRST EDITION

This book is written for the deaf and the hard of hearing and for their families, their parents, their teachers, and their friends. It is written for physicians, for educators, for social workers, and for all who are concerned with the conservation or improvement of remaining hearing or with the approach to normal living for those who have suffered either complete or partial hearing loss. It is written to answer the thousand and one questions that are continually being asked by all sorts of people about the nature of hearing and the problems posed by partial or complete loss of hearing. Many of us who are concerned primarily with these problems have been so besieged with questions over the years that writing this book is perhaps partly a gesture of self-defense. More important, however, we feel that the flood of questions in itself shows the need for and justifies the book.

The reasons for the multiple authorship are explained in the first chapter, but they can be summed up in seven words: *No one person knows all the answers.* The first chapter also discusses the field of "Audiology," which the editor and contributors as a group represent. In fact, the field is well defined by our Table of Contents. The first chapter also contains some information that traditionally belongs in an Introduction—about why the book is written the way it is; and, to assist readers with special interests, there is a paragraph of comment, or preview, of each chapter. In a book that covers such a wide range of subject matter, we think that such a preview will be more useful than any attempt at a final summary.

The authors of the various chapters are listed in the Table of Contents, and their qualifications are indicated by their academic and professional degrees and by the positions that they have held or now hold in organizations and institutes for the hard of hearing and the deaf, in medical schools, in universities, or in the Army and the Navy.

Former, as well as present, positions are included in order to show the breadth of perspective and experience that they represent as a group. The editor believes that this group, acquainted for years with problems of hearing and deafness, best knows what problems are important for those afflicted with loss of hearing and are therefore most able to write with authority about them.

Miss Wright and Miss Hill are among the well-known members of the executive staff of the American Hearing Society, and most of the other contributors have been engaged throughout their professional careers either as otologists or as teachers of the deaf or the hard of hearing. During World War II many of them performed special tasks in relation to problems of the ear or in programs for auditory rehabilitation. Drs. Canfield, Carhart, Fowler, and Morrissett, and Miss Pauls were in uniform. Dr. Ramsdell was a member of one of the Aural Rehabilitation Units, and Drs. Lane and Silverman, as well as the editor, worked on related research projects under the National Defense Research Committee.

All the authors write from their experience, and several of them present some of the specific results of war work on impaired hearing and related problems. One of the objectives of the book is to combine recent war experiences with previous knowledge and give an up-to-date and authoritative survey of what we now call "audiology." Unfortunately, not all of the able contributors to recent knowledge could be included as authors, but we hope that our accounts give adequate representation of current views, either by direct reference or by the modification of the contributors' personal ideas. The emphasis on one of the Army Rehabilitation Centers, for example, by selection of authors, is the result of a combination of circumstances and is by no means a reflection on the important work of the competent personnel of the other units.

Both the contributors and the editor have been assisted by several able critics who have read one or more chapters, offered suggestions, corrected errors, and sometimes even composed differences of opinion between authors. Among these good friends and silent partners we thank particularly Dr. John R. Lindsay, Professor of Otolaryngology at the University of Chicago; Professor S. S. Stevens, Director of the Psycho-Acoustic Laboratory at Harvard University; Dr. Harvey Fletcher and Dr. Rudolph Nichols of the Bell Telephone Laboratories; and Dr. Powrie V. Doctor, Professor of English and History at Gallaudet College and Assistant Editor of the *American Annals of the Deaf*. Our debt to Dr. Doctor is especially great. He has reviewed no less than six of our chapters and has offered innumerable constructive comments and suggestions.

We also thank our friends the manufacturers of hearing aids for their cooperation in furnishing information and for the many illustrations that they have provided. Two individuals, Dr. Fred W. Kranz of the Sonotone Corporation and William E. Snodgrass of Western Electric Company, have been particularly helpful in this respect. Unfortunately, the practical problems of publication have made it impossible to use all of the wealth of illustrative material made available by many manufacturers. The specific credits for the illustrations finally chosen are listed where the pictures appear, but to all we give our thanks.

For the new anatomical drawings we were fortunate to obtain the assistance of Alfred Feinberg, who has long been an expert illustrator of the ear. His artistic talents and anatomical knowledge have added materially to the presentation of the anatomical, medical, and surgical material. And, finally, the editor is also grateful to Miss Violet M. Alford for her patient typing and retyping of mangled manuscript during the successive revisions of many chapters.

HALLOWELL DAVIS

St. Louis, Missouri
September, 1947

PART 1

AUDIOLOGY

AUDIOLOGY: A MEETING OF VARIED SPECIALISTS

Hallowell Davis, M.D.

You who read this book may be deaf yourself; or perhaps your hearing is not as keen as it used to be; or you may have a parent or a friend whose hearing is failing. Possibly your child is deaf and needs special teaching so that he may understand and be understood. Imperfect hearing is so common that sooner or later it comes close to everyone. Perhaps you are beginning your training to become a professional audiologist. But, whether you want to help yourself or want to help others, or are merely curious, you want to know what can go wrong with hearing and what can be done about it.

Five hundred years ago you might have consulted for guidance the writings of St. Albertus Magnus, teacher of Thomas Aquinas and the dominant figure in Latin learning and natural science of the thirteenth century, who wrote: "Lion's brain, if eaten, causes madness; but remedies deafness, if inserted in the ear with some strong oil." [1] And another widely respected authority, St. Hildegard of Bingen (about 1125), held that "deafness may be remedied by cutting off a lion's right ear and holding it over the patient's ear just long enough to say, 'Hear, *adimacus,* by the living God and the keen virtue of a lion's hearing,'" and that "the heart of a weasel, dried and placed with wax in the ear, benefits headache or deafness." [2]

Audiology

This book not only attempts to guide a student in problems relating to hearing and deafness. It also gives a survey of a general field of knowledge and of social endeavor centering around hearing.

[1] Lynn Thorndike, *A History of Magic and Experimental Science* (New York: Columbia University Press, 1923), II, 561.
[2] *Ibid.,* pp. 145–146.

"Audiology," meaning the science of hearing, seems to be a useful name for this field, even though linguistic purists may object to adding a Greek suffix to a Latin root. The word is probably inevitable. We shall use it in a very broad sense. For some purposes it may be helpful to speak more specifically of "medical audiology" when medical aspects of impaired hearing are our primary concern. The government use of the term (as in the title "Consultant in Audiology") is in a definitely medical context. It is particularly useful here, however, because it indicates an interest in the *function* of the ear, and not only in *diseases* of the ear. The diseases of the ear, the recognized province of *otology*, may be a threat to life, and hearing then becomes secondary. *Audiology* considers the ear as an *aid* to life.

Since 1946 audiology has become a profession as well as an area of knowledge. Numerous "clinical audiologists" are engaged in testing hearing in hospitals, in special clinics and other institutions, and in private offices. Many of these men and women are members of the American Speech and Hearing Association. This association has established a Committee on Clinical Certification which sets examinations in Hearing and issues certificates of qualification both in Speech and in Hearing. It is, as a matter of fact, to students beginning their preparation for the profession of audiology that the second edition of this book is primarily addressed.

Clinical audiologists test hearing and may make recommendations concerning the use and choice of hearing aids. They do not, however, sell hearing aids. As a matter of fact, according to the code of ethics of the American Speech and Hearing Association, it is considered unethical for a member to engage directly in the sale of hearing aids or even to test hearing in a center that would benefit directly from the sale of a particular hearing aid. The business of distribution and sale of hearing aids is handled by hearing aid dealers.

The development of audiology and specifically of clinical audiology has led to many and serious discussions of the relations of audiology to otology. How far do the rights and responsibilities of the clinical audiologist, with his special training and experience, go— particularly in the directions of making a diagnosis, in recommending the use of a hearing aid, and in planning a course of education or rehabilitation? In the medical area he is clearly dependent on and subordinate to the physician, but other areas are his own. Where is the boundary?

Probably the best statement of a point of view that seems to be more and more widely accepted was drafted in 1955 by a committee, under the cochairmanship of Dr. Gordon Hoople and Dr.

Raymond Carhart, concerned with this problem. The report of this committee has never been published in full, but permission has been granted to reproduce from it the following "statement of orientation."

A Statement of Orientation

We have learned a great deal during the past quarter century about (1) how to measure sound; (2) how to assess hearing; (3) how to study the physiology, biophysics, and psychophysics of the auditory system; (4) how to deal with hearing impairments by surgical or medical means; and (5) how to educate and to re-habilitate persons with impaired hearing. Representatives from many disciplines are now concerned with the facts of hearing and the problems of hearing loss. Their various activities have come to carry the label "audiology."

Audiology is the science of hearing. In other words, audiology is undergirded by the competences and methods of many fields. Among the contributing fields are (1) physics, which studies acoustic events as one manifestation of matter and motion; (2) medicine, which is concerned with the human organism in sickness and health; (3) psychology, which deals with responses of the organism to stimuli; (4) education, which seeks to modify and guide the behavior of the organism; and (5) sociology, which attacks the problems of fitting the individual into his culture. Audiology, then, is not a par-ticular academic discipline of professional activity. It is the mobiliz-ing of professional skills to cope with the phenomena of hearing. Thus, when an individual concentrates his training, his com-petence, and his experience on problems of auditory communica-tion, he is working in the field of audiology. His interest may be to investigate auditory phenomena, his chosen task may be to train others to work in the field, or his goal may be to serve clinically those persons who suffer impaired hearing.

Current emphasis among those who use the term "audiology" is heavily clinical. Consequently, important problems of inter-profes-sional relationships have arisen. Among these is the question of how to achieve optimal inter-action between otologists and clinical audi-ologists, as we shall in this report designate specialists in managing non-medical aspects of auditory impairment.

The two committees agreed that otology and clinical audiology have distinctive yet related tasks. These tasks may be described as follows:

1. Otology has basic responsibility for the biological function of hearing. *It alone rightfully undertakes the work of diagnosing diseases of the ear, of specifying the causation of hearing impairment, and of treating pathologies of the auditory mechanism.*

2. Clinical audiology deals with hearing as a foundation to the

learning and the utilizing of language skills. *The emphasis is upon understanding the social functions of hearing and upon increasing the ability of handicapped individuals to cope with the communicational demands of everyday life.*

3. The two fields share responsibility for jointly planning the proper sequence in management of the individual patient. Information on the patient should be exchanged freely. Moreover, decisions regarding otological management of the patient should always precede decisions on audiological management, since maximal social efficiency can be achieved only after biological function has been restored as fully as possible.

While the public is coming to expect and to demand audiological services, there exists confusion as to the kind of organization under which these services should be made available. One individual, properly qualified, can perform the tasks of both the otologist and the clinical audiologist. However, the majority of otologists have not undertaken personally to perform most audiological services. Instead, they have depended upon a growing group of nonmedical people to do this work. There has been great diversity in the administrative framework through which audiological services have been developed. Audiological activities have quite often been conducted as part of the program of a university Department of Speech, Education, or Psychology. Again, these activities have frequently been organized as a subdivision of a Department of Otolaryngology. Under these circumstances, clinical audiology has been included within the services of departments of rehabilitation, of public health, or within programs for crippled children, within the services of a hospital, or within the private practice of the otolaryngologist. Finally, clinical audiology has been made an independent enterprise in a few instances.

In view of the many ways in which audiological services are being made available, it is probably unwise to specify any particular organizational or administrative pattern as the only proper one. The contemporary situation is furnishing a trial of the effectiveness of the various patterns. We may expect the most desirable organizational practices to evolve only if we avoid premature opinions and encourage sympathetic insight among all those who have a part in the development and administration of programs in clinical audiology.

About the Book

A COOPERATIVE UNDERTAKING

Many books and many magazine articles have been written about sound, about the ear, about speech, about the education of deaf children, and so on. Many of them have been written by a single author and from a single point of view. But no one is really an expert on all of the scientific, social, and practical aspects of hearing. The subject is too broad for that. A complete audiologist would have to be at the same time a biologist, a surgeon, a physicist, a psychologist, a teacher, an expert on speech, a sociologist, and several more "—ists" besides.

The authors have therefore joined together to write this book. No one author is competent to do it alone, for we are all specialists. We have pooled our experience to try to answer your questions. Each of us, in the field he knows best, has tried to distinguish for you the true from the false, and fact from mere theory; and we have tried to strike a proper balance between the important and the unimportant. In distilling a brief survey from the mass of detailed information it has been as difficult to judge what *not* to try to explain as to explain accurately everything that *is* included.

Each of us, of course, has his own personal enthusiasms and point of view, but each has submitted his manuscript to two or more of the other authors for criticisms and suggestions. Many of the chapters have also been read by other experts in special fields. We have often been severe critics of one another's writing, but as a result many ambiguous statements and doubtful points have been eliminated. The responsibility for all statements, however, naturally rests with the author of each chapter and with the editors. Even with our best collective efforts, we cannot hope that the product is perfect, but perhaps a little more collective wisdom has emerged than would have if each of us had written what was in his mind without the benefit of mutual criticism.

In a field so broad as audiology we have had the advantage that we ourselves are laymen as well as specialists. The surgeon does not teach speechreading nor does the psychologist fit hearing aids. In writing for one another, not merely for our colleagues in our own specialties, we hope that we have made ourselves clear to other laymen. We have often been guided in our choice of topics by the very questions that we ask one another when we meet, and we have learned much from one another in preparing this book.

We have tried not to burden the book with unnecessary mathematical or electronic detail or with unnecessary medical terminology; yet we have not stripped down everywhere to words of two syllables. You probably want to learn the meanings of some of the more common professional and technical terms that you will meet elsewhere. Some of you may be students in one of the specialties and want an introduction to other parts of the field. To help you identify and understand the technical terms more readily, the editors have made free use of italics and quotation marks to tag such words when they first appear and where their meaning is explained or can easily be understood from the context. An appendix elaborates many definitions given briefly in the text.

ORGANIZATION

In the table of contents the chapters have been grouped into six sections. From the titles of the sections it is obvious that the general sequence of the book is from physics, biology, medicine, and surgery to modern studies of impaired hearing and hearing aids, and thence to special education and rehabilitation of adults with impaired hearing. The emphasis then shifts to the problems of the education of deaf and hard-of-hearing children, to organized social efforts on behalf of the aurally handicapped, and finally to employment and vocational guidance. In general, the sequence is from inanimate nature to the individual human to complex social problems.

The sequence is probably as familiar as it is arbitrary. It has a disadvantage in that it places some of the more difficult technical chapters first. We hope that readers with educational and social interests (who may well be a majority) will not be discouraged, but will skip boldly to their own territory at once. After all, something has to come first, and the present arrangement has the advantage of explaining basic terms and ideas, such as the decibel and hearing loss, before they are used in other contexts.

But in spite of the shift from physical to biological to social, there is one theme that runs evenly throughout the book. It could not be concentrated in any one place, and nearly every chapter must be read to learn all we have to say about it. That theme is *psychology*. Hearing, our main topic, is certainly a province of psychology. Communication may use physical tools and have social aspects, but it is basically a psychological process. Tests of hearing are also squarely in the province of the psychologist. The reaction of the individual to deafness and the basic problems of self-adjustment, of education, and of vocational guidance are clearly psychological. At first glance, it may seem that psychology has been slighted and that only one chapter deals with a single and rather special aspect of psychology; on the contrary, the entire book is permeated with it. In fact, the psychological aspects of the various sections give our book its unity.

THE DEPTH AND BREADTH OF EACH CHAPTER

Probably few readers will want to read this book from cover to cover. You will each have your own particular interests, and may rightly hesitate about embarking on a chapter in a new area without knowing something more about it than its title discloses. Our chapters are not all equally "deep." Some, such as the chapters on employment opportunities for the hard of hearing and the use of hearing aids, are almost completely nontechnical. They were written directly for hard-of-hearing men and women. Some of the other chapters, such as those dealing with tests of hearing and with the psychology of the deafened adult, have a clear professional orientation. These two chapters, which also appeared in the first edition, presented for the first time in layman's language information and ideas developed during the war as part of wartime research and rehabilitation. In this revision in the chapters on conservation of hearing, audiometry, special auditory tests, and military standards and medicolegal rules we have included rather extensive direct quotations from certain authoritative statements or reviews that have been published so far only in technical journals. The presentation, which is more detailed and technical than that given some of the more familiar material, was chosen for the benefit of those who are professionally engaged in some branch of audiology. We hope that these more technical chapters will be interesting to casual readers also, but the difference in treatment represents more than the personal caprice of their authors. It reflects the difference in the availability elsewhere of information on these particular topics.

In the following survey of the individual chapters the first paragraph in each case is almost unchanged from the first edition, except, of course, for the new chapters. In almost every case one or more paragraphs have been added to the summary to indicate the substantive changes and additions in this revision. Here the new authors are introduced to our readers and the reassignment of certain material to other chapters is indicated. These added paragraphs as well as the sketches of the new chapters are in themselves an interesting catalogue of the advances made in the intervening twelve years in the area of audiology. They also reflect the change in point of view from "A Guide for Laymen" to a textbook in audiology. For easy identification these new additions are indented.

THE PHYSICS AND THE PSYCHOLOGY OF HEARING

Dr. Davis tells about sound from the point of view of the physicist and the psychologist. The discussion is occasionally technical, notably in dealing with the decibel scale for the measurement of sound. The chapter is written primarily for students, for general readers with some scientific background, and for readers who want

definitions of terms and explanations of ideas that are to be used
later. But the average lay reader will probably be interested in some
description of the sense of hearing, and in knowing how auditory
sensations are related to the physical properties of sound waves, even
if he prefers to skim over a great deal of the specific information about
the range of audible sounds, the measurement of their intensity, the
analysis of complex sounds, and so on.

Dr. Davis now makes no apologies for the decibel scale. In
the second edition he describes the "auditory area" in more detail
and introduces the concept of a "threshold zone" instead of a sharp
threshold of sensitivity. The high-frequency boundary of the
auditory area moves downward as a function of age. He explains that the auditory area for binaural, open-field listening is
not identical with the area of audiometry, which refers to monaural listening under a receiver. The sound level meter and
octave band filters are used to describe noises in terms of their
sound pressure levels in successive frequency bands in much the
same way that hearing is described by an audiogram that shows
a person's hearing-threshold levels at various standard frequencies.
The over-all sound pressure levels of noises may not express
accurately the relative loudness of two noises, however, or the
extent to which they interfere with communication by speech.

ANATOMY AND PHYSIOLOGY OF THE EAR

Dr. Davis's summary of the structure of the ear and how it
works, as presented here, is more detailed and elaborate than has
been customary in most popular treatments. His exposition is helped
by several anatomical drawings that have been made especially for
this book. Dr. Davis combines his descriptions of structure and his
explanations of functions in a kind of functional anatomy. The
chapter should be read by all who are interested in the medical or
surgical aspects of hearing, but other readers may be content merely
to look at the pictures.

Knowledge of anatomy has not changed much in the last
fifteen years but the biophysics and physiology of the inner ear
are better understood. The duplex theory of hearing that involves
a spatial analysis of frequency in the cochlea and also direct
transmission of low frequencies by volleys of nerve impulses is
outlined, as well as the traveling wave pattern of movement of
the cochlear partition. The electrical potentials of the cochlea
and their probable role in hearing and the apparent differences
in function between inner and outer hair cells are described
briefly.

HEARING AND DEAFNESS

This new chapter by Dr. Davis and Dr. Fowler is devoted to a description of the various impairments of hearing and their causes. Much of this information appeared previously in other chapters in the first edition but it has now been unified and amplified. Some new items such as cholesteatoma, serous and mucous otitis, and the toxicity of dihydrostreptomycin have been added. Other topics, particularly the central dysacuses, are discussed in considerably more detail. A slightly different and, we believe, more useful set of definitions for hearing impairments is proposed. "Hearing loss" is retained to designate the symptom of partial impairment of auditory sensitivity or the medical condition that underlies it, but the reading in decibels on an audiometer that measures the impairment is now "hearing level." A change in level, either temporary or persistent, is not a hearing loss but a "threshold shift." "Nerve deafness" becomes "sensory-neural hearing loss." "Deafness" now explicitly implies a peripheral impairment with a loss of sensitivity so severe that sustained communication by the unaided, unamplified voice is practically impossible. Central auditory impairments and some peripheral disorders, such as diplacusis and loss of discrimination, are termed "dysacusis." This broad term includes psychogenic or functional "deafness" and the disorders of perception popularly called "aphasia." All of these conditions as well as congenital deafness, infections of the middle ear, otosclerosis, and, finally, noise-induced hearing loss are described in this chapter. It is both inclusive and detailed enough to serve as a useful summary for physicians.

MEDICAL ASPECTS OF DEAFNESS

Dr. Fowler explains the various things that can go wrong in the ear and how some of them can be prevented or treated medically. The distinction between *conduction deafness* and *nerve deafness* is fundamental, not only in respect to causes, prevention, and treatment, but also in understanding how an impaired ear hears. Dr. Fowler makes clear the importance of preventing common colds and of prompt medical or surgical treatment of infected ears as steps in the conservation of hearing. He also shows how little we can expect from restorative medical treatment once serious damage has been done, and warns against the dangers and deceptions of quack remedies. The discussion of the relation of noise to deafness should clarify (among other points) the question of whether or not noisy surroundings are dangerous to hearing. To answer the question we must know how loud the noise is, how long it lasts, whether the person exposed has an unusual susceptibility to auditory fatigue, and whether he has an impairment of hearing of the conductive or of the nerve type. Dr. Fowler's discussion is also illustrated with original anatomical diagrams and is complete enough to serve as a useful survey and refresher for physicians and surgeons who are not specialists in otology.

In the second edition the nature and causes of hearing impairments are described in the new Chapter 4. In the chapter on the medical aspects of hearing loss (not deafness) Dr. Fowler's discussion of medical treatment and prevention has been brought up to date. Dr. Davis has added an important section on Conservation of Hearing. This section includes extensive direct quotations from the authoritative "Guide for Conservation of Hearing in Noise" recently issued by the Subcommittee on Noise of the Committee on Conservation of Hearing of the American Academy of Ophthalmology and Otolarnygology. This guide strongly recommends "monitoring audiometry" as an essential feature of any program for conservation of hearing in noise, and also describes the hazards to hearing of excessive noise exposure and the value of ear protectors. Dr. Davis explains the difference between screening audiometry and monitoring audiometry.

SURGICAL TREATMENT OF HEARING LOSS

Dr. Walsh explains the surgical procedures that may be necessary when infection of the ear threatens the hearing, the general health, or even the life of a patient. He also describes *otosclerosis,* the disease that causes most of the hearing loss that begins in early adult life. Unfortunately, there is nothing that anyone can do at present to prevent or check otosclerosis. Dr. Walsh explains in detail the "fenestration operation" that may improve the hearing of some sufferers from otosclerosis, and the steps of the operation are illustrated by a series of drawings by Dr. Julius Lempert. The clear explanation for the layman of just what can and what cannot be expected of the operation, and of what kind of cases are suitable for it, is particularly important and timely.

The discussion of otosclerosis as a disease has been moved to Chapter 4, but the alleviation of the conductive hearing loss from otosclerosis by the fenestration operation remains the central feature of this chapter. The operation is now well standardized. The result, in terms of final hearing level for speech, can be predicted with a known degree of accuracy, and the probability of failure is also known, provided the operation is done by a skillful and experienced specialist. The newly revived operation of stapes mobilization, also described by Dr. Walsh, is not yet standardized and perhaps never can be. The final hearing level for speech is sometimes considerably better with stapes mobilization, but the probability of success is much lower than that for fenestration. Dr. Walsh also describes other surgical procedures, such as mastoidectomy to eradicate infection and tympanoplasty to repair certain abnormalities of the middle ear.

TESTS OF HEARING

In this chapter Dr. Davis explains the simple familiar tests of hearing, such as the voice test, the whisper test, and the coin click. He also explains the audiogram, and then the word and sentence tests that were developed and standardized during World War II. He describes in some detail the advantages and the limitations of word tests and "articulation scores." The chapter should be of special interest to all who are concerned with the testing of hearing, and it also gives some insight into the nature of speech and how we hear it. Anyone who is interested in selecting a hearing aid (or in helping someone else select one) should profit by the chapter, although the elaborate apparatus necessary for the most complete and accurate tests is at present available in only a few hospitals and clinics. In the Appendix at the end of the book are given the actual word lists and extensive samples of the sentences that have been developed recently at the Bell Telephone Laboratories, the Psycho-Acoustic Laboratory at Harvard University, and the Army and Navy Aural Rehabilitation Centers. These word lists and sentences may be used to advantage by anyone who desires good practical material for tests of hearing.

In the second edition, this chapter is entitled "Audiometry." It has been expanded by a more complete description of tuning fork tests and their use in diagnosis and also by an assessment, in the light of fifteen years of experience, of speech audiometry. Speech is a complex, labile, and redundant affair and the interpretation of the scores that are obtained on word and sentence tests is still difficult. Tests of "discrimination for speech" are not yet fully standardized. The hearing-threshold level for speech is, however, a well-established and useful measure of auditory performance.

A special appendix has been added concerning the zero reference levels for audiometry. "Normal hearing" has proved to be more difficult to define in principle and to measure in practice than was formerly thought. Certain arbitrary choices as well as careful measurements must be made. There is at present (1959) a difference of approximately 10 db between the American Standard and the British and several European Standards for zero hearing level. The differences are not due to faulty measurements but to the different arbitrary choices that have been made on the two sides of the Atlantic Ocean. The possibility of agreement on a new International Standard is discussed.

"Monitoring audiometry" has developed quite recently in industrial and military contexts. This type of audiometry is more elaborate than simple screening audiometry but is less elaborate than audiometry done for diagnostic purposes. Audiometers have been developed for it that are appropriate in choice of frequencies and in dynamic range. Some of the new audiometers are semiautomatic or fully automatic in operation. Some are individual; others are group audiometers. All of these types of audiometer and their special advantages and limitations, as well as the single-frequency or two-frequency screening audiometer, are discussed. Free use is made here, and also in relation to the problem of zero hearing level, of material developed from a CHABA symposium held in 1955. The principles and perhaps the instrumentation of monitoring audiometry are applicable not only to adult situations but also to the conservation of hearing in children.

SPECIAL AUDITORY TESTS

This chapter is new in the second edition and so is its co-author, Dr. Robert Goldstein. Dr. Goldstein was for several years a member of the Research Department of Central Institute for the Deaf, where he gained special experience with the techniques of electrodermal audiometry and electroencephalic audiometry that he describes and evaluates in this chapter.

The authors consider first the assessment of hearing for a hearing aid or for surgery. This involves the assessment of "cochlear function" in the presence of a conductive hearing loss. Then they describe diagnostic tests other than tests of sensitivity of hearing, such as the loudness balance test, tests of difference limen, of diplacusis, and so on, that are planned to detect and evaluate sense organ impairment of the recruitment type. Considerable attention is given to tests to detect possible malingering.

The second half of the chapter is devoted to educational assessment of children. Here Dr. Goldstein discusses electrodermal and electroencephalic audiometry and also the value of a careful clinical history and of conventional or "behavioral" audiometry in deciding whether a child suffers primarily from a peripheral deafness or from a central dysacusis. No details of technique are given in this chapter or in Chapter 7; the emphasis throughout is on the principles and an evaluation of the particular tests.

MILITARY STANDARDS FOR HEARING AND MEDICOLEGAL RULES

This chapter is another new addition in the revision. In the first part, which deals with "physical standards" for hearing, Dr. Davis summarizes the audiometric standards developed by the Armed Forces as well as a system of classification proposed in 1949 by the Committee on Hearing of the National Research Council. These standards reflect the accumulated experience of otologists and audiologists as to the relation between hearing levels measured on an audiometer and the competence or degree of handicap, particularly for communication by speech, that a person shows in everyday life. For the Armed Forces the very practical criterion is fitness for full or for restricted military duty. The complete classification also considers other forms of service in a national emergency. In the use of physical standards for hearing, the Armed Forces distinguish between fitness to *enter* full military duty and the unfitness of trained personnel to *continue* to perform effectively duties, such as piloting an airplane, that they have already learned.

The practical experience and the logic of military physical standards have now been carried over into the industrial and medicolegal problem of evaluation of hearing impairment for purposes of compensation. The Committee on Medical Rating of Physical Impairment of the American Medical Association defines "impairment" as a medical condition that affects one's personal efficiency in the activities of daily living. The term "disability" is reserved for situations in which the ability to earn wages is reduced because of the physical impairment. Impairment of hearing in this practical and medicolegal sense is not related to hearing for all tones in the auditory area, but to the hearing level for speech. Furthermore, impairment does not begin at zero level but somewhere between the 15 db and the 20 db levels. These are basic concepts for audiology.

Two important statements concerning impairment of hearing published by the Committee on Conservation of Hearing of the American Academy of Ophthalmology and Otolarnygology are reprinted in full. They are "Principles for Evaluating Hearing Loss" and "A Guide for the Evaluation of Impairment of Hearing."

HEARING AIDS

This chapter deals with hearing aids in general, both electrical and nonelectrical, and is intended primarily for users of hearing aids who want to know how their instruments work, what they may be expected to do, and what their limitations are. It may help prospective purchasers to evaluate advertising claims. Dr. Davis's descriptions of a vacuum-tube amplifier, crystal and magnetic receivers, different kinds of batteries, and so on, may be too technical for those who prefer to take their instruments for granted, but many users probably want just this information. Dr. Davis summarizes the principles governing the proper selection or "fitting" of hearing aids, which he helped to develop as part of the war work on aural rehabilitation. He explains why a compromise must often be made between adequate amplification, satisfactory quality, and the maximum loudness that the wearer is willing to tolerate. He believes that the proper solution of this compromise is more important than the time-honored principle of "selective amplification," that is, fitting the instrument strictly according to the audiogram. The technical information in this chapter is the foundation for much of the practical advice given in the following chapter.

The design objectives for hearing aids remain the same in 1959 as they were in 1947, but one of them, namely, light weight, small size, and inconspicuousness, has now been much more fully realized, thanks to the transistor, the mercury battery, and the printed circuit. The transistor has been a major "breakthrough." The principle of its operation is explained in this chapter in the second edition, as well as the all-on-the-head types of hearing aid and the true binaural hearing aids that it has made possible. From this chapter Dr. Silverman, Dr. Davis, and Mr. Taylor have dropped a major section devoted to batteries and some of the details about carbon amplifiers and vacuum-tube hearing aids. The principles of necessary gain, of desirable maximum power-outputs and frequency responses, and of peak limiting and other forms of distortion remain the same, although in advertising less emphasis is now placed on versatility of tone control and on naturalness of reproduction than on inconspicuous appearance or the possibility of binaural hearing.

Some passages in this chapter concerning the "fitting" of hearing aids now begin to sound a little out of date, as the word "fitting" now appears less and less frequently in advertisements and in clinical discussions. In order to maintain historical continuity, the passages have been allowed to stand as they were written in the first edition.

THE CHOICE AND USE OF HEARING AIDS

Dr. Silverman states that the use of hearing aids by those who can profit by them is a social duty. He deplores the hardships and inconveniences on others that may be imposed by the vanity of the hard of hearing. At the same time he points out that elderly people and those who have certain types of nerve deafness may be unable to profit by hearing aids. He explains the importance of training in listening and in speechreading after a hearing aid has been bought. He gives the list of hearing aids that have been "accepted" by the Council on Physical Medicine, and explains the meaning of the "acceptance." He tells in detail how a layman without expert advice should go about the business of selecting a hearing aid, and he describes simple but effective tests that can be administered by a friend. He also gives many practical bits of advice as to cost, availability of service, individual earmolds, batteries, spare parts, and so on. Mr. S. Gordon Taylor is himself a veteran user of hearing aids and has served as a special lecturer at New York University and as a member of the scientific staff of Columbia University in the Division of War Research. For the benefit of actual users he gives full instructions for the home construction of a good battery tester. He also shows how the garments for carrying the hearing aid may be simplified. The condensed Troubleshooting Chart at the end of the chapter was arranged by Mr. Taylor. It will enable the average user of a hearing aid to locate and often to remedy minor troubles, thus avoiding unnecessary trips to the dealer for services.

The problems of the choice and use of hearing aids have not changed, and this chapter stands almost untouched, including its informal conversational style directed to the lay reader, except for the omission of the description of the outdated battery tester. But we do not yet know just how much difference it makes, in terms of practical everyday success in communication by speech, to go through the elaborate "fitting" procedures and comparative trials of hearing aids that are so dear to the hearts of audiologists and hearing aid dealers alike. The practical rules for selection of a hearing aid without expert advice are still valid. The Troubleshooting Chart has been revised to apply to the modern transistor hearing aid.

Dr. Silverman quotes some interesting estimates of the number of hard-of-hearing individuals in this country, both actual and potential users of hearing aids. These estimates are based on a series of "best guesses" made by manufacturers of hearing aids from their own experience and for their own guidance.

SPEECHREADING

Dr. Miriam Pauls explains the principles of speechreading. She shows how much of our speech can be "read" by intelligent attention to the movements of the lips and jaws of the speaker, but she also points out how much information and context can be gained from the expression and gestures of the speaker and attention to the entire situation. It is because of this broader view of the whole process that Dr. Pauls calls it "speechreading" instead of the more familiar "lip reading." Dr. Pauls explains how speechreading is taught. Pupils learn to take advantage of everything that can be seen, anything that can be heard, and even the "feel" of imitating the movements of the talker's mouth. She points out how admirably speechreading and a hearing aid supplement each other if a hard-of-hearing person has any residual hearing. Dr. Pauls illustrates the principles of speechreading and the methods of teaching it by a description of the speechreading unit (under her own supervision) at the Naval Aural Rehabilitation Center at Philadelphia. She emphasizes the importance of combining speechreading, auditory training, and conservation of speech in a single broad concept of "rehabilitation in communication." She closes with a series of practical suggestions for ease of communication that will be useful to all who are hard of hearing.

AUDITORY TRAINING

Dr. Raymond Carhart continues the theme of rehabilitation in communication begun by Dr. Pauls. He discusses the nature of auditory discrimination, pointing out the major types of distinction which must be made if the listener is to get full practical usefulness from his hearing. Dr. Carhart has interesting things to say about the development of the understanding of language, and shows how the ear must discriminate between speech sounds. Learning and practice are much more important for this process than most people realize. Dr. Carhart outlines the influence of types of hearing loss upon auditory discrimination and contrasts the problems of the child with those of the adult. He summarizes and illustrates the principles of auditory training, again contrasting the needs of the young child with those of the person whose impairment arises later in life. Special emphasis is given to the role of the hearing aid in auditory training, and the point is made that such training must include instruction in making discriminations while wearing the instrument. Dr. Carhart emphasizes the value of a hearing aid if a person has any hearing whatever. Even though the patient may never hear well enough to understand speech, the hearing aid can be a great help in keeping his voice normal and pleasing. The discussion includes advice to parents and practical suggestions by which a formal program of auditory training can be supplemented at home.

CONSERVATION OF SPEECH

Dr. Carhart points out that hearing is basic in the normal process of learning and controlling speech, and for this reason an auditory impairment may cause abnormalities in speech. He stresses the fact that speech includes not only vowels and consonants but also nonphonetic elements, such as melody, quality, rhythm, and emphasis. Dr. Carhart discusses the major problems in speech which arise because of hearing loss. Among other things, hard-of-hearing people often have difficulty in adjusting their conversation to the loudness required by the background conditions of the moment. He outlines the methods for teaching speech to the deaf and contrasts these with the methods used for hard-of-hearing children. He also covers the problems and procedures of maintaining adequate speech habits following the appearance of auditory impairment in an adult. Throughout the discussion there appear suggestions regarding the help which parents and friends can give.

These three chapters on speechreading, auditory training, and the conservation of speech all deal with fundamental *techniques* for rehabilitation or conservation. These techniques are the same as they were twelve years ago, and the chapters that describe them are virtually unchanged from the first edition. The later chapters, on the other hand, are grouped around *problems*. The problems differ according to the age at which the impairment occurs and the severity of the impairment.

A particular way of applying the basic techniques of rehabilitation on a large scale was developed during World War II and was described in Chapter 12 of the first edition. The Army centers are no longer in operation, however, and the military problem of rehabilitation has been inherited by the Veterans Administration. Chapter 19, by Mr. Bernard Anderman, has been substituted for the former chapter on military aural rehabilitation by Dr. Canfield and Dr. Morrissett. The major problems of rehabilitation have shifted from a wartime to a peacetime basis.

FROM ARISTOTLE TO BELL

Dr. Silverman introduces the sections on education and socio-economic problems with a brief historical survey. He shows how, through the centuries, the social point of view toward deafness has gradually changed. Once the deaf, particularly those who were born deaf and therefore never learned to talk, were regarded as imbeciles and remained social outcasts for life. Eventually the language of signs, the manual alphabet, speechreading, and the teaching of speech to the deaf brought to these unfortunates the power of communication. The deaf are now recognized as handicapped and in need of special education, but with that education they can and do take their places as fully responsible members of society. Dr. Silverman tells briefly the part played in this social revolution by such pioneers as De l'Épée, Heinicke, Gallaudet, Clerc, Fuller, Yale, Bell, and Goldstein.

History has not changed, and there have been no substantial additions to or deletions from this chapter.

DEAF CHILDREN

Dr. Lane and Dr. Silverman approach the problem of the education of deaf children from the oral point of view. They believe that it is possible, practical, and desirable to teach even totally deaf children to speak and to read speech. If special instruction is begun early enough, at nursery school age, the children learn to communicate very effectively. In fact, if they have the mental capacity and the ambition, they are able to complete high school and college in regular schools for the hearing. Dr. Lane and Dr. Silverman do not (nor do any of our other authors) go into any detail concerning the manual alphabet or the language of signs, useful as these are for the deaf who learn them. It seems to be the consensus that instruction in speech should be given to all deaf children, although opinion differs as to the emphasis that should be placed on the manual methods of communication.

Dr. Lane and Dr. Silverman discuss the problems of testing the hearing of very young children, and also of testing their other abilities. The ordinary "intelligence test," for example, is not applicable to deaf children on account of the importance in it of linguistic ability. The general thesis of the authors is that deaf children suffer from a specific handicap, not from a general mental or physical inferiority, and they discuss the educational methods that they believe are best suited to overcoming the handicap. They point out also the responsibilities of parents and of the general community.

For the second edition Dr. Silverman has entirely rewritten and considerably expanded this chapter on deaf children. It now precedes the chapter on hard-of-hearing children. Much of the new material in this chapter is paraphrased or slightly condensed from Dr. Silverman's chapter in the *Handbook of Speech Pathology* (Lee Travis, ed.). We are indebted to Dr. Travis and to the publishers, Appleton-Century-Crofts, Inc., for their courtesy in allowing this reuse of the substance and often of entire sections. The chapter now deals broadly with the whole problem of the education of deaf children. It reviews several historic controversies between different "schools of thought," and for this, if no other, reason should provide a starting point for any future discussion of methods of education of deaf children, whether by the oral or the manual or the combined method.

Dr. Lane and a new collaborator, Dr. Donald G. Doehring, have reappraised the problem of the mental abilities of deaf children and the methods appropriate for testing them.

HARD-OF-HEARING CHILDREN

Dr. Silverman makes an estimate of the number of children in the United States who, on account of their defective hearing, require preventive or remedial medical or surgical attention, hearing aids, speechreading, or other special education. His estimate is about 1,500,000. This figure is half the figure which has been widely quoted in recent years, but it shows that impaired hearing in children is nevertheless an important social and economic problem. Dr. Silverman's estimate is lower, partly because of differences in terminology and partly because we now have more and better information from systematic tests of hearing in school children. Dr. Silverman tells how such group testing is done and gives practical suggestions as how best to pick out the children who are in need of special attention. Many cases of impaired hearing due to infection of the middle ears can be checked by proper medical care or surgical treatment before further deterioration occurs. With the help of hearing aids and instruction in speechreading, hard-of-hearing children can be educated successfully in our regular schools.

The chapter on hard-of-hearing children has been reduced by the shift to other chapters of some of the material formerly included in it. The estimates of the number of hard-of-hearing children have been revised to match our present definitions of "hard of hearing" and the increased population of the country, but the estimates are still very uncertain.

THE PSYCHOLOGY OF THE HARD-OF-HEARING
AND THE DEAFENED ADULT

Dr. Ramsdell bases this chapter very largely on his experiences as psychologist at the Army Rehabilitation Center at Deshon General Hospital. It is confined almost entirely to the special psychological problems of adults who have been able to hear, have learned to talk, but who then have lost all or a large part of their hearing. Taking his cue from the oft-repeated statement by deafened soldiers that "the world has gone dead," Dr. Ramsdell makes a thoughtful analysis of the psychological importance of hearing for maintaining a normal sense of participation in a living world. To the sudden loss of this normal but unrecognized function of hearing Dr. Ramsdell attributes the characteristic depression of those who become deaf. He finds that, fortunately, an understanding by the patient himself of the source of the trouble goes far to alleviate it. This chapter is Dr. Ramsdell's first formal presentation of the results of his work, and he therefore goes quite deeply into his subject. The chapter should be of great help to the deafened in understanding and overcoming their special psychological problem and to their families and friends in assisting them.

Dr. Ramsdell also shows how deafness tends to accentuate and bring to the surface the personality traits of suspicion, of the feeling of being discriminated against, and of consequent hostility. Deafness does not create these traits but it tends to intensify them.

Psychological deafness in its various forms, particularly hysterical "psychogenic" deafness as it appeared in army patients, is explained. The observations originally made during the war at Hoff General Hospital indicate that psychological factors may be responsible for more deafness than has usually been recognized. Quite unknown to the patient himself, psychological factors may make a deafness much worse than the injury to the ear itself can explain, or they may cause the deafness to persist after the ear has recovered.

The section of this chapter on the psychology of the hard-of-hearing and the deafened adult stands virtually as Dr. Ramsdell wrote it in 1946. Nothing has appeared in the meantime to amplify or controvert his observations and interpretations.

Dr. Davis has revised the section on psychogenic deafness. It now appears as part of Chapter 4.

THE VETERANS ADMINISTRATION'S AUDIOLOGY PROGRAM

Mr. Anderman is able to write authoritatively about this program, for he is Chief of Audiology and Speech Correction in the

Veterans Administration. He tells of the objectives, the size, and the general plan of the program, with its ten Veterans Administration Audiology Clinics distributed over the country, reinforced by numerous university and hospital clinics that cooperate on a contract basis. He notes the special interest, including a research interest, of the Veterans Administration in "nonorganic deafness" and in the most efficient large-scale procurement and individual distribution of hearing aids. This chapter, new in the second edition, thus forms a sequel to Chapter 4 with respect to psychogenic deafness and to Chapters 10 and 11 on hearing aids. It is also an appropriate introduction to the general topic of organizations of or for the benefit of the hard of hearing and the deaf. The Veterans Administration training program in audiology may also interest students who intend to become audiologists.

ORGANIZATIONS AND AGENCIES FOR THE AURALLY HANDICAPPED

Miss Wright gives a very useful series of thumbnail sketches of the leading national organizations of and for the deaf and the hard of hearing. The objectives of each organization are given, as well as a brief account of their histories, publications, present headquarters, membership, and activities. We hope that the information will help the organizations in their work by making them known to some who may not have been acquainted with them but who are eligible to join and wish to do so. Miss Wright, as Director of Field Service for the American Hearing Society, writes with special authority and enthusiasm about the work done by that society for the benefit of the hard of hearing.

Both this chapter and the next chapter on employment for the hard of hearing have been brought up to date by Miss Hill. This chapter has also been extended in the second edition by Dr. Silverman to include mention of the subcommittees of the Committee on the Conservation of Hearing of the American Academy of Ophthalmology and Otolaryngology and also of the Armed Forces–National Research Council Committee on Hearing and Bio-Acoustics, among others.

EMPLOYMENT FOR THE HARD OF HEARING

Miss Hill, another enthusiastic worker in the American Hearing Society, has brought together in a brief but useful chapter a survey of the problems of employment for the hard of hearing. The topics include the types of work suitable for the hard of hearing, the principle of selective placement, and compensation insurance. She makes a number of practical observations that will be read with interest by the hard of hearing themselves, their parents, their teachers, and prospective employers.

Dr. Myklebust, as Director of Research at the New Jersey School for the Deaf, is one of the country's leading authorities on vocational guidance in general as well as on the special problems of the deaf. He explains some of the basic problems of vocational guidance, what it is, and what it attempts to do. He deals particularly with the psychology of deaf youth—children and young adults who are a little older than those discussed by Dr. Lane and Dr. Silverman. He points out the importance of personality and social maturity in addition to intelligence, aptitudes, interests, and special skills. The deaf as a group are quite normal in the last four categories. Dr. Myklebust suggests that more attention be given by parents and educators to the development of social maturity, for a retardation here and in general education is the most common shortcoming of deaf youth. He believes that the job should be chosen to fit the intelligence, competence, and interests of the young man or woman; and also that the ambitions and desires of the young man or woman should be realistically adjusted to his or her abilities, with a frank recognition of the handicaps of deafness. This thesis should command the attention of all readers, no matter how good their hearing.

The original chapter by Dr. Myklebust has been replaced by an entirely new chapter on the same subject written by Mr. Boyce R. Williams. Mr. Williams is a particularly appropriate addition to our list of authors. He is himself deaf and, as Consultant, Deaf and the Hard of Hearing, in the Office of Vocational Rehabilitation, Department of Health, Education, and Welfare, holds an important government position concerned with vocational guidance for the deaf. He therefore writes with special enthusiasm, authority, and understanding of the subject.

Mr. Williams surveys vocational guidance services currently available to the deaf, emphasizing the team approach as represented in the actively coordinated joint thinking and action of interested and responsible agencies. Working definitions of vocational guidance, the deaf, and the team are offered. He describes the vital and often continuing role of the school for the deaf in the vocational guidance process. The functions of team members of the state vocational rehabilitation agency and the state employment service are identified and described. Two important aspects of vocational guidance work with the deaf, specifically, counseling and psychological evaluation, are discussed. He presents an overview of the deaf at work, including guides to their placement and orientation. Finally, some suggestions are made about better jobs for deaf people.

SUGGESTIONS FOR READING

We have adopted the policy of avoiding detailed documentation of our statements. A complete list of references would run into the hundreds. This book is intended to be a survey, not a textbook. For the benefit of those who wish to read more widely in any area and to find more detailed information and evidence for our statements, we have placed at the end of each chapter a brief list of a few additional books or articles on each subject. In some cases we have ventured a comment or two to guide the prospective reader in his choices.

In this second edition we have expanded some of our lists of suggested readings in accordance with our objective of providing a textbook on the principles of audiology. But in keeping with our desire to emphasize principles and not details of fact or of technique, we have listed very few primary scientific articles in technical journals. We do not attempt to document every statement in detail, except to give the source of direct quotations. We have tried to select, instead, the best books, monographs, and review articles that deal more fully with particular phases of our subject matter. Through these secondary sources, students who so desire can easily find their way to the original sources or to detailed treatises on techniques.

In the same spirit we have avoided reference by name to many distinguished workers in the cause of the deaf and the hard of hearing. Except for those who are named by virtue of the place that they hold in some organization, we have not named any of those who are still living, although we are aware that in the perspective of time some of them will take their places with Helmholtz, Clerc, Gallaudet, and Bell, among the immortals.

PART 2

HEARING AND
HEARING LOSS

2

PHYSICS AND PSYCHOLOGY
OF HEARING

Hallowell Davis, M.D.

"Sound is what we hear." So says the man just in from the street.

"No," says a physicist, "sound is a form of energy. It is an organized movement of molecules; it is a series of waves of pressure in the air or water or whatever medium is transmitting the sound."

"Yes," says a psychologist, "but you should add that sound is a sensation, something that exists only within ourselves. The sensation is aroused when sound waves tickle our ears and send nerve impulses running to the brain along the auditory nerve. We all know what sound is like in experience. It is real but intangible. We can't weigh it in a pair of scales, measure it with a meter, or even take it out and look at it."

And while the physicist glares at the psychologist, the man from the street raises the old question: If a bomb explodes in the midst of the Sahara Desert or at the South Pole with no man or other living creature there to hear, will there be any sound?

"Of course there will," says the physicist.

"Impossible," says the psychologist. "Didn't I tell you . . . ." And so it goes.

What Is Sound

The sort of argument recorded above was once taken quite seriously, until it was realized that words and their meanings are not created in Heaven but are consciously or unconsciously made by man for his own use. And often very clumsy, foggy, and ambiguous he makes them! The word "sound" is used, and we shall so use it, to mean *both* the physicist's pressure waves and moving molecules and the

29

psychologist's subjective sensation in the mind of the listener. And now that we realize that the word has a double meaning, there need actually be no confusion. Which meaning is meant is usually quite clear. The physicist's sound can be measured by apparatus, and it can do work; it can push small objects back and forth or generate heat. The other kind of sound is all in our minds and may be high-pitched or low-pitched, loud or faint, pleasant or unpleasant. These attributes cannot be measured by thermometers or voltmeters, but they can be appreciated by a listener; and a listener can tell us a lot about his sensations and about the relations among them: which of two sounds is louder, which is higher in pitch, and so on.

Between the physical sound of pressure waves and our insubstantial but intensely real sensations lie our ears, our nerves, and our brains. The physiologist, who thinks of sound in the physical sense, studies how the sound waves are gathered by the external ear, conducted by the middle ear, and concentrated and analyzed in the inner ear, as well as how they set up nerve impulses in the auditory nerve. He follows the nerve impulses up to the gray matter of the brain and can tell us something of how their pattern in time (and in distribution among the thousands of nerve fibers in the auditory pathways) corresponds to the original pattern of the physicist's sound waves. But no one can say how the patterns of nerve impulses generate our subjective sensations.

The psychologist who wants to relate sensations to objects and events in the physical world gets little help from the physiologist. He must go back to the beginning and compare the loudness, the pitch, or the unpleasantness of the sensations as reported by his subjects with the intensity, the frequency, the wave form, the temporal pattern, or other measurable attribute of the physical sound. This sort of study is known as *psychophysics*, and much of what we shall have to say about sound and hearing will be statements of just these relationships between the objective and the subjective aspects of sound. The relationships are not properties of physical sound but the relation between physical sound and the properties of human beings, particularly of their ears and their brains.

The physicist's sound is a form of energy. It can be "created" only by transformation from another form of energy, and it in turn can do work and be transformed into still other forms. Specifically, it is an organized movement to and fro of the molecules of a gas or liquid or solid. Small solid objects, such as particles of dust in the air, move bodily with the air molecules and help us to visualize the organized movement of the molecules.

Solid objects may "vibrate," one part moving back and forth in relation to other parts. The to-and-fro motion of the vibrating part is much the same as the motion of the air molecules in sound waves except that the molecules of the bell, the tuning fork, or the violin string are stuck together and must move as a mass.

THE PHYSICAL NATURE OF SOUND

The commonest source of sound waves in the air is a vibrating solid body. As the air molecules fly about and collide with one another in their random dance, they are pushed back by the solid body when it starts to vibrate, just as a jostling crowd of spectators awaiting a parade is pushed back by a cordon of police. The molecules, or spectators, in the front ranks collide more powerfully with their neighbors and push them back; and so the wave spreads through the crowd. Then each molecule (or spectator), bumping and jostling, takes advantage of the reverse movement of the solid body (or a relaxation of the cordon), and they surge back to or beyond their original positions, only to be pushed away once more. Among the molecules, as in the crowd, there are zones of denser pressure which move away from the source of the disturbance. These are the *sound waves*. The waves of pressure travel slowly in a New Year's Eve crowd, but they go at about a thousand feet a second in air. (The velocity of sound in air or "mach 1" is about 760 miles an hour at sea level and is now familiar as a unit of speed of jet planes and rockets.) Each molecule moves only a very short distance, however, and then returns to or beyond its original position. The air movement does not become a wind. The crowd is still in Times Square, not charging down Broadway. And anyone who has been a "molecule" in a large crowd will recall the "pressure waves" that made him surge back and forth.

Most solid objects vibrate when they are suddenly set in motion or suddenly stopped. Their *inertia* keeps them from starting all at once. Their *momentum* keeps parts moving even after one portion has met an obstacle. The momentum makes the wood, metal, or whatever it may be stretch until the attractions that hold the molecules together finally stop the forward movement. Now, if the object has only stretched out of shape and not shattered to bits, the elastic forces restore it to shape. Usually they restore the shape so rapidly, however, that it overshoots in the opposite direction, like the swing of a pendulum, and it may take many swings to come to rest. Each swing pushes out a sound wave in the surrounding air. The vibration may be kept going by some continuing force, like wind flapping a flag; or the original event may be repeated, like a clock striking twelve. And air itself becomes turbulent when it moves rapidly, and its eddies and surges generate the sound waves that we hear as the wind whistles through a crack, around an airplane, or in our own ears.

Nature is as full of sound as it is of wind, of splashing water, and of hard vibrating objects. It is a rarity to find a really silent event, except for those that take place so slowly that we can hardly even see them happen. Few objects are so soft and spongy as to be noiseless; although skin, flesh, and fur qualify as well as any. Nature, particularly inanimate nature, is noisy.

THE SENSITIVITY OF THE EAR

When we say that nature is noisy we do not mean that nature's sounds are unpleasantly loud; we merely mean that they are audible. The sound waves have enough energy to stimulate the ear, and if nature is noisy, it is partly because our ears are so sensitive. The human ear is actually so sensitive that at its best it can almost hear the individual air molecules bump against the ear drum in their random thermal flight. The distance that the eardrum moves in and out with each wave when we just hear the faintest audible tone at the most favorable frequency is less than one tenth of the diameter of a single hydrogen molecule. This distance is, of course, far less than anything that we can see under the best microscope. As a matter of fact, it is about one thousandth of the wave length of light. We cannot easily think of it in terms of inches, for it is less than a hundred-millionth of an inch. If the capital I at the beginning of this sentence were enlarged to the height of the Empire State Building, a hundred-millionth of an inch would correspond to about the thickness of a piece of cigarette paper.

The extraordinary sensitivity is due to the highly specialized structure of the ear. The outer ear of man, to be sure, is not as efficient as the ear of the dog or the rabbit in collecting sound energy. Cupping the hand behind the ear or inserting an ear trumpet causes an appreciable over-all gain in sensitivity for sounds coming from the proper direction. But the inner ear, where the delicate sensory cells lie protected in their special chamber within the hardest bone in the body, is just about as sensitive as it could usefully be. If the cells were stimulated by the random thermal motion of molecules, we would hear a continuous meaningless rattle or hiss and could not distinguish sounds any fainter than the best human ears can now detect. Nature has apparently gone the limit in developing an organ sensitive to the telltale sound waves given off by most events around us. Small wonder, then, that so delicate an organ may sometimes be injured by very intense blasts of sound or degenerate when affected by disease. The wonder is not that our ears sometimes fail us, but rather that they stand the racket as well as they do.

Intense sounds can be felt, either as a single blast or as vibration, by the sense of touch. Our hairs may be set in vibration by the sound waves of the air and tickle the *touch corpuscles* at their roots. (A hair and its touch corpuscle is, as we shall see, a crude large-scale model of the actual sense organ in the inner ear.) Or with the tips of our fingers we may feel a piano case vibrate. We may even distinguish with our fingers, although crudely, whether the piano is vibrating rapidly (when a medium or high note is struck) or slowly (when one of the lowest notes is sounded). The sense of vibration, which is really the sense of touch, and the sense of hearing merge into one another in two ways. From the point of view of evolutionary development, the inner sense organ of hearing is a highly specialized organ of touch, specialized to be "touched" only by vibrations of the air and never by a solid object. Secondly, when we "hear" the very lowest notes of a pipe organ we are probably *feeling* the vibration quite as much as we are *hearing* it. As tones get lower and lower in frequency, the ear is less and less sensitive to them and the tones must be stronger, with larger vibrations, in order to be heard. Finally, the point is reached at which the pressure waves begin to stimulate the skin of our hands, the linings of our noses and throats, the hairs of our heads, and even our bones, joints, and inner organs. The senses of hearing and touch merge as imperceptibly as do smell and taste. But touch, like taste, cannot distinguish the fine differences for which hearing (like smell) is specialized. Therefore, although we may, for example, perceive the *rhythm* of a piece of music as accurately by touch as by ear, we cannot feel the *tune,* because touch is so poor at discriminating the frequencies that give us our sense of musical pitch. Likewise, the tempo and stress of very loud speech can be felt, but only in the most favorable *context* can words ever be understood through touch alone.

MEASURES OF SOUND: FREQUENCY AND INTENSITY

Two kinds of measurement are enough to define a *pure tone* completely. One is *frequency,* usually measured in cycles (complete swings or double vibrations) per second. In these days of radio and its kilocycles we should all be accustomed to the idea of frequency. The other measurement is *magnitude,* or *intensity,* and may be measured as the alternating *pressure* of the sound waves, as the *velocity* with which air particles move to and fro, or as a *flow of energy* in horsepower or watts.

We are all accustomed to steady pressures, such as thirty pounds per square inch in a tire, and to steady velocities, such as 1000 feet per second, approximately the velocity of sound in air. Alternating pressures and velocities are less familiar. They bear the same relation to steady pressures and velocities that an alternating electric current bears to direct current. Both kinds can do work, but one of them is continually reversing its direction. The concept of power, illustrated by the horsepower of our automobiles or the watts of electric power consumed by our electric light bulbs, is familiar to us; and acoustic power, although the quantities are extremely small, can be measured in the same units. Thus the physicist says that the acoustic power of the faintest 1000-cycle tone that can be heard by a good ear is about 0.000 000 000 000 000 1 watt or, in a more familiar unit, 0.000 000 000 000 000 000 13 horsepower per square centimeter. Noise becomes uncomfortable, as in a boiler shop, at 0.0001 watt and sharply painful at 0.01 watt.

Numbers of this sort, consisting chiefly of a decimal point followed by a string of nothingness, are more impressive than convenient. Moreover, the range that is covered between the faintest audible and the sharply painful sounds is tremendous. The latter are ten million million times as powerful as the former. It helps a little, but only a little, if we talk about the pressure, which is what the acoustics engineer actually measures with his sound level meter, instead of the power, because the pressure is proportional to the square root of the power and fewer zeros are required. (The faintest audible 1000-cycle tone has an acoustic pressure of about 0.0002 dyne per square centimeter; the painful tone, 2000 dynes per square centimeter.) Even so, our calculations consist chiefly of locating the decimal point correctly.

To deal conveniently with such an unwieldy range of values, a logarithmic system has been universally adopted in acoustics and in electrical engineering. The system has no fixed unit, like the pound or the centimeter, but deals only in ratios, like double, tenfold, or hundredfold. One logarithmic unit (to the base 10) of the ratio (of one acoustic power to another) is known as a *bel*, in honor of Alexander Graham Bell, who invented the telephone. Thus one bel means tenfold the power, two bels means tenfold and tenfold again, that is, a hundredfold the power. The bels count the number of steps the decimal point takes along the chain of zeros.

To avoid inconvenient fractional values of the bel, the *decibel*, which is one tenth of a bel, is usually employed instead. It is abbreviated *db*.

Unfortunately there is the slight additional complication that we usually deal with *pressures* whereas the decibel is defined as a ratio of two *energies* or powers. Acoustic pressures are proportional to the square root of the corresponding power. The ratio of the *squares* of the acoustic pressures corresponds to the simple ratio of the acoustic powers, and therefore the logarithm of the pressure ratio is *double* the logarithm of the power ratio. Thus tenfold (for acoustic pressures) is 20 db, a hundredfold is 40 db, and double pressure turns out to be almost exactly 6 db.

The decibel scale is logarithmic. This means, among other things, that when we add decibels we *multiply*. We cannot perform the operation of adding sound pressures, as when sounds from two sources are present at the same time, without first translating to actual intensities in watts per square centimeter. We then add the watts arithmetically and translate back into decibels relative to the reference level. For example, two sounds measure 74 and 77 db (relative to 0.0002 dyne per square centimeter) respectively. Their combined sound pressure is *not* 151 db! 74 db correspond to 1 dyne per square centimeter or 2.5×10^{-9} watt per square centimeter, as shown by the scales in Figure 2-4. 77 db correspond to 5.0×10^{-9} watt per square centimeter. Their sum is 7.5×10^{-9} watt per square centimeter. On the decibel scale this is about 78.8 db relative to 0.0002 dyne per square centimeter. (Such calculations are readily made with the help of tables, rather like the familiar tables of logarithms.)

A decibel has no fixed absolute value or any units. It is simply a ratio, telling by what proportion one value is greater or less than another. To give the decibel scale an anchor, so to speak, we conventionally assume certain reference levels that are understood unless otherwise specified. For acoustic pressures the *standard reference level* is 0.0002 dyne per square centimeter. This value is conveniently close to the intensity of the faintest sound that can be heard by the best ear. Sound that is painful, at 140 decibels, exerts a pressure $10^{(14 \div 2)} = 10^7 = 10,000,000$ times as great. And the increase in absolute pressure from 140 to 141 db is 10,000,000 times as great as the increase from 0 to 1 db.

It might seem inconvenient to have the absolute value of the decibel change as we go up and down the intensity scale, but actually it is a convenience because the just noticeable difference that the ear can detect in the intensity of a sound stays nearly constant in terms of decibels. The just noticeable difference varies only from 3 or 4 db for very faint sounds to about 0.3 db for very intense sounds. We can easily hear a pin drop if the room is almost quiet; but if an airplane engine is warming up nearby, a ten-pound box of pins might fall unheard. But the ability of the additional decibel of sound intensity to attract our attention varies little. There is also another way in which the logarithmic decibel scale corresponds approximately to the way in which the ear hears sounds. A sound that is 10 db more intense than another sound of the same frequency sounds about twice as loud. Thus if a sound 40 db above the standard reference level is increased to 70 db, it sounds $2 \times 2 \times 2$ or 8 times as loud. This is a very convenient approximate rule. Unfortunately, however, if two sounds are of different frequencies, the rules for predicting their combined loudness when they are sounded simultaneously are much more complicated.

The frequency in cycles per second and the intensity in decibels are enough to define a *pure* tone, that is, a tone with the simple

-A-
A PURE TONE

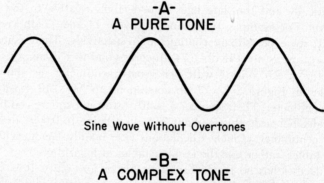

Sine Wave Without Overtones

-B-
A COMPLEX TONE

Tone of an Oboe at 256 Cycles Per Second

-C-
STREET NOISE

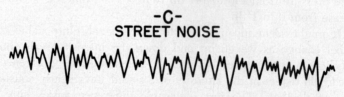

Fig. 2-1. See text for explanation. Curve *B* is redrawn after D. C. Miller, *The Science of Musical Sounds* (by permission of The Macmillan Company, publishers). Curve *C* is a draftsman's copy of an original illustration by Fletcher. The fine detail of the original is not reproduced. The drawing serves, by contrast with *A* and *B* above, to show the mixed and irregular character of noise. (*After Fletcher, Speech and Hearing, D. Van Nostrand Company, Inc.*)

smooth wave form known as the *sine wave*. The tone produced by a violin or clarinet is complex, but it can be analyzed by acoustic filters into its component pure tones, each with a definite frequency and intensity. In such a musical tone the various additional frequencies are known as *overtones* or *harmonics,* and their frequencies are simple integral multiples of the frequency of the lowest tone, or *fundamental.* The frequencies and intensities of the harmonics are represented in the form of a *line spectrum* of the sound, as in Figure 2-2. The relative strengths of the higher harmonics give a *quality* to the tone that is characteristic of the particular instrument. For the human voice the components of higher frequency are responsible for the differences between the different vowel sounds when all of them are sung or spoken at the same pitch.

NOISE

Most of the sounds we hear are neither pure single-frequency tones nor even musical tones containing only one fundamental frequency and its higher harmonics. Instead, they are a scramble of many frequencies that may or may not stand in any simple numerical relation to one another. In fact, one very familiar noise, the hiss of an air jet or escaping steam, is completely random in its wave form. If we analyze such a random noise, we find equal amounts of energy in a given band width (range of frequencies), whatever part of the spectrum we examine. High, low, and middle frequencies are equally represented, and, because the spectrum is a continuous band of equal intensity, none stands out from the other. Since there is an obvious analogy to white light, such a noise is often called *white noise*. It is a useful tool for the acoustic physicist and fortunately is easily generated by merely amplifying the background hiss produced in certain electronic vacuum tubes. Other noises have a predominance of high or low frequencies, and although their pitches may be very vague, we can recognize that one such noise is higher pitched than another. The noises may be thought of as more or less "colored." The pure tone with its line spectrum corresponds to a pure color. A noise may be a mixture of a line spectrum, like the hum of an airplane motor, with a more or less uniform band spectrum, like the wind noise around the wings of the plane. Of course, unless the line spectrum (of the motor or from any other source) is more intense than the band spectrum at that particular frequency, the pure tone will be submerged in the noise and the ear will be unable to detect it. The pure tone is then said to be "masked" by the noise. The masking of speech by traffic noise is very familiar to all of us.

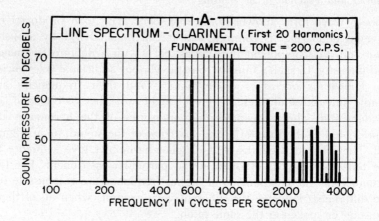

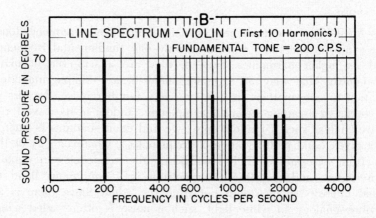

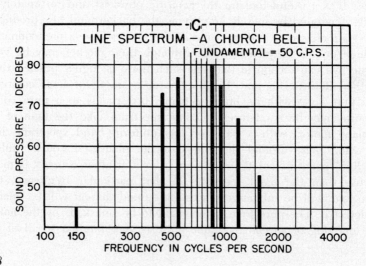

THE SOUND LEVEL METER

We have mentioned the sound level meter. This is a basic tool for the acoustic engineer. The sound is converted into a corresponding electrical signal, which is then amplified and measured with a meter. The meter gives directly the *sound level* in decibels relative to the standard reference level. The ear, as we shall see, is more sensitive to sounds of some frequencies than to others, but the sound level meter is so constructed as to be equally sensitive to all frequencies from 20 to 10,000 cps unless special "weighting networks," to be described later, are employed. When more than one frequency is present, the meter reads the total acoustic pressure as an *over-all sound level*. This over-all sound level is understood when we say, for example, that the noise in a weaving room is 100 db and on a busy street is 70 db (See Figure 2-3).

Another basic acoustic instrument is the electrical filter which rejects signals that are above or below a desired *pass band*. If desired, the pass band can be made very narrow, only a few cycles per second in width. The filter is then said to be sharply "tuned" to a desired frequency. With such a filter the engineer can measure separately the components of a complex tone such as a musical chord. The line spectra illustrated in Figure 2-2 were obtained in this way. Or the pass band can be made wider, say a third of an octave or half an octave or, most commonly, a full octave in width. With such an *octave band filter* the sound pressure level of each octave band of a complex noise, such as street noise or airplane noise, can be measured separately. In this way the band spectra illustrated in Figure 2-3 were obtained. The band spectrum is a very useful way of describing a complex noise and gives the acoustic engineer part of his fundamental data if he needs to design, for example, an audiometric booth to exclude the noise in question. High frequencies are, in general, easier to exclude than low frequencies; hence it is

Fig. 2-2. In the clarinet spectrum (A) the second and fourth harmonics (400 and 800 cps) are more than 30 db below the intensity of the fundamental tone. The sixth harmonic is also very weak. In the violin spectrum (B) the second, fourth, and sixth harmonics are the strongest and the odd-numbered harmonics are weak. The "overtone structure" gives the characteristic quality of each instrument. The strength of each harmonic is easily measured with the help of electrical filters that allow only a very narrow band of frequencies (a constant number of cycles per second) to pass through. The sound of a bell also has a line spectrum (C), but the energy is very irregularly distributed among a few of the higher harmonics. In the sounds of many bells inharmonic frequencies are also strongly present. (*All from H. Fletcher, American Journal of Physics, 14: 215–225 [1946].*)

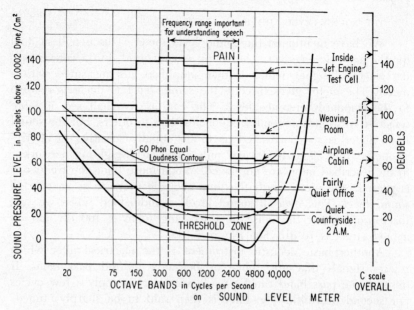

Fig. 2-3. **The auditory area and octave band spectra of five steady background noises.** The threshold zone and the threshold of pain are the same as in Fig. 2-4. It is not strictly logical to plot data based on pure tones, such as thresholds and equal-loudness contours, on the same scale of sound pressure levels that is used for octave band analyses. The error is not large, however, in relation to the dynamic range of the sounds represented here, and it does not affect the comparisons of one noise with another. The 60-phon equal-loudness contour is at a comfortable listening level. It lies entirely above the spectrum of the quiet office but below the spectrum in the airplane cabin. The top spectrum was measured inside a typical jet-engine test cell with the engine operating at military power. The peak of acoustic energy is in the 300–600 cps band. The weaving room had mechanical looms; the floor was wooden. These two spectra are fairly "flat." The airplane spectrum was taken at the last window seat while the plane was climbing. It is a sharply sloping spectrum. Notice that its over-all sound pressure level (right) is higher than that for the weaving room because of the large contribution of the lowest, 20–75 cps, band. Speech is better understood in the airplane noise, however, because in the 600–1200 and 1200–2400 cps bands the sound levels are lower than those in the weaving room. (The levels are nearly equal in the 300–600 band.) In the "fairly quiet office" there were no business machines. Its over-all sound level of 64 db is deceptively high because of the sloping spectrum. The spectrum of the quiet countryside at 2 A.M. lies almost entirely within the threshold zone, i.e., some people with normal hearing would hear only a very faint rustle (600 to 4800 cps), although the over-all sound level is 50 db. The noise in the jet engine test cell is above the threshold for pain. (*Adapted from a figure by J. R. Cox, Jr., in Industrial Hygiene and Toxicology. New York: Interscience Publishers, 1958, Vol. I.*)

40

important for him to know not only the over-all level, but also how much energy is present in each octave band.

SOUND POWER

The acoustic engineer finds it very convenient to calculate the total acoustic power-output of sound sources, such as jet engines, automobiles on the highway, ventilating fans, or the human voice. The sound power is expressed in watts, but here again it is convenient to use the decibel scale and to talk about the "power level" (PWL). Unfortunately, this additional use of the decibel leads to much confusion. The *power levels* are, of course, always much higher than the *sound levels* that the same sources produce at the ears of the listeners. The power level is a measure of all of the watts of acoustic energy radiated in all directions by the source. The sound level is only the number of watts that flow through one square centimeter at the position of the sound level meter. Thus a full symphony orchestra may generate 140 db PWL (relative to 10^{-12} watt per square meter but the listener may receive only 90 db SL (relative to 10^{-16} watt per square centimeter) at his seat in the balcony.

The usual reference for power level is the same as for sound level. For power it is usually expressed as 10^{-12} watt per square *meter*, which is the same physically as 10^{-16} watt per square centimeter. The sound power level is conceived as a flow of acoustic energy through an area of one square meter that forms the surface of an imaginary spherical source. Only a tiny fraction of this power reaches a distant listener. Our principal present concern with sound power is to avoid being misled when we encounter this other use of the decibel scale.

RESONANCE

In describing the electrical filter, we referred to "tuning" the filter to a desired frequency. The idea of a tuned circuit should be familiar to everyone who "tunes" his radio or television circuit to a desired broadcast frequency or who tunes acoustical devices such as musical instruments. We know that a violin or piano string vibrates at a higher frequency when it is pulled tighter as in "tuning up," or when, on the violin, the vibrating part is shortened by the player's finger. And we have probably noticed that the bass strings of these instruments are thicker and heavier than those in the treble.

In general, any mechanical system that is free to vibrate tends to vibrate at a *natural frequency* that is determined by the mass of the vibrating parts and their stiffness. It is easier to set the system vibrating or *oscillating* at this frequency than at any other, in the sense that for a given amount of alternating pressure the vibrating system will build up a greater amplitude of movement. The system tends to move of itself or "oscillate" exactly in step with the driving force and does not tend either to lag behind or to creep ahead. This relation of tending to move exactly in step with the driving force is called *resonance*.

Energy tends to be stored in a resonant system, whether it be acoustic or electric. This energy is continually being changed back and forth from kinetic energy to potential energy. In a typical mechanical system these forms of energy are represented by the momentum of a moving mass and the elongation of a spring, repectively. Energy is removed from the system by doing work elsewhere or by being dissipated into heat by friction. Frictional dissipation of the energy is called *damping*. If a system is too heavily damped it will not vibrate at all but when displaced will simply creep back slowly to its position of rest without overshoot. Imagine a violin string vibrating in molasses!

For our purposes it is important to recognize that air in a container that has one or more openings is a resonant system. Air has mass and it acquires momentum as it moves in and out of the container. The air is also compressible, so that it acts both as the mass and the spring. The natural frequency or frequencies of an air-filled system depend on the volume of the container, on the size of the openings, and, in more complicated ways, on the shape of the cavity. We know that the trombone player lengthens his "pipe" to reach a low note and that if we blow across the mouth of an empty bottle it resonates at a lower frequency (lower pitch) than if it is half full, and so on. We shall see that the resonances of air-filled cavities enable them to store energy at certain frequencies and also to transmit these frequencies more effectively than others from one end to the other. This principle was utilized in the construction of nonelectrical hearing aids. The same principle in electrical circuits is the basis of most electrical filters.

THE TIME-PATTERN OF SOUNDS

To describe music or speech, the physicist tells how the frequencies and the corresponding intensities vary from moment to moment. The rhythm (*stress-pattern*) and the tempo, whether regular or irregular, are essential features that we learn to recognize as well as the sequence of different pitches. Speech and music are not static but are patterns that change from moment to moment.

Biological and Psychological Aspects of Hearing

Sound is produced incidentally by almost all events in nature that involve the rapid motion of air or water or even moderate movement of solid objects. It is very difficult to make any sort of machine run without some noise. Sound is one of nature's surest signs of activity, and therein lies its primitive biological significance. Hearing keeps us *informed* of activities going on at some distance from us and *gives us warning* if that activity becomes more powerful or approaches very close. The important psychological consequences of loss of the primitive awareness and warnings of hearing are discussed in detail in a later chapter. Sight, to be sure, also informs us of distant events, but hearing is the true "watchdog" of the senses. (A watchdog should really be called a "harkdog," for he hears the stranger approach by night before he sees him.) The sun never sets for hearing, and sound waves come to us around corners and reach our ears whichever way our heads are turned. No "earlid" covers the ear in sleep. Experiments on the electrical activity of the brain show that the sleeping brain is at least partially aroused by sounds, even by rather faint sounds if they are unusual or if we have learned that they are warning signals for us.

When we recognize a warning sound, we usually also have some sense of the direction whence it comes. The sense of direction—*auditory localization*—is usually good enough to cause us to look in more or less the right direction. Both ears are necessary for this localization, or *stereophonic effect,* and we must admit that we are often misled by the curved path of sound around corners and by its reflection as an echo from any large flat surface. It is interesting, however, that bats have developed to an extraordinary degree the power of locating distant objects by the reflection of high-pitched chirps that the bats themselves emit. Nature developed this sonar principle (like radar, but using sound) long before World War II! The blind can learn to make practical use of it, just as the deaf learn speechreading to replace a lost auditory function.

The highest level of audition lies in the recognition of the nature of distant activity. We know what is going on when we hear footsteps, traffic noise, barking dogs, and the like. And, above all, man, by his ability to distinguish and recognize the meaning of sounds, together with his ability to produce a great variety of them with his voice, has developed a system of communication with his fellows that far outdoes the communication between any other animals. The practical and social importance of speech and the hearing of speech need no elaboration. Probably the greatest prehistoric invention of the human race was not fire or the wheel or even the weapon but *language,* for language gave man not only the ability to share experience but a tool for abstract thinking.

FREQUENCY LIMITS OF AUDIBLE SOUND

The range of audible frequencies extends from about 20 to about 20,000 cps. Neither limit is at all precise. Not only the frequency but the intensity of a sound determine whether or not we can bear it. The ear is limited, like a radio receiver, to a band of frequencies. For the ear the most sensitive range is from 500 to 4000 cps, approximately the same range of frequencies, by the way, that is most important for understanding speech. Above 4000 and below 500 cps the sensitivity of the ear declines more and more rapidly, but the tones can still be heard at comfortable intensities by normal young ears. Another uncertainty about the limits arises from individual differences in ears. The child may be able to hear the "inaudible" dog whistle at about 20,000 cps, whereas the old man may no longer hear even the overtones of the human voice at about 5000 cps. And for the low tones, there is still a lively debate as to whether we really *hear* through the auditory nerve a tone as low as 20 or 30 cps or only *feel* it through the nerves of touch while we hear its higher harmonics.

Below and above the range of frequencies that the ear can detect lie the *subsonic* (vibration) and the *ultrasonic* frequencies, respectively. The ultrasonic frequencies used to be called *supersonic;* but present usage is to speak of "ultrasonic frequencies" (by analogy with ultraviolet light) and "supersonic speeds." The ultrasonic waves can be compared to the short-wave radio broadcasts, which cannot be picked up by an ordinary radio receiver. The physicist with his instruments cares little for the arbitrary limits imposed by human ears. The limits of hearing are certainly higher for dogs, cats, rats, and probably all small mammals. The physicist's instruments carry him on up into the ultrasonic region of high frequencies where blasts of air, crackling of twigs, the chirping of many insects, the cries of bats, all produce pressure waves in air of the same kind as ordinary sound, but inaudible to us because of their high frequency. Actually, these ultrasonics in nature are never very intense and would probably not be very important to animals of our size, even if we could hear them. They do give fairly accurate information as to the direction of their sources, for they travel in straighter lines, bend less around corners, and consequently cast deeper "sound shadows" than do the lower frequencies. However, as a general rule, ultrasonics are generated by *small* objects and are not transmitted so well through the air as are the longer wave lengths. The air is partially opaque to the ultrasonics, and, even if fairly intense at their source, they can be detected only at relatively short distances. The near ultrasonics in the first octave or so above the human limit may be important for small animals, but not for us. We need not fear them, as some people have suggested, as possibly injurious, for they are feeble. Theory and experience agree that they are practically quite harmless.

THE SOUND RANGE OF THE EAR

The psychophysicist is interested in the relations between our sensations and the dimensions and magnitudes of the changes in the external world (the stimuli) that arouse them. We know that the dimensions of physical sound are frequency and intensity, measured, respectively, in cycles per second and in decibels. On a chart scaled off in these two dimensions we can map the *area of audible tones* (Figure 2-4). It is bounded at the bottom by the *threshold of hearing.* The "threshold" is the faintest sound of a given frequency that can just be heard. This curve expresses the *acuity* of human hearing, although the term "acuity" is slightly ambiguous and is sometimes misunderstood as referring instead to the ability to discriminate between two tones that are nearly the same. It is therefore safer to say that the curve in question represents the *threshold of sensitivity* of human hearing or the "threshold of detectability" of pure tones. Tones above threshold are audible, those below are inaudible.

In Figure 2-4 we have represented the threshold by a shaded area instead of by the conventional black line. We have done so because not all persons have the same thresholds and also because one person's threshold varies somewhat from day to day and even from moment to moment. Above all, the threshold depends on how the signals are presented, how much effort the listener is making to listen carefully, how much practice he has had in such listening and what percentage of success in repeated trials he must achieve for us to credit him with being able to "hear" a particular test signal. (Fifty per cent correct is the usual requirement.)

The lower edge of the shaded boundary in Figure 2-4 represents the average performance of a group of practiced, well-motivated young adults, listening with both ears. It represents reasonably the "best" threshold of human hearing, although some members of the group did consistently better than others and all members did better on some trials than on others. Of course, the tests were carried out

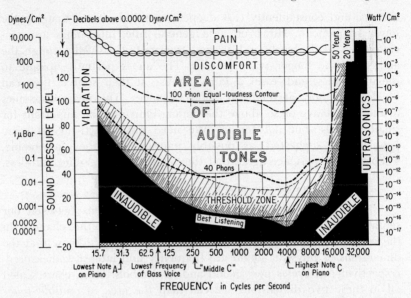

Fig. 2-4. The auditory area for listening with both ears in an acoustic field, as in everyday listening, is bounded below by the threshold zone, by vibration on the low-frequency side, by ultrasonics on the high-frequency side, and, practically, by the threshold of pain in the direction of high intensity. Below the threshold zone, tones are inaudible. None of the boundaries are sharp. Even under the best listening conditions, normal well-motivated young listeners may differ by 15 db. The lower edge of the zone, labeled "best listening," represents the median sensitivity of a group of otologically normal young ears listening in a free acoustic field. The dips at 4000 and 12,000 are due to resonance effects in the ear canals, diffraction patterns around the head, etc. (The acoustic field is measured before the head is placed in it.) The high-frequency boundary becomes progressively lower with age. Two equal-loudness contours are shown for tones judged to sound as loud as 1000 cps tones at 40 db and 100 db SPL, respectively. Sound pressure levels (SPL) are given at the extreme left in dynes per square centimeter or microbars (μ bar), next in decibels above the standard reference level, and at the right in watts per square centimeter. (*Data from D. W. Robinson and R. S. Dadson, Journal of the Acoustical Society of America, 29:1284–1288* [1957].)

in very carefully sound-treated rooms where "background" noise and echoes were so faint that they did not interfere with or "mask" the faint test tones. The listeners were listening with both ears to a sound coming from the front. (The dips and peaks in this contour are due, at least in part, to the pattern of reflection of the sound waves around the head and ears of the listeners. They are not present when the same kind of test is made with earphones instead of, as we say, in an "acoustic field.")

The threshold boundary of the auditory area is broad. The shaded zone extends from the "best" threshold to the thresholds typical of the least sensitive young adults who have had no training in careful listening and who, although honest enough, are not particularly interested in making any special effort to listen. Yet none of these poorer listeners have anything *wrong* with their ears. Their eardrums look normal to the examining physician and they have never had any trouble with their ears or their hearing. They simply represent the upper limit of the range of normal auditory acuity. People vary considerably in their acuity just as they do in height or intelligence. Of course, the distribution covers the entire range of the threshold zone, and many more people have thresholds near the middle than at either the upper or the lower limit of this zone.

For all listeners the threshold curve rises quite sharply in the high frequencies. The tones must be made much stronger in order to be heard at all; finally they cannot be heard at any practical intensity. This nearly vertical part of the curve separates the inaudible ultrasonics from the area of audible tones. Here, too, the zone of normal acuity is wide, and above 2000 cps the *age* of the listener becomes more and more important. Old ears do not hear high frequencies as well as young ears hear them.

For low frequencies, thresholds also rise, but not as abruptly as for high frequencies. Below about 30 cps it is difficult to be sure that we are really *hearing* the sound and not simply *feeling* the vibration. This question is not of much practical importance, however. Moreover, it is hard to generate really pure tones at these very low frequencies. We can hear the higher harmonics easily even though they may have less than one ten-thousandth of the acoustic energy of the fundamental.

The auditory area is bounded at its upper edge, for practical purposes, by the thresholds of discomfort, of tickle, and, finally, of pain. These thresholds also vary from person to person and with the attitude of the listener toward these very loud sounds and toward the tests. There are also problems of just what the words "discomfort," "tickle," and "pain" mean. Many listeners are likely at first to report pain for a sensation that they later call merely "tickle" after they have once felt the sharp stab of true auditory pain. If prolonged, such very intense sounds are dangerous to hearing as well as painful, so the practical upper limit of the auditory area at about 135 db sound level is very real. As it happens, these thresholds of discomfort, tickle, and pain are pretty nearly constant, regardless of frequency. Only the first unpleasantness, the "discomfort," is a truly auditory sensation. Actually the *loudness* of the sounds keeps on increasing as the intensity is increased, regardless of discomfort, tickle in the ear, or pain.

HEARING LOSS AND THE AUDIOGRAM

The most common impairment of hearing is a loss of sensitivity for some or all frequencies. A full discussion of the several varieties of hearing loss is given in Chapter 4. The amount of "hearing loss" or "shift of threshold" is measured in decibels by means of an *audiometer*. Details of this instrument and its use are given in Chapter 7, but the nature of the measure that it gives us is of interest here because of certain parallelisms and certain contrasts between the sound level meter and the audiometer and because of the relation of "hearing loss" to the threshold zone of hearing that bounds the auditory area.

For practical reasons the audiometer employs a pair of earphones for the listener and not the acoustic field that was used to define the auditory area. The acoustic problems are far simpler with earphones; moreover, it is possible to test each ear separately. Two new problems are introduced, however, which concern the relation between the measurements of hearing made with an audiometer and the measurements of sound made with a sound level meter. One problem is the relation between field listening and earphone listening; the other is the problem of monaural versus binaural listening.

The problem of hearing with one ear rather than with two is not a serious one. Careful tests, both in an acoustic field and with earphones, show that two ears are better than one and that the gain in sensitivity is about 3 db. This seems reasonable because 3 db represent a doubling of acoustic power, although the physiologist finds it a little difficult to explain just how the two ears manage to interact to do a better job than either one can do alone. But when we compare the pressure level of the minimum audible field with the minimum audible pressure (at the entrance to the ear canal) under an earphone, we find that hearing, even for one ear alone, seems to be 6 db more sensitive for field listening than for earphone listening. The methods of measuring both the hearing and the sound pressure levels have been examined and re-examined, but so far no one has solved the mystery of "the missing 6 db."

For this reason, among others, we must start all over again with the audiometer and determine experimentally the auditory area for earphone listening. The best threshold that we now find with trained, well-motivated, and otologically normal young listeners we call the "minimum audible pressure" (MAP) instead of the "minimum audible field" (MAF). The whole auditory area is displaced upwards about 6 db. Actually, the best measurements of the thresholds of discomfort, tickle, and pain have been made with earphone listening. They are therefore directly applicable to the problem of hearing aids.

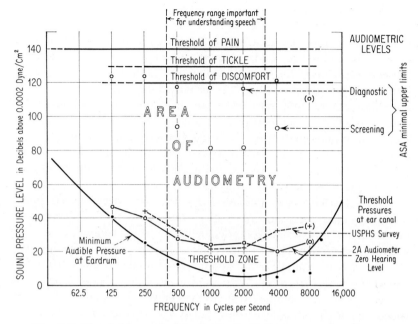

Fig. 2-5. **Threshold sound pressure levels in the ear canal under an earphone (monaural), and the SPL specifications for American Standard audiometers.** The minimum audible pressure close to the eardrum membrane can be measured by a probe tube. This threshold curve, originally determined at the Bell Telephone Laboratories, is quite well established. The British audiometric zero (solid circles) lies very close to it. The two other lower curves are based on pressure measurements under the earphone near the *outer* end of the canal. The pressures here differ appreciably at 4000 and at 8000 cps from those deep in the canal. This difference is important at high frequencies and accounts in part for the lack of parallelism among the three curves above 2000 cps. The values at 8000 cps, in parentheses, are questionable. The USPHS survey data (Beasley) are the basis of the American Standard zero hearing level. (*Calculations of ear-canal pressures for these and the 2A audiometer data are by J. E. Steinberg, et al., Journal of the Acoustical Society of America, 11:270 and 12:291 [1940].*) The sound levels corresponding to the thresholds of discomfort, tickle, and pain (measured at Central Institute for the Deaf) are the levels in a NBS-9A coupler. These thresholds have not been adequately explored below 250 or above 5000 cps except for the threshold of pain at low frequencies. The open circles near the threshold of discomfort are the maximum output levels required in the American Standard for Audiometers for General Diagnostic Purposes (Z24.5-1951). Actually, many makes of audiometer provide levels 5 or even 10 db higher in the middle-frequency range, i.e., about 120 to 125 db SPL at all frequencies except 8000 cps. The open circles nearer the middle of the area are the corresponding ASA requirements for the maximum output of "screening" audiometers (Z24.12-1952). The solid circles represent the British Standard for normal threshold of hearing, transferred to an American earphone (705A) and coupler (NBS-9A). (*Transfer based on data of J. P. Albrite, et al., courtesy of National Bureau of Standards.*) The deviation of the points at 4000, 6000, and 10,000 cps from the solid curve is probably due in part to the resonance of the ear canal.

49

The audiometer is designed to tell the tester how much the hearing of the ear under test differs from a standard "normal" value. The difference is expressed as a ratio in decibels. The reason for looking only at the differences and not at the absolute values is to discount the curved shape of the threshold shown in Figure 2-5. The curvature is normal, but the audiologist is usually interested in possible abnormalities. A straight zero reference line shows up deviations most effectively. The audiometer is calibrated so that zero on its intensity scale corresponds to "normal" hearing (by earphone listening). More details about this zero reference level are given in Chapter 7, but this difference between the actual threshold level and the normal reference level is the value we want. We call it the *hearing level*.

The hearing level measured by the audiometer corresponds broadly to the sound pressure level measured by the sound level meter. Each is expressed in decibels and each represents a ratio with respect to a rather arbitrary reference level. The acoustic reference level is the same for all frequencies, but the audiometric reference level varies from one frequency to another. The hearing levels are conventionally plotted octave by octave, like the octave band spectrum measured with a sound analyzer. This graphic representation of the hearing levels for pure tones is the *audiogram.*

The otologist habitually thinks of the hearing level as a deviation from normal. The traditional name for it has for years been "hearing loss." The reasons for using the relatively new term "hearing level" are given in Chapter 4. The audiogram is conventionally plotted with the zero reference level as a straight horizontal line near the top. Here positive values of hearing loss (hearing level) are plotted downward to convey the idea of impairment, as in Figures 7-6 and 7-7. Notice that this is opposite to the convention used for plotting the auditory area. There we plotted the actual sound pressure levels, and a low value for threshold (downward on the chart) meant *more sensitive* hearing.

The audiometer has been described at this point to emphasize that it is a fundamental tool of the audiologist and is very much like the sound level meter and sound analyzer of the physicist. The latter measures acoustic energy in the form of sound pressure levels, the audiometer measures auditory sensitivity in the form of hearing levels. Unfortunately, however, the differences in reference levels as between earphone listening and field listening ("the missing 6 db") make it impossible to relate the sound pressure levels (sound level meter) to hearing levels (audiometer) in any simple way, even though both are expressed in decibels. Part of the task of the audiologist, the psychologist, and the acoustic engineer is to understand and to explore further just these relationships.

THE SPEECH AREA

A particularly important part of the auditory area is the range of frequencies most important for the understanding of speech. This range extends from roughly 400 to 3000 cps. Speech contains frequencies both above 3000 cps and below 400 cps but they are not necessary for almost perfect intelligibility of everyday conversational speech. The importance of the speech range will appear later in relation to the design of hearing aids and to the problem of auditory handicap. The part of the auditory area that is important for speech is further bounded at the top by the thresholds of tolerance, and at the bottom, for practical purposes, by the background sound level against which we are likely to hear faint everyday speech. Practically this is at an octave band level of approximately 30 to 40 db. Figure 2-6 shows the range of frequencies most important for good understanding of everyday speech. It also shows the approximate distribution with respect to frequency and intensity of the actual sounds of conversational speech.

Auditory Sensations

PITCH

Pitch is a subjective quality of sound that is most clearly recognized for pure tones. It is a quality by which we can arrange sounds on a scale from "low" or bass to "high" or treble. It is the quality that enables us to play a tune. The musical pitch of a note depends chiefly on the physical frequency of the sound waves and also, to a very limited extent, on their intensity. The positions of the lowest and the highest notes of the piano and of its middle C (261.6 cps) are shown in Figure 2-4. The relation of the musical scale to simple numerical ratios of the frequencies of the sound waves is too familiar to need elaboration. We need only mention the particularly close musical relation between two frequencies that are an octave apart. The higher frequency is exactly double the lower frequency. The musical scale is thus related to the *logarithm* of frequency even more closely than loudness is related to the logarithmic decibel.

The pitch of a pure tone is clear and definite, and so is that of a fundamental and its series of harmonics (Figure 2-2). We hear the pitch of such a complex tone as the same as that of its fundamental, although its musical quality is different. The pitch of musical chords is harder to specify. Sometimes they sound single; sometimes the components are heard separately. Even noises that have a large part of their acoustic energy concentrated in one part of the spectrum have more or less pitch, although the pitch produced by striking two

Below 1000 cps is power of speech — vowel sounds.

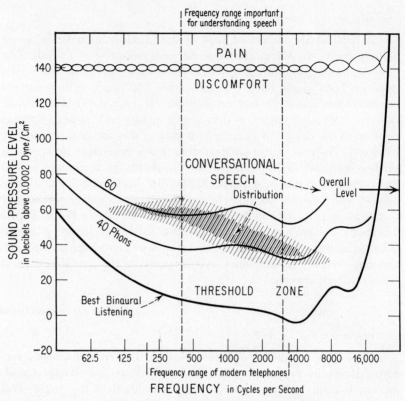

Fig. 2-6. **The speech area.** Speech is a mixture of complex tones, wide band noise, and transients. Both the intensities and the frequencies of speech sounds change continually and rapidly. It is difficult to measure them and logically impossible to plot them precisely in terms of sound pressure levels at particular frequencies. This figure shows the approximate distribution of sound pressure levels with respect to frequency that would occur if brief but characteristic bits of phonemes of conversational speech were actually sustained like pure tones. The density of the shaded area represents roughly the probability of finding in a sample of speech the particular combinations of intensity and frequency. Individual voices differ, however, and obviously the boundaries of the speech area are not sharp.

The over-all sound pressure level of the stronger vowels in conversational speech at 1 meter is about 72 db. The fundamental frequency of a deep bass voice is about 100 cps, but the fundamental frequencies of most women's and children's voices are about 250 cps. The strongest individual sounds in the frequency range below 1000 cps are louder than 60 phons while the weakest significant elements are about 30 db below the strongest. The weaker elements are very often masked by background noises. Modern telephones transmit the frequency range from 200 to 3400 cps, but for good understanding of everyday speech the range from 400 to 3000 cps is sufficient. This range includes almost all of the "formant" frequency bands of speech which distinguish the vowels and many consonants. See "Man's World of Sound" by Pierce and Davis for a good acoustic description of speech.

52

kinds of wood together, for example, may not be appreciated until two other pieces of wood are struck together and we begin to play a tune with them. "Pitchness" grades without boundaries from the pure musical tone to the complete randomness of white noise.

LOUDNESS

Loudness is the psychological attribute of sound that is most closely related to intensity. As the intensity of a pure tone increases, so does the loudness that we hear, and we have mentioned that the just noticeable steps of loudness are (very roughly) constant in terms of decibels. But a given physical intensity (in dynes per square centimeter) may sound much louder if the tone lies near the middle of the range of audible frequencies than it will if its frequency is very high or very low. In fact, a tone at 30 db above the standard reference level is well heard at 1000 or 2000 cps but is inaudible at 200 and at 10,000 cps. On the other hand, if the sound is very powerful, say at 100 or 120 db, it seems almost equally loud at all audible frequencies. The loudness of a very high-pitched or very low-pitched tone must therefore grow more rapidly than the loudness of a tone of middle pitch as its intensity is increased from just audible up to 100 db, because its just audible intensity (or threshold) lies *higher* on the decibel scale and the tone reaches the *same* loudness at 100 db. In Figure 2-4 are two curves labeled "equal-loudness contours." They lie above the threshold curve, but they are straighter, and the upper curve is straighter and more horizontal than the lower. These two curves represent a whole family of equal-loudness contours that can be drawn across the auditory area. Each curve connects the tones of different frequency that sound equally loud. An understanding of the change from curved to straight in the equal-loudness contours will help in understanding some of the problems of partial hearing loss, particularly of the so-called sensory-neural deafness described in Chapter 4. Notice in Figure 7-11 (sensory-neural deafness) that the equal-loudness contour at about the 100-db level is only slightly displaced upward, in spite of the very great elevation of the threshold. Contrast this with the great elevation of the equal-loudness contour in Figure 7-10 (conduction deafness). The practical significance of this difference will be explained later.

At the top of the area of audiometry shown in Figure 2-5 are three horizontal lines labeled "Threshold of Discomfort," "Threshold of Tickle," and "Threshold of Pain." These contours were determined by increasing the intensity of tones by small steps and asking a listener to report. These *thresholds of tolerance*, as they are called, seem to be straight lines, like the upper equal-loudness contours, over the frequency range where it has been possible to map them accurately. The shape of these curves means that for the average listener and for earphone listening, tones become uncomfortably loud, begin to tickle, and begin to hurt at about 120, 130, and 140 db, respectively, regardless of their frequency. Most of the individual end points scatter over a range of 10 db above or below the medians for the group. It is both interesting and important to know that with a little experience in listening to these very loud sounds, the thresholds of tolerance rise by as much as 10 or 15 db, so that tones which at first were considered "uncomfortable" or "painful" are later tolerated and found to be painless. A series of wartime experiments at the Central Institute for the Deaf showed that both normal and hard-of-hearing listeners could increase their tolerance in this way. There is an obvious moral here for those who find on first trial that a hearing aid sounds uncomfortably loud and may therefore deprive themselves of the benefit from it that they might comfortably attain with a little systematic practice.

EXAMPLES OF LOUDNESS

Loudness and pitch are sensations. What is meant by speaking of a given degree of loudness or the position of pitch can be illustrated by familiar examples. On the pitch scale such examples are easy to find, for our musical scale is well established and is built into many of our musical instruments. We can strike A above middle C on a piano and immediately illustrate what we mean by the pitch of a note of 440 cps. But it is not easy to cite familiar useful examples of loudness to give a meaning in experience to the decibel scale. For one thing, most familiar sounds are complex and contain many frequencies, and the acoustic energy at these various frequencies may add together quite differently for the sound level meter and for the ear. For example, the ear is much less sensitive to the 60-cycle hum that is usually present to some extent in the music that comes from our radios but it is very sensitive to frequencies from 800 to 4000 cps in the upper part of the musical range. If the music is soft we may hear it and it alone, even though the hum is physically more intense than the music. But the over-all level in decibels measured by the sound level meter will in this case be determined chiefly by the hum. In this situation there is simply no practical relation between the loudness that we hear and the decibel reading on the meter. In other words, *the sound level meter is not a loudness meter.* The acoustic engineer can calculate approximately from the band spectrum levels of a noise how loud it will sound in relation to a standard tone of 1000 cps at a sound level of 40 db, but the rules are rather complicated and have not been fully standard-ized. He does not express the answer in decibels but in a sub-jective unit of loudness called the *sone,* i.e., the loudness of a 1000 cps tone at 40 db. But in everyday life we are not accustomed to thinking in sones.

When the sound level meter was first devised it was called a noise level meter and its designers tried to make it deal with sounds in approximately the same way the ear does, so that its readings (in decibels) would correspond to the loudness (sones) that we hear. Two sets of filters (the so-called A network and B network) were provided. Their pass bands corresponded roughly to the shapes of the human equal-loudness contours for faint and for moderate sounds, respectively. For loud sounds like factory noise or heavy traffic, the "flat" or "C" setting (no filter) was to be used. For a number of years the meter was used consistently in this way and many characteristic "noise levels" in decibels were published. Some of these were cited in Figure 6 (page 45) of the first edition of this book. But since 1940, when octave band filters came into general use, the A and B networks have been used less and less and the early noise levels measured with them are now usually confused with over-all sound levels measured without any network. The result is that the old levels given for "quiet dwellings," "rustling of leaves," "whisper," and the like, look ridiculously low. We have therefore omitted any tabulation of such decibel levels from the present edition. Instead, we give in Figure 2-3 the octave band analyses of five noises, all relatively steady and easy to measure. The corresponding over-all levels are also given. Perhaps in the future, when band spectra of various kinds of noise have become more familiar and when the rules for calculating loudness have be-come better standardized, a new table can be prepared. For the present, a few approximate rules, in terms of *over-all sound level,* must suffice:

> A broad-band noise like most aircraft or factory noise is very loud at 90 db and is definitely uncomfortable at 120 db.
> A shout at 1 foot from the ear is about 100 db, but the highest level that can be maintained for long is 90 db.
> Conversational speech at 1 yard is about 65 db.
> Faint but intelligible speech in a quiet room is about 40 to 45 db.

In the above rules we have put some numbers on the *sound level of speech.* This introduces a new difficulty. The sound pressure level of speech varies from instant to instant, from one word to the next and from sound to sound within the word. The momentary instantaneous peaks of pressure are 10 to as much as 20 db above the over-all long-time average. The needle of the sound level meter dances up and down, and we must be content to settle for its "average maximum swing." A rather vague rule indeed! Abrupt brief sounds like a pistol shot or a hammer blow give particular difficulty. Certain special meters called *impact meters* deal with them better than does the simpler sound level meter, but even these are not yet fully satisfactory and the measurements made with them are not easy to interpret. For all of these reasons it requires some special instruction and training to use even the ordinary sound level meter properly and to interpret the measurements made with it.

Finally, our own sense of the loudness of a sound is not constant. We may consistently judge a given tone louder or softer, depending on whether we have just been listening to loud or to faint sound. If a sound is rather strong, it sounds less loud after we listen to it for a few moments. Previous experience with very loud sounds (over 120 db) makes them less unpleasant and uncomfortable and even raises the level at which a listener says that they are actually painful. We are accustomed to the idea that our eyes adjust to the level of illumination. We expect to be temporarily blinded when we first enter a movie house but we know that in three or four minutes we will see the aisle and the seats fairly well, and we are not surprised when we are painfully dazzled on coming out into the afternoon sunshine. Our ears sometimes adapt more rapidly than our eyes but sometimes much more slowly. We are only just learning how dynamic and labile our sense of loudness actually is. The idea of temporary auditory fatigue or "threshold shift" is a relatively new one in the laboratory and the clinic even though workers in noisy places have known about it for a hundred years.

OTHER QUALITIES OF SOUNDS

Loudness and pitch are the two chief subjective qualities of pure tones, and they correspond, approximately at least, to the physical dimensions of intensity and frequency, respectively. Tempo and time-patterning of pitch and loudness obviously correspond to the pattern in time of the changes in frequency and intensity of the physical sound waves. Several other psychological attributes of sounds include "timbre," "brightness" or "brilliance," "roughness," "density," and "volume." All of them apparently depend on the composition of complex tones or else on particular combinations of frequency and intensity. The details of these attributes need not concern us in our rapid survey.

A musical instrument such as the clarinet or the violin tends to strengthen all the harmonics that fall in a particular frequency range, whatever the fundamental of the note that is being played. This range of reinforcement is called a *formant* and gives distinctive character or quality to the sound. The vowels of speech differ from one another in the formants that are imposed by the resonant cavities of the mouth and pharynx. The formants change with different positions of lips, tongue, and jaw, and are independent of the fundamental frequency of the voice that is determined by the vibration of the vocal cords in the larynx.

SENSATIONS AND NERVE IMPULSES

So far we have considered the over-all relationship between sound waves in the air around us and our sensations of hearing. Two major steps are involved in going from the physical level to the psychological: first, the translation in the ear of the pattern of sound waves into a pattern of nerve impulses, and then the translation of the nerve impulses in the brain into sensations. We know something about how the sound waves set off nerve impulses. We know more about how the impulses travel along the nerves and to what parts of the brain they go; but as to *how* nerve impulses "set up" sensations we know almost exactly nothing. We hardly even know how to phrase questions that could be given meaningful answers. All that we can do at present is to describe the same sort of laws of correspondence between nerve impulses and sensations that we have described between sound waves and sensations.

THE SPECIFICITY OF SENSORY NERVES

The first law of psychophysiology in general is the *specificity of the sensory nerves*. Only by means of nerve impulses in specific auditory pathways can auditory sensations be aroused; and however impulses are set up in those pathways, the sensation is always one of hearing and not of any other sense. We never see or taste with our ears. If we seem to feel tickle or pain with our ears, it is because nerve fibers of touch and of pain also run to the ear as they do to nearly all parts of the body. And if, by touching with a probe or by applying an electric current, we stimulate the auditory nerve directly, we do not feel a touch but instead hear some sort of noise, just as we "see stars" from the mechanical stimulation of the optic nerves by a violent blow on the head.

No exceptions to the law of specificity of sensory nerves are known, and we must accept the practical consequence that when, from accident or disease, the auditory nerve degenerates, no direct substitute for it can be found. And, unfortunately, the highly specialized auditory nerve tends to degenerate rather readily after injury to its delicate terminations in the sense organ. A violent explosive sound can cause such injury. Neither the fibers of the auditory nerve nor the specialized sensory cells that excite them regenerate after they have been seriously injured. Therefore we do not waste time chasing rainbows in efforts to restore hearing once we are sure of a diagnosis of nerve degeneration.

A more restricted proposition in the psychophysiology of hearing has recently passed from the realm of theory into the class of well-established generalizations and may now properly be called a scientific "law." It states that *one basis for the sensation of pitch is the transmission of nerve impulses by specific auditory fibers.* Stimulation of certain fibers causes us to hear a high-pitched tone; stimulation of others, a low-pitched tone. The sense of pitch is distributed, so to speak, among the fibers of the auditory nerve just as the sense of touch is distributed over the body. In this analogy, hearing a high-pitched tone corresponds to feeling a touch on the face; a low-pitched tone, a touch on the foot. White noise depends on a simultaneous all-over massage. Actually, we shall see that the ultimate sense organ of hearing deep within the ear is a long line of tiny individual sensory cells side by side on a flexible vibrating membrane. The individual fibers of the nerve of hearing run to these cells. When one part of the membrane vibrates, those particular sensory cells are stimulated to set up impulses in the few fibers connected directly with them. The impulses run to several parts of the brain and somehow or other "arouse the sensation" of a particular pitch.

Sound waves of different frequencies cause the long, narrow membrane to vibrate most strongly in different regions and thus stimulate different groups of sensory cells and their nerve fibers. We now have a fairly complete physical and mathematical model and theory as to how this selective "tuning" of the membrane is brought about. It depends on the details of the anatomy of the inner ear, on the size and density and elasticity of the various structures. Direct measurement of the physical properties of the different parts is almost impossible because of their small size and inaccessible location, but great advances in our knowledge have been made in the last twenty years, thanks especially to the experimental genius of George von Békésy.

The *law of neural specificity of pitch,* formerly known as "the place theory of hearing," has recently been demonstrated by a very direct experiment. The nerve impulses in single nerve cells of the auditory system of an anesthetized animal were recorded by appropriate (and, we may add, complicated) electrical apparatus. Only when tones in a particular narrow band of frequencies were delivered to the animal's ear did nerve impulses appear in a particular cell, and different cells responded to different bands of frequencies. Of course, the louder the tones, the wider was the band of frequencies to which each cell responded; but until the tones were made very loud indeed, each cell responded to only a small fraction of the entire audible range. The "tuning" of each unit, like the tuning of a radio set, is fairly sharp but not absolutely selective.

The place theory is not the whole story of pitch, however. For tones that are not too high in frequency, which means for tones below about 1000 cps, information as to the frequency is sent up the auditory nerve in the form of a time-pattern of the discharge of the nerve impulses. Volleys of impulses reproduce directly the frequency of the sound waves because each wave tends to trigger a group of impulses in several fibers. Above approximately 1000 cps the nerve fibers cannot keep up with the frequency of the sound waves and the impulses in neighboring fibers get more and more out of step with one another. Below 500 cps, however, the *frequency principle or volley principle of neural action* contributes significantly to our sense of pitch. Its relative importance is probably greater the lower the frequency.

It seems odd that pitch, which our musical experience leads us to think of as a simple, single attribute of a sound, should depend on two different kinds of information carried to the brain: the activity of certain fibers stimulated by a mechanical sound analyzer and also the frequency of nerve impulses in a rather large nonspecific group of fibers. But the nervous system apparently uses all of the information that its sense organs place at its disposal. With proper acoustic stimulation we can manipulate separately the two aspects of nerve activity. Either way we can play a tune that is easily recognized by the listener, although a clear, pure, fully musical tone with sharply defined, unambiguous pitch is produced only when both forms of activity are set going at once, as they are when a pure, steady sine-wave tone is the stimulus.

The auditory nerve is the essential pathway to the brain, and its 30,000 fibers (a small number compared with over a million in the optic nerve from the eye) are the bottleneck through which, in the dot-dot-dot code of nerve impulses, the entire variety of our auditory experiences must pass.

The experiments in which the impulses from single nerve cells were recorded separately also tell us a great deal about how information concerning loudness is carried by the auditory nerve impulses. The louder the tone, the more impulses traversed each fiber every second, until the fiber was working at its maximum rate. Also, the louder the tone, the more sensory cells and their nerve fibers were stimulated. The total number of nerve impulses delivered to the brain per second was increased in two ways: more impulses per fiber and more fibers active. (The strength of the individual impulses, we should add, remained constant, in accordance with the well-known behavior of all nerve fibers. A nerve fiber works something like a repeating rifle. It can be fired slowly or rapidly, but its caliber and the size and speed of its bullets remain the same.) Apparently, too, some fibers are held in reserve, so to speak, and are not stimulated by tones of any frequency until the intensity becomes quite high. These fibers of high threshold help us to understand how loudness can keep on increasing over the tremendous range of intensity between the threshold of acuity and the threshold of pain.

Suggested Readings

cox, j. r., jr. "The Measurement of Industrial Noise," in *Industrial Hygiene and Toxicology*, Leslie Silverman, ed. 2d ed. New York: Interscience Publishers, 1959, Vol. III, chap. 8.
   This chapter describes fully the use of the octave-band filter from the point of view of an acoustic engineer.

fletcher, h. *Speech and Hearing*. Princeton, N.J.: D. Van Nostrand Company, 1929.
   A classic, now out of print.

———. *Speech and Hearing in Communication*. Princeton, N.J.: D. Van Nostrand Company, 1953.
   A rather extensive revision of his earlier monograph.

pierce, j. r., and e. e. david, jr. *Man's World of Sound*. New York: Doubleday & Company, 1958.
   A very readable and informative introductory treatment.

rao, v. v. l. *The Decibel Notation*. New York: The Chemical Publishing Company, 1946.
   Mathematically oriented but relatively simple.

stevens, s. s., ed. *Handbook of Experimental Psychology*. New York: John Wiley & Sons, Inc., 1951.
   Chapter 25 ("Basic Correlates of the Auditory Stimulus," by J. C. R. Licklider) and Chapter 26 ("The Perception of Speech" by J. C. R. Licklider and G. A. Miller) are especially pertinent.

stevens, s. s., and h. davis. *Hearing: Its Psychology and Physiology*. New York: John Wiley & Sons, Inc., 1938, Pt. I.
   This is a monograph for advanced students. The second part, physiology, is now rather out of date.

3

ANATOMY AND PHYSIOLOGY
OF THE EAR

Hallowell Davis, M.D.

Concerning the structure of the ear and how it gathers sound waves and brings them to the sensory cells we can be rather definite. And some understanding of both the structure and the function of the various parts of the ear is needed to understand the different types of deafness and the means of preventing or circumventing them.

THE OUTER EAR AND THE CANAL

We need not describe the outer ear. Look at your neighbor or get a mirror and you will do better than we can do with words or diagrams. The external ear, the *pinna* or *auricle,* is not very important, except perhaps for ornament. Man has lost or never acquired the three main functions of the external ear of most animals: (1) to collect and focus the energy of a large area of sound waves; (2) to make possible precise judgments of the direction of sound by turning the ears (instead of the whole head) until the sound becomes loudest; and (3) to keep water and dirt out of the ear canal, as seals and moles do, by special valvelike movements of some of the external parts that for us are rudimentary rigid structures.

The human ear canal is irregularly oval in cross section and varies from man to man in details of size and shape quite as much as does the external ear—to the distress of those whose task it was during World War II to devise a simple ear plug for all ears to protect them against the blasts of heavy artillery and antiaircraft batteries. Sometimes the canal is nearly round; sometimes it is little more than a vertical slit. The canal runs nearly horizontally toward the center of the head for a little less than an inch (2.5 centimeters) as shown in Figure 3-1, and there it dead-ends at the eardrum,

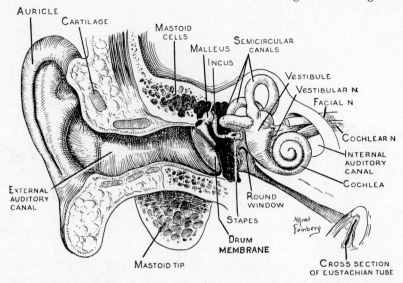

Fig. 3-1. In this semidiagrammatic drawing of the ear, the inner ear is shown with the temporal bone cut away to reveal the semicircular canals, the vestibule, and the cochlea. The cochlea has been turned slightly from its normal orientation to show its coils more clearly. The opening for nerves through the bone to the brain cavity of the skull is quite diagrammatic. The Eustachian tube actually runs forward as well as downward and inward. The muscles of the middle ear, shown in Figures 3-2 and 3-3, are omitted.

or *tympanic membrane*. The skin of the outer portion of the canal secretes a dark, bitter-tasting wax that as a rule discourages the entry of insects and keeps the skin of the canal and the drum from drying out.

THE MIDDLE EAR

With proper illumination and when the canal is straightened by pulling the pinna gently backward and upward, the eardrum can be seen as a pearl-gray wall at the end of the canal. The thin, tough, flexible fibrous membrane is attached to the bony wall of the canal by a tough ring of fibrous tissue and forms a diagonal partition as shown in the diagram in Figure 3-2. It is not stretched flat across but points inward and upward, like the cone of a loud-speaker, into the middle-ear cavity behind it. Its area is about a tenth of a square inch on the average. Through the translucent drum can sometimes be seen, like the hour hand of a clock at 11 o'clock (in the right ear), the "handle" of the hammer (the *malleus*), the first of the chain of three tiny bones (*ossicles*) that transmit the vibrations of the drum to the inner ear. The malleus serves also to keep the membrane stretched tight and cone-shaped under the influence of a small muscle, the *tensor tympani,* that attaches to it near the base of the handle.

The enlarged round head of the malleus nestles into a well-fitting socket in the anvil (or *incus*), the second of the ossicles, and for sounds of ordinary intensities the two move together as a single unit. They execute a rocking motion as the drum vibrates, turning around a horizontal axis just behind the upper edge of the drum and perpendicular to the external canal. The axis on which they turn is formed by a short axlelike projection of the malleus and another from the incus. The projections are attached by firm but flexible ligaments to the walls of the middle-ear cavity. The bony mass of the ossicles is delicately balanced around the axis so that the inertia (or, more accurately, the *turning moment*) of the system is very small and the ossicles do not tend to strain and rattle when the drum vibrates. The incus ends in a long slender curved tip near the center of the middle-ear cavity and in contact with the tiny head of the stirrup (*stapes*), the last of the three ossicles.

The stirrup is well named from its shape, and its oval foot-plate is sealed by the *annular ligament* into the *oval window* that looks into

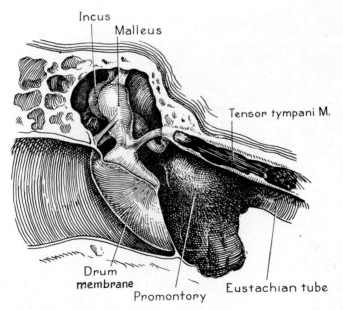

Fig. 3-2. This view of the drum membrane (partly cut away) and the middle ear is from a slightly more lateral angle than that in Figure 3-1. The tensor tympani muscle lies in a separate canal (partly cut away) just above the Eustachian tube. Its tendon turns at nearly a right angle in the tendinous sheath from which it emerges. In the text the drum membrane is still called the eardrum, according to popular usage, but technically eardrum means the entire middle ear.

the inner ear. The stapes rocks like a bell crank as the drum vibrates because the annular ligament is thick and snug at one end of the oval window and more slack and flexible at the other. The tendon of another tiny muscle, the *stapedius,* attaches to the neck of the stapes. It pulls the stapes outward and backward, thus counteracting the opposite pull of the tensor tympani. The two muscles work together to take up any slack in the ossicular chain and to stiffen the whole system. The balance between them is so good that the drum membrane itself scarcely moves at all when they contract.

The middle ear is a narrow cleft between the slanting eardrum and the irregular bony wall opposite it, and is nearly filled by the ossicles. Its capacity varies from one to two cubic centimeters. However, it opens directly into the air cells of the temporal bone behind,

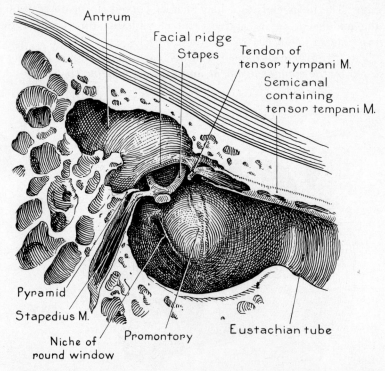

Fig. 3-3. The middle ear is here viewed from the external canal, with the drum membrane, the malleus, the incus, and some of the surrounding temporal bone cut away. The tendon of the stapedius muscle turns at an angle as it emerges from the tip of the "pyramid." When the stapedius contracts, the stapes rocks on the posterior (left in this figure) end of its footplate so that the footplate swings outward like a door into the cavity of the middle ear. The facial nerve runs in a bony canal in the facial ridge just above the stapes.

and the *Eustachian tube* opens into its anterior wall about midway between floor and roof. The two muscles that we have mentioned are not located in the middle-ear cavity itself. The tensor tympani lies alongside the Eustachian tube and the stapedius in a little bony tunnel all its own. The longest dimension of the cavity—the vertical dimension—is about half an inch, and a magnifying glass is required to appreciate the fine mechanical architecture of the ossicles with their balanced suspensions and their adjusting muscles.

Another opening between the middle ear and the inner ear is the *round window*, located just under the oval window. It is closed by an elastic membrane rather like the eardrum, but thinner, much smaller, and stretched flat. This opening serves as an elastic termination of the acoustic pathway in the inner ear, as shown in Figures 3-4A and 4B. If the walls of the inner ear were completely rigid, the stapes could not move in the oval window, because the fluid within is practically incompressible. Pressure could be transmitted, but the mechanical movements would be negligible, and it is mechanical movement that ultimately stimulates the sensory cells.

The air-filled cavity of the middle ear and the mastoid air cells that lead off from it as a blind alley are ventilated periodically through the Eustachian tube. The tube connects the middle ear with

Fig. 3-4A. **Schematic diagram of the tympanic membrane, the ossicles, and the basilar membrane.** The solid figures of the ossicles and the solid lines for the tympanic, the basilar, and the round-window membranes show the positions of these structures at rest. The broken outlines of the ossicles and the broken lines for the membranes show their positions following inward displacement of the tympanic membrane by a sound wave. The cross shows the axis around which the ossicles rotate. The dot shows their center of gravity. The stapes is drawn at right angles to its true position in order to show its rocking motion. It rocks around an axis through the posterior (not the inferior) edge of the round window. Its plane of motion is at almost right angles to that of the other two ossicles. (*Modified from Stevens and Davis, Hearing.*)

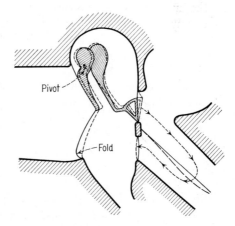

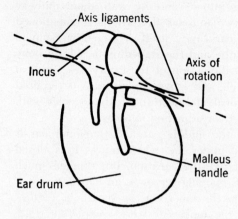

Fig. 3-4B. **Diagram of the axis of rotation of malleus and incus.** (FROM *Békésy and Rosenblith in Introduction to Experimental Psychology, John Wiley & Sons, Inc.*)

the back of the nasal cavity, called the *nasopharynx*. The first half inch runs through the temporal bone. It is permanently open, like a funnel, in contrast to the longer wider portion toward the pharynx, whose walls are composed of cartilage and flexible membrane, and which is normally collapsed. The Eustachian tube enters the nasopharynx diagonally under a valvelike flap of tissue that closes the orifice except during certain movements, such as swallowing and yawning. Sometimes, also, the tube opens during a sneeze or a cough or when the air pressure is increased by blowing the nose.

The function of the Eustachian tube in equalizing the air pressure inside and outside the eardrum is described more fully later. Immediate equalization of small changes, such as are caused by contraction of the tensor tympani muscle, is provided by a small slack segment of the eardrum itself, at its top and above the axis of rotation of the malleus. Longer-term equalization is needed, however, because any air bubble left in the tissues of the body is gradually dissolved and absorbed by the blood: first the oxygen and then, slowly, the nitrogen. The air in the middle ear must therefore be replenished periodically.

The middle ear with its drum and ossicles increases the sensitivity of hearing for air-borne sound. The drum receives energy from a relatively large cross section of light, tenuous, highly compressible air. The energy is delivered through the ossicles to the smaller footplate of the stapes, about one thirtieth the area of the drum. This reduction of area favors the efficient transfer of the energy to the dense, almost incompressible fluid that fills the inner ear. Thereby the drum and ossicles appreciably increase the sensitivity of the ear. Loss of drum and ossicles causes some hearing loss, but not by any means a very serious one. Simple interruption of the train of ossicles reduces the sensitivity by about twenty-five decibels. And a simple hole in the drum may cause only a five- or ten-decibel loss.

The middle ear and its drum and ossicles probably serve also to protect the inner ear from injury by loud sounds. The air enclosed in the rather small middle ear must exert some cushioning effect for low tones, because loud tones of low frequency have a very appreciable amplitude of movement. Just how important this effect may be has not yet been determined. The contractions of the muscles of the middle ear stiffen the drum and ossicular chain and thereby further resist the transmission of low tones. Contraction is set off automatically by unconscious reflex action from the lower centers of the brain a few hundredths of a second after a loud sound first reaches the eardrum. The increased tension of the drum also raises the "natural period" of vibration of drum and ossicles. The net result is a rather considerable loss of sensitivity for low and for high tones and rather slight loss for the middle range. The most important practical result is probably the protection it affords both the middle and the inner ear against possible damage by very loud low tones. The joint between the malleus and the incus also yields elastically, when the sound waves become very powerful, before the stapes is pushed bodily through the oval window. Also, the stapes begins to rock in a different and less efficient direction, sideways instead of lengthwise of the footplate.

THE INNER EAR

The inner ear is a series of channels and chambers in the temporal bone that are so complicated in shape that they are known as the labyrinth. In these bony canals, filled with clear watery fluid, lies a corresponding series of delicate membranous tubes and sacs, filled also with a similar watery fluid and containing sensory cells and their supporting structures. The central portion, the *vestibule*, of the labyrinth joins the snaillike coil of the organ of hearing, the *cochlea*, and the loops of the three *semicircular canals* that form the sense organ for turning in space. In the vestibule itself lie the *utricle*, sensitive to the pull of gravity and to acceleration (as in an elevator or automobile), and the *saccule*. The latter apparently shares the functions of the utricle, although in fish, which have no cochlea, it seems to be the sense organ for vibration and whatever true hearing the fish may have.

These very different senses, hearing and movement, have very similar sensory cells that are specialized organs of touch. The cochlea "feels" the mechanical movements caused by sound waves. Gravity

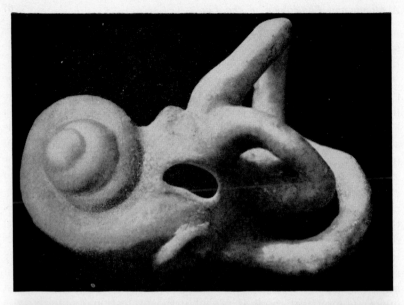

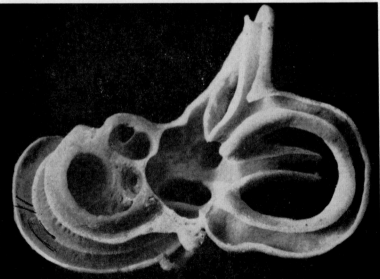

basilar
memb.

Fig. 3-5. In the top photograph the left bony labyrinth of an infant has been removed from the substance of the temporal bone. The oval window appears clearly in the center. Below it, seen obliquely, is the protruding rim of bone around the opening of the round window.

In the bottom photograph the right bony labyrinth, viewed from within the head, has been opened to show the hollow vestibule and canals. Notice the spiral shelf of bone that partly subdivides the canal of the cochlea (lower left). The hollow central core of the cochlea, through which the nerve emerges, is clearly shown, and also the round window, with rim partly cut away, opening into the canal of the cochlea (lower center). (*Rüdinger.*)

is "felt" by the utricle as it pulls on tiny grains of calcium carbonate attached to microscopic hairlike extensions of the sensory cells. The cells at the enlarged ends of the semicircular canals "feel" the pressure of the fluid within the canals as it tends to lag behind, because of its inertia, when we turn our heads. Two practical consequences of the close anatomical association are, first, that the symptom of dizziness (vertigo) is often associated with certain forms of deafness and, second, that the surgeon can make the bony channels of the vestibule and semicircular canals alternative pathways for sound. Other details of this part of the labyrinth need not concern us here. The opening of a new oval window by the fenestration operation for the restoration of hearing in otosclerosis will be described in Chapter 6.

The cochlea is coiled like a snail in a flat spiral of two and a half turns. The canal within is a little over an inch (35 millimeters long) and ends blindly at the apex. The canal is partly divided into upper (*vestibular*) and lower (*tympanic*) galleries (*scalae*) by a spiral shelf of bone protruding outward from the inner wall of the

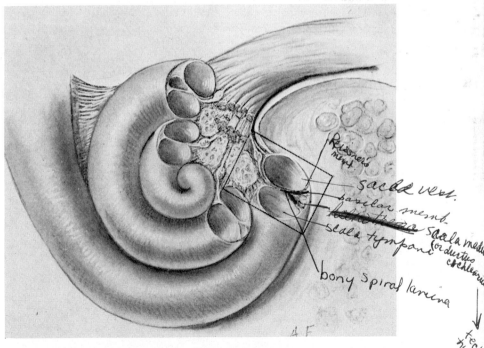

Fig. 3-6. The cochlea has been opened to show cross sections of its turns and also the distribution of the nerve to the turns. The area in the rectangle is shown enlarged in Fig. 4-7.

passage like a shelf along the inner wall of a circular staircase. The division of the two galleries is completed by a fibrous flexible membrane, the *basilar membrane,* that stretches across from the lower edge of the bony shelf to the spiral ligament that attaches it to the outer wall. The basilar membrane and the shelf both terminate a millimeter or two short of the end of the galleries so that the two galleries join at the apex of the cochlea. On the vestibular surface of the basilar membrane lies the membranous tube that contains the sensory cells and their supporting structures, known as the *organ of Corti.* The basilar membrane is just over an inch long (32 millimeters) and tapers in width from about half a millimeter near the apex down to a twentieth of a millimeter at the base of the cochlea near the oval window. The oval window opens into the vestibule near the end of the vestibular gallery and the round window opens into the tympanic gallery beneath at the base of the cochlea. When the fluid in the vestibule is pushed by the stapes into the vestibular gallery, it makes the basilar membrane bulge into the tympanic gallery; and, in turn, the membrane of the round window bulges into the air-filled middle ear.

The sensory cells, called "hair cells" because of the dozens of microscopic hairs, or *cilia,* that each one carries on its upper end,

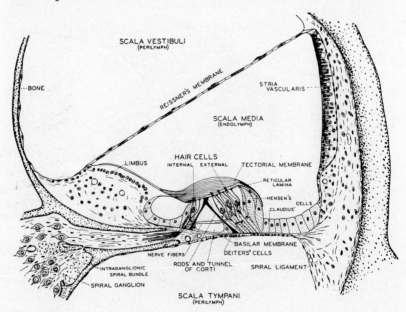

Fig. 3-7. Cross-sectional drawing of the canal in the second turn of a guinea pig's cochlea. The human cochlea is very similar to this. The position corresponding to this section is shown by the rectangle in Fig. 3-6.

are arranged in four parallel rows along the basilar membrane near its attachment to the central bony shelf. About 3500 hair cells stand side by side in an inner row, and about 20,000 slightly smaller hair cells are evenly spaced in orderly arrangement in three outer rows. Figures 3-7 shows a typical cross section of the organ of Corti and gives an idea of the rather complicated supporting structures. The heavy *pillars of Corti*, braced together at their tops to form a triangle with part of the basilar membrane, give stiffness to this part of the organ, and it apparently rocks as a unit, as shown in Figure 3-8, when the basilar membrane bulges upward or downward. The ends of the hairs of the sensory cells are imbedded in the *tectorial membrane* that lies in contact with the upper surface of the organ of Corti (Figure 3-9). The tectorial membrane is composed of a rather viscous, slow-flowing jelly stiffened by a system of fibers that arise from its attachment to the outer edge of the solid *limbus*. The limbus in turn is based on the bony inner shelf of the modiolus. The tectorial membrane is thus a long ribbon attached to the limbus along one edge. It can move up and down rather stiffly, like the cover of a book. It is loosely attached to the organ of Corti along its outer edge and also again near the limbus. The organ of Corti and the tectorial membrane must slide past one another slightly as they move

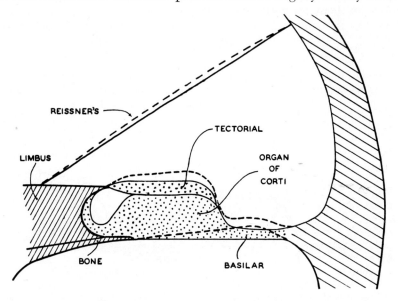

Fig. 3-8. The organ of Corti and the tectorial membrane form a relatively stiff section of the cochlear partition. Most of the bending takes place in the more flexible portion of the basilar membrane between the organ of Corti and the spiral ligament.

up and down together. This movement bends the hairs, as shown in Figure 3-9.

Somehow the bending of the hairs in the proper direction sets off nerve impulses in the nerve fibers that terminate around the opposite ends of the hair cells. Our best present theory is that the bending of the hairs controls the flow of a current of electricity through the hair cell to the nerve ending. We do know definitely that the hair cells, like most other living cells, are electrically charged inside and can act as batteries. The cochlea also seems to be provided with an additional biological battery located in the *stria vascularis*. This battery keeps the entire interior of the inner tube (*scala media*) of the cochlea electrically charged. The organ of Corti forms part of the wall of this tube and some current apparently leaks through it continually. The sound waves cause more or less current to flow, and the additional current presumably stimulates the nerve fibers. The electrical charges and currents of the cochlea have been much studied recently, and it has also been found that the chemical composition of the fluid inside the membranous labyrinth differs from that of all other body fluids. The significance of the chemical difference is unknown, however.

The nerve fibers run from the hair cells through tiny holes in the spiral bony shelf into the central core of the cochlea. There they join, like the strands of a rope, to form the auditory nerve and pass through a channel in the temporal bone to the base of the brain. Within the spiral of the cochlea, forming a bulbous enlargement on each nerve fiber, are the nerve cell bodies. The cell body is the housekeeping center for the nerve cell as a whole, and it nourishes the long threadlike fiber that reaches from the cochlea to the brain.

There are 25,000 to 30,000 nerve cells in each ear, about one for

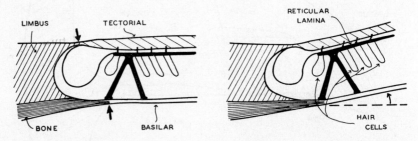

Fig. 3-9. At the left the organ of Corti and tectorial membrane are in the position of rest. Their respective "hinge points" where they attach to the limbus and the bony lamina are shown by the heavy arrows. At the right the partition has moved "upward." Because of its different hinge point the tectorial membrane must slide past the reticular lamina and bend the hairs.

each hair cell; but the connections to the hair cells are not quite so simple. Each hair cell connects with several nerve fibers and each fiber connects with several cells in neighboring but overlapping zones. Some fibers run for a millimeter or more along the basilar membrane connecting with numerous external hair cells. This arrangement suggests that no single hair cell or nerve fiber is individually essential but that there is a liberal factor of safety in the design. Several cells and fibers work together, sending impulses even when only a very small area of the basilar membrane is agitated by a faint pure tone.

ANALYSIS OF SOUNDS BY THE EAR

The over-all "tuning" of the basilar membrane, which leads to the place principle of hearing, has already been mentioned in Chapter 2. The cochlea does in fact act as a mechanical analyzer of sounds. For high-frequency tones only the part of the basilar membrane in the basal turn nearest the stapes and round window vibrates. With middle-frequency tones the middle part of the basilar membrane in the second turn also vibrates and vibrates more vigorously than does the basal turn. Low-frequency tones cause all or nearly all the membrane to vibrate and the greatest amplitude of movement is near the apex. Thus the place principle is not a matter of either-or, but rather of how much of the membrane is vibrating in response to a particular frequency and where the maximum amplitude and the cut-off point are. The ear seems to be sensitive, in the detection of differences of pitch, to a shift in the position of maximum and cut-off of about one fifteen-hundredth of an inch or about 0.02 millimeter.

The "map" shown in Figure 3-10 gives the approximate locations of the positions of maximum movement. Curiously, the low-frequency octaves below middle C of the piano (262 cps) are packed closely into a short bit of cochlea near the apex while the high-frequency octaves occupy much more length in the basal turn. This makes some sense, however, if we recall from Chapter 2 that for frequencies below 500 cps the frequency principle becomes more and more important. The basal turn is not idle with low-frequency stimulation, except very near threshold. The nerve fibers respond and their impulses contribute to the recognition of the pitch by the frequency principle and probably also to the over-all loudness. For high-frequency tones, however, the frequency principle cannot operate and the basal turn receives no help from the apical region. This unsymmetrical relation helps us understand certain features of high-tone hearing loss that are otherwise rather puzzling.

The most important anatomical feature of the cochlea that brings about the "tuning" of the basilar membrane so that it can act as an acoustic analyzer is its tapering width. The dimensions are given in Figure 3-10. The greater width at the apex than at the base is actually exaggerated in the drawing for emphasis. The basilar membrane is a continuous structure, not a series of strings, and is not "stretched" in the sense of living under tension. Any comparison to a series of tuned strings (as in a piano or harp) is therefore misleading, but the principle of "resonance" and the dependence of the natural period of vibration of the cochlear partition on the elasticity and the mass of the moving parts are nevertheless correct. The mass in this case is the mass of the organ of Corti and of the fluid so close to the membrane that it must move with it. The elasticity is the stiffness of the membrane, which is much greater where it is narrow at the base than where it is wide at the apex.

Two other important features of the movements of the cochlear partition are also well known. First, the ear is almost "dead beat" (that is, critically damped), which means that its movements cease immediately or within one or two vibrations after the air ceases to vibrate. It also starts vibrating strongly with equal promptness. An acoustic or an electric resonant system can be tuned sharply only by reducing the damping, and good damping can be obtained only at the expense of selectivity. It seems that Nature has compromised in the ear by giving us nearly critical damping. The ear can follow the changes of intensity of sound quite accurately, but at the expense of the sharpest possible tuning.

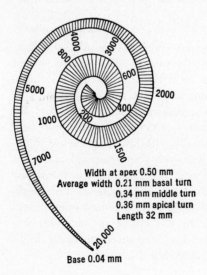

Width at apex 0.50 mm
Average width 0.21 mm basal turn
0.34 mm middle turn
0.36 mm apical turn
Length 32 mm

Base 0.04 mm

Fig. 3-10. In this diagram the width of the basilar membrane is exaggerated relative to its length to show more clearly its progressive widening as it approaches the apex. The approximate positions of maximum amplitude of vibration in response to tones of different frequency are also indicated. (*From O. Stuhlman, Jr., An Introduction to Biophysics, John Wiley & Sons, Inc.*)

Second, although the movements of the basilar membrane and its selective tuning are direct consequences of the principles of resonance, the pattern of movement of the membrane is quite complex. The various parts do not move in step (in "phase") with one another. The wider, more apical region always lags more or less behind the narrower part. On the other hand, the membrane is continuous, so the lag must develop gradually. The result is a pattern of *traveling waves* that seem to move along the membrane from the stiffer and narrower toward the more flexible and the broader part. The waves get bigger as they approach the resonant region but beyond this point they shrink, and then shorten and die out in a short distance. Figure 3-11 illustrates this pattern.

Over all we see that the inner ear acts as a sound analyzer as well as a frequency repeater. The various frequencies, harmonic or otherwise, in a complex sound are sorted out and cause the basilar membrane to vibrate in an equally complex pattern. Each frequency stimulates a corresponding group of nerve fibers to deliver

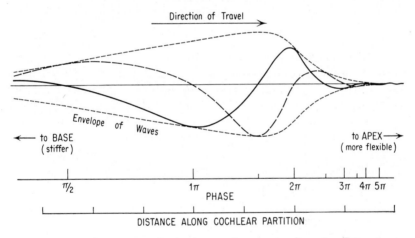

Fig. 3-11. The waves in the basilar membrane move from base toward apex. Their velocity becomes progressively slower and their wave length shorter. The solid curve shows the pattern of displacement at the instant that the upward displacement at the basal end is maximal. The dashed curve shows the pattern a quarter of a cycle ($\pi/2$) later. The phase differences are relative to the extreme basal end. The dotted lines are the envelopes of the displacement patterns. The envelope increases slowly, goes through a maximum between $3\pi/2$ and 2π and then falls off rapidly. The position of the maximum along the membrane is a function of frequency, as shown in Fig. 3-10, but the relation of maximum to phase lag is constant. The small short waves beyond about 3π are probably of no physiological importance. In this diagram the vertical dimension of displacement is exaggerated to show the patterns more clearly. The formation of traveling waves depends on the gradient of stiffness along the cochlear partition. (*After Békésy.*)

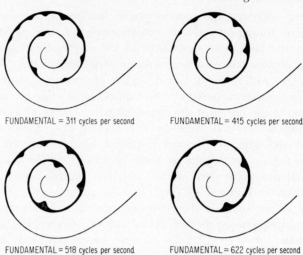

FUNDAMENTAL = 311 cycles per second   FUNDAMENTAL = 415 cycles per second

FUNDAMENTAL = 518 cycles per second   FUNDAMENTAL = 622 cycles per second

Fig. 3-12. Auditory patterns for four notes of bugle playing taps. The width of the black area is proportional to the loudness contributed by that particular bit of the organ of Corti. (*Courtesy of H. Fletcher, Bell Telephone Laboratories.*)

impulses in proportion to the intensity of each part of the pattern. In this way the pattern is translated and transmitted to the brain. In Figure 3-12 is a graphic representation of such a pattern of activity on the basilar membrane. The width of the dark band is proportionate to the contribution to the total loudness made by different parts of the organ of Corti when the note of a bugle is sounded. The pattern of the various harmonics is seen as a series of broad peaks of activity of different intensities spaced in a definite sequence along the sense organ of hearing.

BONE CONDUCTION

Any vibration of the basilar membrane will stimulate the sensory cells and give rise to the sensation of sound. It makes no difference how the vibrations in the cochlea may have been set going. Ordinarily the pathway for sound is through the external ear and across the chain of ossicles, but sound waves may also be transmitted directly through the bones of the skull. A vibrating tuning fork may be heard by air conduction if it is held opposite the open ear or by bone conduction if its stem is applied to the top of the head, to a tooth, or to the mastoid bone behind the ear. Transmission is not so efficient across the skin and through the bone as it is by the normal route, but if the normal route is obstructed, as in certain forms of deafness, bone conduction may be put to great practical use. Its diagnostic importance will also be discussed in later chapters.

The sound waves traveling in the skull probably set up mechanical movement of the fluid relative to the bone in several ways. For one thing, the membrane of the round window is more flexible and yielding than is the footplate of the stapes, so that when the labyrinth as a whole is compressed by a sound wave reaching it through the bone, the round window is the most yielding of the various outlets. The fluid from the vestibule and the semicircular canals, as well as that within the cochlea, is therefore driven toward the round window. This fluid movement is exactly like that normally set up by the vibrations of the footplate of the stapes and is analyzed by the cochlea and heard in the brain exactly like air-borne sound. For another thing, the head is vibrated as a whole by sounds below about 800 cps. The ossicles tend to lag behind because of their inertia. The resulting relative movement of skull and ossicles is exactly equivalent to vibrations set up by air-borne sound. Fortunately, this effect is minimized by the dynamic balance of the malleus and incus around their axis of rotation described earlier in this chapter.

These are two of the most important but by no means all of the mechanisms and pathways of bone conduction. Of course, any very intense sound in the air will set the skull vibrating to some extent; a telephone receiver held tightly against the ear may do so even more effectively. Our own voices generated inside our heads reach our ears by bone conduction as well as by air conduction. But it is air conduction that gives the ear its great sensitivity, particularly for the higher audible frequencies.

ELECTRICAL STIMULATION OF HEARING

If an alternating electrical current of a frequency in the audible range is passed through the head in the neighborhood of the inner ear and adjusted to a suitable intensity, it is sometimes possible to hear a tone corresponding to the frequency of the alternating current, or at least a noise. (The current is most effectively applied by filling the external ear canal with salt solution and immersing the end of one wire in it. The circuit is completed through a metal plate on the forearm.) The strength of the current must be carefully adjusted because at only a few decibels above the threshold of hearing, the current may begin to be felt as a tickling, burning, prickling, and, finally, painful sensation.

In spite of the lack of purity of the sounds heard by this "electrophonic effect," some hope was aroused by its original announcement that useful hearing might be obtained by electrical stimulation of the auditory nerve even after the sense organ itself had degenerated from disease or old age. Unfortunately, this hope cannot be realized for several reasons. In the first place, the fibers of the auditory nerve often degenerate once the sensory cells to which they attach have been lost. In the second place, it is now known that the hearing of anything resembling a pure tone by the electrophonic effect depends upon the existence of an intact cochlea. The electric current by one sort or another of electrical attraction and repulsion sets the fluid of the cochlea in motion very much as it does in bone conduction. It is true that the auditory nerve may be stimulated by the current, but in that case the analyzing function of the cochlea has been bypassed, and the nerve fibers are stimulated indiscriminately by the current. No high-frequency pitches are heard, only noises. Low pitches become rough buzzes instead of clear tones. Thus even if the current were to be applied directly to the auditory nerve (as has recently actually been done) the electrophonic effect offers no hope for any useful alleviation of deafness.

Suggested Readings

DAVIS, H. "Biophysics and Physiology of the Inner Ear," *Physiological Reviews,* 35: 1–49 (1957).
This article contains an extensive bibliography as well as an exposition of the author's electromechanical theory of cochlear function.

FLETCHER, H. *Speech and Hearing in Communication.* Princeton, N.J.: D. Van Nostrand Company, Inc., 1953.
This is a logical historical successor to the author's classical monograph of 1929, "Speech and Hearing." It deals with speech and hearing from the point of view of the communication engineer but also contains information and discussions relevant for understanding the process of hearing.

FOWLER, E. P., JR. *Nelson Loose-Leaf Medicine of the Ear.* New York: Thomas Nelson & Sons, Inc., 1939.
A standard reference book for otolaryngologists.

POLYAK, S. L., G. MCHUGH, and D. K. JUDD. *The Human Ear in Anatomical Transparencies.* Elmsford, N.Y.: Sonotone Corporation, 1946. (Distributed by T. H. McKenna, Inc., New York.)
A unique and very effective presentation of the anatomy of the ear accompanied by an excellent text.

Proceedings of the International Conference on Audiology, St. Louis, May, 1957. *The Laryngoscope,* 68: 209–682 (1958).
This volume contains a planned symposium on the physiology of the auditory system and also many contributed papers. It is probably the best summary of several aspects of audiology in the English language as of 1957. The articles are written at a professional level suitable for audiologists and otologists.

STEVENS, S. S., ed. *Handbook of Experimental Psychology.* New York: John Wiley & Sons, Inc., 1951.

Chapter 27 ("The Mechanical Properties of the Ear," by G. von Békésy and W. A. Rosenblith) and Chapter 28 ("Psychophysiology of Hearing and Deafness," by H. Davis) are particularly pertinent.

WEVER, E. G., and M. LAWRENCE. *Physiological Acoustics.* Princeton, N.J.: Princeton University Press, 1954.

This book deals authoritatively with sound conduction in the middle ear.

4

HEARING AND
DEAFNESS

Hallowell Davis, M.D.,
and Edmund Prince Fowler, Jr., M.D.

Definitions and Distinctions

The word "deafness" has been used to mean either partial or total loss of hearing. In French the word "surdité" and in Spanish the word "sordera" have just this broad meaning. In English, however, the term "hard of hearing" has been introduced to replace the phrase "partially deaf." Unfortunately we have no corresponding noun, "hardness of hearing," equivalent to the German "Schwerhörigkeit," to replace "partial deafness." Our nearest equivalents are "impairment of hearing" and "hearing loss."

The medical and social problems of hard-of-hearing patients are quite different from those of the totally deaf and therefore the two should not be grouped together indiscriminately. The psychological value of this point is discussed at some length in later chapters. But there is still some confusion resulting from old habits of speech and from the necessity of distinguishing between two or three terms.

The introduction of new terms and the change in the meaning of old ones depend on the gathering of new information, the development of new insights, and the formulation of new purposes. We believe that the time has come to repeat some old definitions, carefully worded and phrased, and to introduce certain new or nearly new additional terms. A change in terminology involves, of course, the rejection of some old terms and the restriction of the meaning of others.

DEAFNESS, HEARING LOSS, AND DYSACUSIS

The simple, everyday concept of "deafness" is a total or severe impairment of hearing, and in this book we shall continue to use "deafness" to include total loss of hearing, whatever the cause. Impairment of hearing of the sort that simply requires the other person to talk louder we shall call a "hearing loss," and we shall avoid the term "partial deafness." Hearing loss and deafness both imply a loss of sensitivity of hearing, presumably in the peripheral hearing mechanisms. Both lie along the same dimension, and the question is where to draw the line between "hard of hearing" and "deaf."

The usefulness of a criterion depends on our purposes, and the important purposes for which these terms are useful are social, educational, and medical. We shall adopt a social criterion for *deafness*, namely, that *everyday auditory communication is impossible or very nearly so.* In terms of decibels we find a zone of uncertainty from 60 to 80 db hearing level for speech in which some individuals are socially deaf while more of them are merely very hard of hearing. The frequent successful use of hearing aids makes it undesirable to include this "gray area" automatically under the term "deaf," as has often been the custom in the past. *We propose to confine the term "deafness" to hearing levels for speech of 82 db or worse.* A good reason for selecting this particular boundary is that the most authoritative medical rule for estimating the handicap imposed by hearing loss (see Chapter 9) reads "the handicap [for the hearing of everyday speech] is considered total at 82 db hearing loss for speech." Our criterion thus has a medical sanction in a social and economic context.

We do not here propose any educational criterion for deafness. Whether a child is judged to be "educable" or not may involve his visual skills, his intelligence, his emotional stability, and so on, perhaps in addition to handicaps other than deafness. Most deaf children, as well as hard-of-hearing children, can be educated, although the methods may differ, as we shall see in Chapters 16 and 17.

The successful use of a hearing aid may make the difference between being socially "deaf" or being merely "hard of hearing" even for some persons whose hearing levels for speech are 82 decibels or higher. For them "hard of hearing" is a better practical designation than "deaf." This is true even though in the context of accidental injury or industrial hearing loss their handicap for hearing everyday speech is considered total. In assessment of handicap for purposes of compensation the evaluation is made without the use of a hearing aid.

So far we have considered only the dimension of sensitivity of hearing. On this dimension the zone of normal includes hearing levels for speech from −10 to +15 db. The condition known as "hard of hearing" begins at 16 db and "deaf" begins at 82 db (see Chapters 2 and 9). There is, however, another dimension or, rather, several other dimensions, of hearing which may be impaired. For example, a person may say "Don't shout. I hear you but I can't make out the words." Then it is his "discrimination for speech" that is faulty. Or he may be unable to attach meaning to auditory signals because of a failure of understanding of the type we call "auditory agnosia." And there are other kinds of impairment, all of which we shall consider in more detail later in this chapter. All of these many types of impairment of hearing have one feature in common which makes it desirable to have a single term to include all of them. The common feature is that *they are not simple losses of sensitivity of hearing.* These impairments cannot be measured properly in decibels. *The inclusive term that we shall use for all of these other impairments of hearing is "dysacusis."*

"Dysacusis" is not a new word in the medical vocabulary, but it is not widely used. It means, however, just what we want to say: "faulty hearing." "Acusis" (or acousis) refers to hearing, as in the more familiar terms "presbycusis," "diplacusis." "Dys-" as a prefix may mean "ill" or "painful," but it also means "difficult," "faulty," "impaired," or "abnormal."

Dysacusis (also spelled "dysacusia" and "dysacousia") may be due to malfunction of the sense organ or it may be due to abnormal function of the brain. Thus we will call certain forms of diplacusis, presbycusis, and discrimination loss "peripheral dysacusis" and we will use the term "central dysacusis" for such various conditions as psychogenic or hysterical block of hearing, auditory agnosia, phonemic regression, and so on.

A point that must be emphasized immediately is that *deafness or hearing loss* on the one hand *and dysacusis,* both peripheral and central, on the other hand *are not mutually exclusive.* A patient may have both a hearing loss, measurable in decibels, and a dysacusis in the form of a loss of discrimination or some phonemic regression, or the like. In case of doubt, "dysacusis" should be considered the broader term equivalent to "impairment of hearing" of all kinds, two or three of which may be present at the same time, while "hard of hearing" *implies specifically one kind of impairment,* the one that is best understood and most readily measured, namely, *simple loss of sensitivity,* presumably in the ear itself or in its nerve. "Deafness" will remain the general term for the symptom of total or nearly total loss of hearing, but we shall avoid the term "central deafness." Of course, before a diagnosis is made we may use the terms "deaf" and "dysacusic," or "hard of hearing" and "dysacusic" pretty much interchangeably. "Dysacusis" is the word to use when we wish to emphasize either (1) that the symptom is not merely a partial loss of sensitivity of hearing, or (2) that the trouble may lie in the central nervous system rather than in the ear.

For those who enjoy complete, well-rounded systems of nomenclature there are the terms "anacusia" (or "anacousia") and "hypoacusia" (or "hypoacousia"), which can be used as exact synonyms for deafness and hearing loss, respectively.

VARIETIES OF DYSACUSIS

From the medical and anatomical point of view there are three major types of impairment of hearing: poor conduction of sound to the sense organ, abnormality of the sense organ or its nerve, and impairments that result from some injury to or failure of function in the central nervous system. The problem of otological and audiological diagnosis is to assess correctly the part played by each type for each particular patient. The terms that the diagnostician should use to describe the patient's difficulty are clear for two but only for two of the three anatomical types.

The common mild or moderate impairments that are due to failure of normal physical conduction of sound to the sense organ are "hearing losses" and the people who suffer from them are "hard of hearing." If the impairment is only to physical conduction the loss automatically cannot be more than about 60 db because at this level bone conduction takes over and the sound is heard, provided the sense organ is still intact. Really loud speech can still be understood and the successful use of a hearing aid is easy. We shall therefore speak of "conductive hearing loss" and give up the old term "conductive deafness."

Auditory agnosia, phonemic regression, and hysterical or psychogenic dysacusis are very clearly the result of some abnormal functioning of the central nervous system. The patient may or may not respond to a test with an audiometer, and he may give very different results on different trials. He is, however, unable to understand speech, or does so only in a very limited way, even though he may "hear" something on the audiometer.

The real difficulties of definition appear when the trouble lies anatomically in the sense organ of the cochlea or in the central auditory connections or both. For this group of disorders we shall use either "dysacusis" or "hearing loss," depending on whether we wish to emphasize loss of discrimination or loss of sensitivity. We shall lean toward the medical tradition in our basic classification and usually speak of *sensory-neural hearing loss*. Sometimes we want to distinguish between disorders of the sense organ and degeneration of the auditory nerve. Modern diagnostic tests are making this distinction possible and, as we shall see, the accurate diagnosis of the site and type of the trouble is of great importance for prognosis and, above all, for treatment. We shall then speak of "sense-organ dysacusis" or "sense-organ hearing loss" on the one hand and "neural hearing loss" (or sometimes "neural dysacusis") on the other. We shall avoid the familiar but less grammatical form "nerve deafness," and particularly the pernicious term "perceptive deafness." The latter is a wastebasket term once much used by otologists to catch everything that is not conductive. They disregard the prior use of the terms "perception" and "perceptive" by psychologists. If the term ever had a proper logical meaning it should have meant approximately what we now call "auditory agnosia" or "central perceptive dysacusis," but it was for a long time a synonym for "nerve deafness."

Still another term is necessary to describe the common combination of conductive and sensory-neural hearing losses. For this we shall use the familiar term "mixed hearing loss," but it will not include impairments that lie central to the auditory nerve.

When, as also may happen, a person has some conductive or sensory-neural or mixed hearing loss and also some *central* difficulties of the central perceptive or of the psychogenic variety, we shall speak of a "combined dysacusis" or perhaps of a "peripheral hearing loss" with a "psychogenic (or central or agnosic) overlay."

The proper antonym for "central" is "peripheral." "Peripheral" hearing loss means "conductive or sensory-neural or mixed" hearing loss. The otologist may sometimes use the word "retrocochlear" to cover the anatomical areas beyond the cochlea, i.e., auditory nerve, brain stem and beyond, or, practically speaking, everything outside the primary domain and responsibility of otology. "Retrocochlear" or "retrolabyrinthine" includes tumors of the auditory nerve but excludes sense-organ impairment.

A pair of contrasting terms in common use are "organic" and "functional." "Organic" implies that the difficulty is caused by an anatomical injury or abnormality which a pathologist could identify if he looked in the right place. "Functional" may mean either "nonorganic" or "physiological" or "with no visible pathology" or "better understood on a psychological than on an anatomical basis." An objection to these terms, in addition to the vagueness of "functional," is the implication that they usually carry that a difficulty is exclusively organic *or* functional, whereas, more often than not, anatomical, physiological, and psychological factors are all significant.

HEARING LOSS AND HEARING LEVEL

The term "hearing loss" has carried a heavy burden for the last three decades. In the medical and social senses in which we have used it here it has served to mean "an impairment of hearing that does not entirely prevent practical communication by speech." But "hearing loss" has also been used to mean the number of decibels by which the threshold of hearing is elevated above normal. Here "normal" really means the zero level to which the audiometer is calibrated at each frequency. "Hearing loss" has also been used to mean a change for the worse or shift of threshold from one level to another. Thus, terms are sometimes confusing, as in the following statements, which might have been made in a court or before an industrial commission.

> This employee suffered a hearing loss of 40 decibels from exposure to noise. He had a hearing loss of 15 decibels before employment, which, however, is just within normal limits. His actual hearing loss was 55 decibels when he was examined the day after stopping work. Of this loss, 10 decibels later proved to be a temporary hearing loss, so his permanent hearing loss now appears to be 45 decibels. This is not a conductive but a pure sensory-neural hearing loss.

In Chapter 2 we introduced the relatively new term "hearing level" to take some of the load off "hearing loss." "Hearing level" is the number of decibels that a person's threshold of hearing lies above the standard zero of the audiometer for that particular frequency (or for that particular speech test). In short, hearing level is measured on an *audiometer*. It is analogous to sound pressure level, which is measured with a *sound level meter*. The American Standards for Audiometers have required that the intensity dial be labeled "hearing loss," and most audiogram charts are marked the same way, but here we shall use "hearing level" instead.

Furthermore, when there is any possibility of ambiguity we shall call a shift or change of threshold a *threshold shift* and not a hearing loss. The least one can do to avoid confusion when referring to a change of level is to speak of a "loss of hearing" and not a "hearing loss."

In sum, we shall use (1) *hearing level* to designate the status of hearing, as measured in decibels on an audiometer, and (2) *threshold shift* for any change in the hearing level; and we shall reserve (3) *hearing loss* for the general condition of impaired hearing or the process that causes it. The implications of "hearing loss" are of a partial handicap or of an abnormality of structure or function. "Hearing level," however, carries no implication of handicap or even abnormality. It simply states the result of an objective psychophysical measurement. A practical rule to keep the usage of these terms straight is: "If decibels are involved, the term isn't 'hearing loss;' it is either 'hearing level' or 'threshold shift.'"

Another rule to which we shall return in Chapter 9 is: "There is no such thing as percentage of hearing level or even percentage of hearing loss." Occasionally we talk of percentage of handicap or of an index of adequacy, and a lawyer may talk about percentage of disability, but these values are calculated by arbitrary rules and only for particular purposes, such as compensation.

Now with our new terms to help us, let us try again that statement made in court by the examining physician. He now says:

> This employee suffered a loss of hearing from exposure to noise. The threshold shift was 40 decibels. His hearing level before employment was 15 decibels, which is just within normal limits. His actual hearing level the day after he stopped work was 55 decibels. Of this, 10 decibels proved to be a temporary threshold shift, so his final and presumably permanent hearing level now appears to be 45 decibels. He does not have any conductive hearing loss; he has a pure sensory-neural loss.

Peripheral Hearing Loss

A few moments' study of the anatomy of the ear, shown in Figure 4-1 and described in Chapter 3, will make clear the distinctions between conductive and sensory-neural hearing loss. The distinction is important because the prognosis and the treatment, as well as the causes of the two types, differ considerably. It is sometimes very simple to distinguish between the two by tests of hearing, but it is always possible and even probable that any case is really a mixture or combination of the two types.

CONDUCTIVE HEARING LOSS

Conductive loss may be caused by plugging the external canal, damping the free movement of the drum, or restricting the movements of the ossicles. Any of these will reduce the intensity of the air-borne sound that finally reaches the inner ear. Wax impacted in the canal is the commonest form of plug, and wax in contact with the drum or the scars of old healed perforations of the drum may restrict its vibrations. Adhesions of scar tissue on the ossicles or a bony new growth of otosclerosis around the edge of the stapes in the oval window may restrict the normal movements of the ossicles.

The classical test to distinguish conductive hearing loss from sensory-neural loss also illustrates clearly the fundamental difference between the two. In conductive loss the audiometer may show a hearing level for air-borne sound as high as 50 or possibly 60 db. The patient may be quite unable to hear a vibrating tuning fork held close

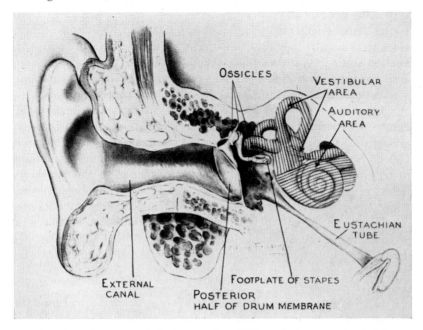

OSSICLES

VESTIBULAR AREA

AUDITORY AREA

EUSTACHIAN TUBE

EXTERNAL CANAL

FOOTPLATE OF STAPES

POSTERIOR HALF OF DRUM MEMBRANE

Fig. 4-1. This anatomical diagram has deliberately been made slightly inaccurate in order to represent all of the important parts of the ear more clearly in a single diagram. (See legend for Fig. 3-1.)

beside his ear. Thus, his "air conduction" is said to be "reduced." But if the shaft of the vibrating fork is now applied to his skull, or the bone-conduction vibrator of the audiometer is placed on the mastoid bone just behind his ear, he may be able to hear the sound as well as a normal person does in the same test. There is then no reduction in his "bone conduction." If he can hear normally by bone conduction, we infer that his sense organ and auditory nerve must be normal and that his difficulty in hearing depends only on some obstacle to the conduction of air-borne sound. Audiograms showing hearing levels by air conduction and by bone conduction in sensory-neural loss and in conductive loss are shown in Chapter 7, where the audiogram will be explained in detail.

It is tempting to assume that if bone conduction is reduced, there must be a corresponding degree of sensory-neural hearing loss. The principle is correct, but there are practical pitfalls. Some skulls and the skin and soft tissues over them do not conduct sound well. Or another example, when the footplate of the stapes is firmly fixed in the oval window by otosclerosis, the fluids in the inner ear can no longer move so freely under the influence of bone-conducted acoustic energy. This makes the hearing level at 2000 cps for bone conduction 10 to 15 db poorer than it would otherwise be. At 500, 1000, and 4000 cps the threshold shift is usually only 5 to 10 db. The resulting dip in the bone-conduction audiogram is sometimes called the "Carhart notch." Following a successful fenestration operation or stapes mobilization the bone-conduction threshold shifts back toward normal by this amount.

In addition, there are special technical difficulties in obtaining accurate measurements of hearing level by bone conduction, such as the presence of too much background noise in the test room. These will also be considered in Chapter 7, but in general the otologist hesitates to conclude, without supporting evidence, simply on the basis of a report of poor hearing levels by bone conduction, that he is dealing with sensory-neural hearing loss. The other difficulties in obtaining reliable measurements of hearing by bone conduction, do not need to concern us here in detail; but in general, without supporting evidence, it is unsafe to conclude that we are dealing with a neural hearing loss purely on the basis of an apparent loss of sensitivity to bone-conducted sounds.

Conductive hearing loss is not much of a handicap to hearing in a noisy place. In fact, a man with pure conductive hearing loss of moderate degree can hear conversation just as well as the average person can (and better than a great many) in traffic, in airplanes, and in similar noisy surroundings. Under these conditions he simply does not hear, or hears only faintly, the noise that disturbs his normal companion and masks any speech at ordinary conversation levels. But in noise, all of us automatically talk louder—loud enough so that we can hear ourselves above the noise. The loud speech overrides a moderate conductive hearing loss. The problem for our hard-of-hearing listener is no longer that of *hearing* the speech but only of *distinguishing* it from as much of the noise as also succeeds in reaching his inner ear. Since he does not hear much of the noise and his inner ear is normal, he can distinguish and understand the loud speech as well as anyone. Furthermore, the training in understanding speech that has been forced on him by his hearing loss is likely to give him an actual advantage over a person with normal hearing. This ability to hear in noisy places as well as, or better than, normal persons has been given the impressive name of *paracusis Willisii* and is characteristic of conductive hearing loss.

SENSORY-NEURAL HEARING LOSS

Sensory-neural hearing loss is most often caused by a degeneration of some of the sensory cells of the inner ear or of their nerve fibers or both. The hearing levels for different frequencies are usually, although not always, unequal. *Hearing for high tones is most likely to be lost.* Occasionally, however, notably in Ménière's disease, the sensory-neural loss may be greater for low tones than for high. Sometimes the transition from good hearing to poor extends over several octaves, and we speak of a "gradual high-tone hearing loss." Sometimes, however, the transition is very abrupt. Obviously, when there are parts of the frequency spectrum that are never heard, regardless of the intensity of the sound, the quality and character of complex sounds, such as those occurring in speech, are altered. The high-frequency components that give character to most of the consonants are lost, and with them the possibility of distinguishing one consonant from any of several others. A *complete* absence of hearing for high tones may quite logically be called "high-tone neural deafness" or "abrupt high-tone deafness." Persons with such a high-tone neural hearing loss are dependent, for the understanding of speech, on very small differences among the sounds that they actually do hear, just as a normal listener is dependent on small differences when the speech can just be heard above a background of noise. With some effort and attention, the man with a high-tone loss may understand speech in quiet surroundings where there are no other difficulties to contend with; but if noise is mixed with the speech, it may mask some of the small differences on which he relies, and he is totally at a loss. Even when the speaker raises his voice, as he normally does in the presence of noise, the listener with a neural loss is as badly handicapped as he is in quiet surroundings, and usually more so. He is likely to become confused or exhausted by the additional strain of discriminating the speech from the noise.

To make matters worse for those with sensory-neural losses, they are not protected from the annoyance of loud speech and noise as are those with conductive hearing losses. It is a curious fact that although the sensory-neural group may not be able to hear high tones at all when the tones are faint, the really powerful tones are as loud for them as for anyone else. For these individuals the transition from hearing little or nothing to having sounds come through very loud is abnormally abrupt. With sensory-neural hearing loss the range of comfortable hearing between the inaudible and the too loud—the zone in which we like to listen—is likely to be greatly narrowed. This effect of abnormally rapid increase in loudness is known as *recruitment of loudness*, and it may be very annoying. "Recruitment" means that faint or moderate sounds cannot be heard, but at the same time there is little or no loss in the sense of loudness for loud sounds. It explains why many people whose hearing loss is sensory-neural complain one moment that they cannot hear a speaker and the next moment, when he raises his voice a little, complain that he is shouting too loudly at them.

Recruitment, then, showing itself as a normal hearing of (and even intolerance for) loud sounds, is a distinguishing feature of sensory-neural hearing loss as opposed to conductive hearing loss or central dysacusis and points toward an abnormal condition of the sense organ itself rather than to a simple degeneration or block of nerve fibers. Recruitment is one reason why it is often harder to learn to tolerate a hearing aid and use it successfully when the hearing loss is sensory-neural, and particularly when it is a sense-organ impairment, than it is when the loss is conductive.

OTHER INDICATIONS OF SENSORY-NEURAL HEARING LOSS

Several other features of the hearing loss tend to differ, depending on whether the loss is primarily conductive or primarily sensory-neural. For example, if the hearing level is very high, there must be considerable involvement of the inner ear or the nerve, because, as noted in Chapter 2, even the most complete stoppage of the external and middle ears alone cannot elevate the hearing level by more than 55 or 60 db. The skull as a whole is set in vibration by air-borne sound waves more powerful than this and the vibrations are then transmitted to the inner ear by bone conduction, so if the hearing level is worse than 50, or at most 60 db, there must be some neural or central impairment.

The part of the inner ear that makes us sensitive to the direction of gravity, of turning, and of being moved (or rather accelerated) in space is a sense organ that is older in our evolutionary history than the cochlea. This is called the *vestibular mechanism* and is made up of the semicircular canals, the utricle, and probably the saccule (see Figure 3-5). It seems to be a general biological law that older and more primitive organs are more rugged and less susceptible to degeneration than are more recently developed, highly differentiated, and specialized organs of the same general sort. However this may be, medical experience tells us that if there is complete degeneration, shown by loss of its function, of the vestibular portion of the inner ear (recall Figure 4-1), it is almost always accompanied by very severe or total neural hearing loss. Any infection, toxin, or other unfavorable condition that so seriously affects the more rugged part of the inner ear almost invariably damages the more susceptible neighboring auditory portion quite as seriously. Some exceptions may occur with mild streptomycin poisoning, influenza, meningitis, and tertiary syphilis. Any abnormality in the so-called *vestibular reactions* concerned with the sense of balance is, as a rule, presumptive evidence that any accompanying dysacusis is at least in part sensory-neural. The abnormality may be a loss of normal sensitivity to turning, or it may be an irritation or supersensitivity and cause vertigo or feelings of dizziness.

Tinnitus is the technical term for head noises and ringing in the ears. Sometimes, particularly in conductive hearing loss, it is a mixed, hissing sound, somewhat like the "white" noise described in Chapter 2, in which all the frequencies of the audible spectrum are present at once. This type of tinnitus implies that the organ of hearing in the inner ear is being stimulated throughout its entire length by some general irritative process. Just why wax impacted in the external canal, for example, should occasionally cause such a general irritation in the inner ear is not clear, but a tinnitus occurs nevertheless and sometimes a mild vertigo also.

Most often, and particularly in sensory-neural hearing loss, tinnitus is a high-pitched ringing or a whistle at a pitch that corresponds to the border line between sounds well heard and sounds heard poorly or not all. But tinnitus is not necessarily high-pitched. Sometimes, particularly in Ménière's disease, it is a low-pitched roar or buzz. Sometimes it is steady, sometimes intermittent. The high-pitched variety associated with high-tone hearing loss probably represents a local irritation, the first stage of a degenerative process that has already destroyed some of the neighboring sensory cells.

CHANCES OF IMPROVEMENT

The division of hearing loss into the conductive and the sensory-neural types is important for predicting the future course of the condition. *Conductive hearing loss, especially in its early stages, can often be arrested, improved, or circumvented. Sense-organ hearing loss may sometimes be helped medically or show spontaneous improvement, but only if it has not been present for any considerable length of time. Neural hearing loss, which implies degeneration of delicate but essential elements of sense organ or nerve, can rarely if ever be improved by medical treatment.* Unfortunately, sensory-neural hearing loss is much less favorable than conductive hearing loss for fully satisfactory use of a hearing aid.

Causes of Hearing Loss and Dysacusis

In this section we shall review the causes of various types of impairment of hearing. The nature of the medical and surgical problems of prevention and cure will become apparent, but the details of programs of conservation of hearing and of medical and surgical treatment will be reserved for the two following chapters.

CONDUCTIVE HEARING LOSS

Congenital malformations. Although cupping the hand behind the ear will amplify the sound reaching the eardrum by about ten decibels, the pinna, or auricle, is not very important acoustically. Congenital malformation or absence of the external ear is likely, however, to be associated with malformations in deeper structures, and these may cause a severe loss of hearing. One such malformation is closure or *atresia* of the external canal. If normal hearing by bone conduction shows that the inner ear is intact, an operation to relieve atresia of the external canal is occasionally successful. Usually, however, it is found at operation that there are also malformations of the drum and ossicles, and in this case the best result that can be attained is a hearing level for speech of about thirty-five decibels.

Impacted wax. Except for congenital malformations, diseases of the external canal rarely produce permanent hearing loss. The most common cause of hearing loss from the external canal is wax (cerumen), which may harden in the canal and become *impacted,* so that it prevents the sound waves from reaching the drum and the middle ear. Blockage of this type is often first noticed after swimming, washing the hair, or bathing. A droplet of water suddenly closes the last tiny hole which was sufficient for the normal reception of ordinary sounds, and only then does the victim know that something is amiss.

External otitis. Occasionally changes occur in the skin of the external canal which permit the growth of bacteria and fungi. Infection of the skin and inflammatory changes involving other structures produce a condition called *external otitis.* This occurs most commonly in hot, wet climates. Our troops were bothered by it in World War II when stationed in the southern states or in the Pacific. One type of external otitis is like a pimple or sty in the skin of the external canal, usually near the outer end. It may be produced by scratching the skin of the canal with a fingernail or some instrument, such as a hairpin or toothpick. It is usually caused by one of the organisms that are commonly found on human skin and which cause no harm unless they invade one or more hair follicles.

External otitis may cause symptoms that suggest middle-ear infection (otitis media) and mastoiditis, but it differs from otitis media in often producing no hearing loss unless the swelling of the skin or the trapped secretions completely close the ear canal. The most prominent symptom is pain on manipulation of the auricle.

Otitis media. The middle ear is an air chamber containing the mechanism that conducts sound from the air in the external ear to the fluid in the inner ear. This mechanism comprises the drum, the ossicles (malleus, incus, and stapes), and their ligaments. When they produce a hearing loss, the diseases of the middle ear involve one or more of these structures and produce a conductive hearing loss.

Inflammation in the middle ear is the most common cause of conductive hearing loss. This inflammation is called *otitis media* and usually develops from a cold in the head. The nasal secretions pass backward and infect the Eustachian tube, as shown in Figure 4-2. The infection then travels along the tube itself or along the lymphatic vessels surrounding it until the middle ear is reached. When the lining of the Eustachian tube is inflamed, the tube cannot be opened by swallowing, and the air pressure in the middle ear is no longer equalized. The oxygen in the air of the middle ear is absorbed by the blood that nourishes its mucous lining, and a partial vacuum is produced. The eardrum is forced inward, producing fixation of the ossicles, and clear tissue fluid exudes from the mucous lining. The condition is called *nonsuppurative* otitis media as long as bacteria do not invade the cavity.

INFECTION OF THE MIDDLE EAR. Occasionally otitis media is produced by puncturing the drum from the outside with a dirty instrument, such as a toothpick or a hairpin, and transplating an external otitis in this way. With few exceptions, however, otitis media starts with a common cold. Indeed, since the middle ear is actually another

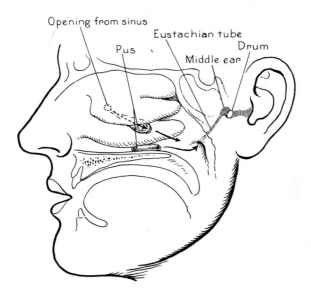

Fig. 4-2. Secretions of pus from the maxillary sinus, and from other sinuses also, easily travel along the floor of the nasal cavity to the mouth of the Eustachian tube and can infect the middle ear.

air cavity leading off from the nose, otitis media can be considered as a cold in the ear. Furthermore, the middle ear is directly connected in turn with the mastoid air cells, as illustrated in Figure 4-3. Middle-ear and mastoid cells form a single air-filled cavity that is only partly sub-divided. Each chamber, large or small, is lined with mucous mem-brane and is connected with the others. With every otitis media there is bound to be some inflammation of the lining of the adjoining mastoid air cells. It is the tremendous surface of the mastoid cells that accounts for most of the secretion of fluid present when the middle ear becomes infected.

It will be remembered that in the early stage of a cold the secre-tion from the nose is watery. In the ear, this stage is properly called *nonsuppurative, or serous, otits media.* As the disease progresses, the watery secretion thickens into pus. Now, when the material in the middle ear has become infected, the disease is said to be in the *sup-*

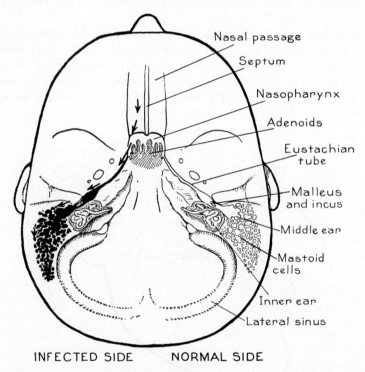

Nasal passage

Septum

Nasopharynx

Adenoids

Eustachian tube

Malleus and incus

Middle ear

Mastoid cells

Inner ear

Lateral sinus

INFECTED SIDE   NORMAL SIDE

Fig. 4-3. In this section the head is viewed from above. The dark shading on the left indicates the extent of the air-filled system of middle ear and mastoid cells that is ventilated by the Eustachian tube. Notice also how close these cavities, which may become infected, come to the brain cavity and large blood-filled channels, such as the lateral sinus.

purative, or *purulent,* stage. There is usually excruciating pain until the drumhead breaks or is opened by a surgeon, or until the growth of bacteria is checked by medication. Often there is pain and tenderness behind the ear over the mastoid.

When properly treated, these conditions usually subside, with or without transient deafness, and should then be designated as *healed.* A mild but long-standing otitis media is occasionally called *subacute.* (It is hard for people to think of the word "acute" without considering it as "severe," but severity is not implied in the medical meaning of the word. Nevertheless, a popular misunderstanding persists.)

If an ear discharges pus for more than two or three months, and especially if it has a bad odor, the condition is called a *chronic otitis media.* There is another misunderstanding concerning the term *chronic catarrhal otitis media.* The words distinctly mean a long-standing watery secretion in the middle ear, but the term is often wrongly applied to a "healed" otitis media that has the scars and adhesions which produce hearing loss. In an effort to avoid this error, some authors have made matters even worse by calling healed otitis media a "dry catarrh"—a direct contradiction in terms. Many such inconsistencies occur in medical terminology. This discussion of terms has been included because these old terminologies persist and unfortunately can still be found in modern classifications of disease for purposes of record and also in popular parlance.

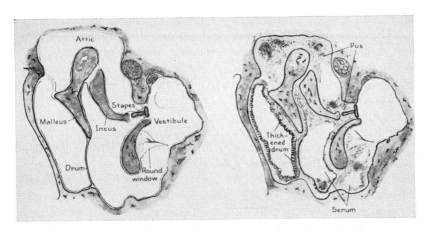

Fig. 4-4. At the left is an enlarged drawing of an actual section through a normal middle ear. At the right is a corresponding section through a middle ear in conductive deafness. The drum is thickened, and the middle ear is filled with pus and serum, which restrict the movements of the ossicles. Pus in the middle ear is a more frequent cause of hearing loss than any other except perhaps senility.

Nonsuppurative otitis media. AERO-OTITIS MEDIA. The best example of uninfected watery effusion into the middle ear occurs during airplane flight if the Eustachian tube is not opened frequently during descent. Eventually the differential in pressure between the middle ear and the surrounding atmosphere, increasing as the airplane approaches the ground, becomes greater than the strength of the muscles that open the tubes. When the tube is not opened, the relatively thin air of high altitudes in the middle air is not replaced by the heavy air near the earth. Uncomfortable pressure and often pain is felt in the eardrum as it is forced inward by the increasing pressure, and fluid collects in the middle ear. This is called *aero-otitis media,* or otitis media due to *barotrauma* (injury from change in barometric pressure). Similar nonsuppurative otitis often occurs among caisson workers and submarine crews. Diving, especially high diving and skin diving, may also produce effusions of fluid.

SEROUS AND MUCOUS OTITIS. A subacute form of nonsuppurative otitis media has recently become very prevalent throughout the world. Why it was previously rare no one knows. When the fluid in the middle ear is thin and watery, the disease is called *serous otitis* or middle-ear effusion or (formerly) catarrhal otitis media. When the effusion is thick, the condition is called *mucoid* or *mucous otitis* or even "glue ear." Some otologists deny that there is any inflammation involved. They therefore object to the suffix "-itis" and prefer to speak of "otic transudates." However, the cellular and chemical content of the fluids of the middle ear in such cases both indicate that there is inflammation, so we shall class this condition as a nonsupperative otitis.

The cause or causes of serous and mucous otitis are not clear. The most common appears to be the treatment of supperative otitis with antibiotics or other biochemicals but without adequate drainage. The bacteria are destroyed or held inactive but the fluid in the middle ear remains. Another cause is allergy. Some cases are certainly allergic in origin but it is impossible to explain all cases on this basis. Another suggested cause is a virus infection of the middle ear.

The fluid that collects in the middle ear causes a hearing loss. The loss may vary all the way from a mild gradual high-tone loss to a very considerable loss for all tones. When thick mucus is present, the hearing loss is most severe and may resemble that seen with otosclerosis. Some surgeons have actually performed fenestration surgery on such cases. Actually, of course, it is quite sufficient to remove the effusion from the middle ear by puncture or incision of the drumhead. The consequent relief of hearing loss is one of the most dramatic affairs in otology.

Since the use of antibiotics for treatment of acute otitis media has become so popular, many physicians not in the specialty of otology have felt complacent when the pain and other symptoms of otitis media disappear following the use of antibiotics. They may have neglected to inspect the ear carefully or may have failed to incise the drumhead in spite of the possibility that some fluid remained in the middle ear. The only remaining symptom is the hearing loss, which may be noticed by the parent or detected by routine testing of hearing in schools. The diagnosis is not always easy, but characteristically the drumhead has a creamy, thick appearance with some slight bulging in the posterior half and it does not move when positive and negative pressure are applied through a pneumatic otoscope.

In these cases a wide incision should be made in the drumhead because it is sometimes peculiarly difficult to evacuate the thick glue-like material from the middle ear. If this mucoid material is not removed by the surgeon it will remain, as it is obviously impossible for it to drain spontaneously through the Eustachian tube. The conductive hearing loss will persist, and the condition may in time lead to the formation of adhesions in the middle ear which firmly fix the ossicular chain with bands of fibrous tissue.

Cholesteatoma. Another important cause of hearing loss, and an important cause of more serious complications as well, is cholesteatoma. This is simply a cyst that is lined internally with skin. This cyst grows from the upper part of the drumhead as a pouch within the middle ear.

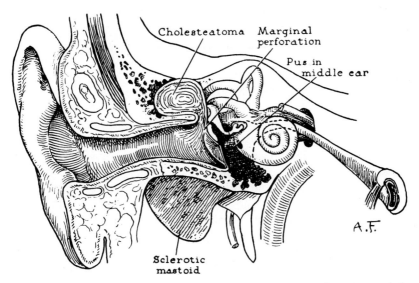

Fig. 4-5. A cholesteatoma forms as an inpocketing of skin at the margin of the drum membrane.

It seems to originate from chronic wetting of the deep parts of the external canal or from inflammation of the middle ear. In any case, a pouch forms and then the lining desquamates into the pouch. It will be remembered that the outer heavy layers of the human skin come off in thin, tiny sheets. As these cornified layers of skin come off in the pouch the cyst becomes larger and larger. Eventually such a soft-tissue cyst may erode away the ossicles or other bony structures and cause symptoms. It constitutes a foreign body in the middle ear and favors suppuration.

The degenerative products formed in such a cyst include a fatty substance called cholesterol. This is the basis of the name cholesteatoma. Usually the patient complains of an intermittent discharge from the ear that has a peculiarly foul odor. The hearing level may be quite good, either within normal limits or within 15 or 20 db of normal threshold. Examination of the ear usually shows a small perforation at the margin of the eardrum, usually at the flaccid upper part.

Other abnormalities of the middle ear. It is not necessary for us to include in this general discussion of medical problems the numerous rare conditions which may involve either the external, the middle, or the inner ear. Tumors, syphilis, tuberculosis, bullet wounds, fractures of the skull, and a variety of other medical and surgical conditions may involve the ear as well as other parts of the body. It is not the problem of the audiologist but of the otologist to diagnose these conditions, and a description of them would be out of place here. By far the most important causes of conductive hearing loss in order of numerical occurrence are (a) inadequate attention to normal function of the Eustachian tube and inadequate treatment of infections of the middle ear and (b) the special disease of the middle and inner ear known as *otosclerosis*.

Otosclerosis. Otosclerosis is a common disease in the white race. *The characteristic bony changes seen under the microscope have been estimated to occur in about one of eight white women and in about one of fifteen white men.* These bony changes are much rarer, about one of a hundred, in Negroes, and little is known about their prevalence in the red, yellow, and brown races.

Otosclerosis is a unique bone disease that affects the bony capsule surrounding the inner ear. This bone, normally the hardest in the body, becomes invaded by a different kind of softer bone which grows intermittently and then becomes hard again, i.e., "sclerotic." The commonest site for the growth of this new bone is in the region just in front of and below the oval window. Sometimes the cochlea itself is involved, and a neural hearing loss develops; but the most common effect of the new bony growth, if it does anything at all, is to fix the footplate of the stapes firmly in the oval window, so that the stapes no longer moves freely. The effect is much like that of some forms of arthritis which limit the movements of fingers, the knee, or the spine; in fact, the two diseases have many points in common. When the stapes becomes fixed, the vibrations carried to it from the eardrum through the malleus and the incus are not effectively transmitted to the fluid of the inner ear. The resulting hearing loss is obviously conductive.

Fortunately, *otosclerosis causes fixation of the stapes and hearing loss in only about 10 per cent of the cases in which it occurs;* and when it does, the fixation occurs only gradually over a period of years. As the hearing loss comes on, more and more powerful sound is required to overcome the increasing resistance to movement, but with the help of a good hearing aid speech may be understood almost perfectly. Ultimately, however, in most cases of otosclerosis in which the hearing loss is severe, there is, in addition to the conductive hearing loss, some sensory-neural loss as well. It is not clear whether this sensory-neural loss is really due to the otosclerosis or is merely a coincidental complication. Sometimes, however, the loss of hearing becomes very severe.

Otosclerosis is a hereditary disease and is passed down in families, although some generations may apparently be skipped. If we recall that the abnormal bony growth does not cause impairment of hearing in 90 per cent of cases, the skipping of generations is easy to understand. Otosclerosis cannot be recognized during life unless there is impairment of hearing, although it can be diagnosed definitely by microscopic examination following an autopsy. It is easy to understand why in this situation we do not know the exact laws of its inheritance.

Otosclerosis is a disease of youth. There have been cases presenting the clinical picture of otosclerosis in young children four, five, and six years of age, and fixation of the stapes has been observed at operation as early as the seventh year, but these fixations are more probably congenital than otosclerotic. The hearing loss of otosclerosis is *usually* first noticed at adolescence or in the early twenties. Nearly always the hearing loss is evident before the thirtieth year, although in a few cases it makes its appearance when the patient is still older. Otosclerosis may become worse during pregnancy, but since the disease is often progressive during early adulthood in any case, until the hearing loss reaches the 40 or 50 db level, and since pregnancy by no means always accelerates the process, *otosclerosis should not be considered a deterrent to the bearing of children.*

When the hearing loss first appears, the patient is often much troubled by *tinnitus,* or ringing in the ears. This ringing may be like a high-pitched whistle or like the sound of a bell. It is much more troublesome at night or when the surroundings are quiet. Sometimes the sound may resemble a rushing of air or water and be synchronous with the pulse. A few patients may also have brief spells of mild dizziness.

In its early stages, the hearing loss of otosclerosis is purely conductive. The bone conduction is normal, or nearly so, but air conduction is impaired. At first the middle range of tones, 1000 and 2000 cps, are often less affected than the lower tones. As a rule, the highest tones, 4000 cps and above, are still less affected at first. As the disease progresses, however—and in a few cases it progresses very rapidly—there is a greater and greater hearing loss for the higher tones by air conduction and the loss of sensitivity by bone conduction centering at 2000 cps, mentioned on page 88, begins to appear. It is when these hearing losses for the higher tones appear that the tinnitus is likely to become severe. Its high-pitched, musical character is evidence of a localized irritation (and perhaps also degeneration) in the sense organ.

We have also mentioned the symptom of *paracusis Willisii*, which is characteristic of conductive hearing loss in general. The patient with otosclerosis seems to hear better in a noisy place, for example, in an airplane, in an automobile, or in a factory. The reason is that people with normal hearing naturally raise their voices to overcome the surrounding noise. The man who has only a partial conductive hearing loss can discriminate the voice from the noise as well as anyone else, if only the voice is loud enough to reach his inner ear. He also hears fairly well over the telephone. But as the otosclerosis progresses and sensory-neural difficulties are added to the mechanical obstruction at the stapes, the patient can no longer so easily distinguish conversation, and he is much handicapped at a party where more than one person is speaking. The more he tries to hear, the less he hears. When he becomes fatigued or nervous, his hearing becomes appreciably worse.

DIAGNOSIS OF OTOSCLEROSIS. The chief points on which a diagnosis of otosclerosis is made are (1) a progressive but moderate loss of hearing, particularly in a a young person; (2) a history of hearing loss in the family; (3) no previous infections of the ear that might account for the hearing loss; and (4) normal eardrums. The drum membrane may perhaps show a pink glow (Schwartz's sign) during the active period or there may be several small atrophic areas like healed perforations, but nothing more.

The hearing levels by air conduction are about equal for all frequencies, or, in the early stages, a little worse for the low frequencies. By bone conduction hearing is substantially normal or a little depressed from 1000 to 4000 cps. Otosclerosis may, of course, be combined with other types of conductive hearing loss, such as those due to chronic infection of the middle ear. In such cases it may be very difficult to decide how much of the hearing loss may be due to the otosclerosis and how much to the chronic otitis media. It is also true that otosclerosis may be combined with some degree of neural degeneration, in which case the audiometric tests show a worse hearing for the high frequencies.

THE COURSE OF OTOSCLEROSIS. Otosclerosis rarely progresses to very severe hearing loss. To call otosclerosis "progressive deafness," as it was once known, is therefore misleading. Many patients believe that this diagnosis means that they will soon be totally deaf. For this reason the term should never be used. Usually there is very little, if any, further loss after the hearing has reached a level of 40 to 50 db below normal. The hearing may stay the same for twenty years or more with a gradual additional loss occurring when the high-tone neural hearing loss of old age adds itself to the conductive hearing loss of otosclerosis.

For many years it was believed that inflation of the Eustachian tubes and pneumatic massage of the drum would loosen the bony fixation of the stapes and improve the hearing in otosclerosis. This has been proved false. The improvement reported by some patients was apparently purely illusory or psychic in origin.

Since the hearing loss of otosclerosis in its early stages is a conductive loss, the patient can anticipate good results with a hearing aid; but, because of the ever-present possibility that neural loss may also develop, the study of speechreading is a very desirable added precaution. If the inner ear is still intact, it is legitimate to consider also the possibility of overcoming the mechanical barrier at the entrance to the inner ear by means of surgery, employing the so-called "fenestration operation" or the "stapes mobilization" described in Chapter 6.

SENSORY-NEURAL IMPAIRMENTS

Presbycusis (Presbyacusis, Presbyacousis). Loss of hearing due to abnormality or disease of the inner ear is almost by definition a sensory-neural hearing loss. *By far the most common cause of sensory-neural hearing loss, and probably of all hearing loss, is advancing age.*

Some atrophy of the organ of Corti and of the auditory nerve is very common after the age of forty. Indeed, *the development of a certain amount of high-tone sensory-neural hearing loss seems to be part of the natural course of growing older.* Such hearing loss is known as *presbycusis* or *presbyacousis.* Figure 4-6 shows a series of composite audiograms. A large number of subjects were grouped according to age and their audiograms averaged. The increasing severity of high-tone hearing loss on the average is perfectly clear. On the other hand,

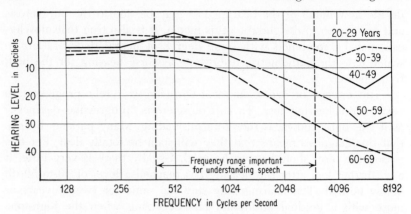

Fig. 4-6. A series of composite audiograms for different age groups shows a progressive loss of sensitivity for the high frequencies. Individuals in the age groups may, of course, vary widely from the averages. (*Data from C. C. Bunch.*)

not every old man or woman becomes hard of hearing. Many who have been examined, even up to the age of eighty, have been found to have nearly perfect hearing; but the majority show a significant loss with age, just as most people begin to suffer from hardening of the arteries and need to put on reading glasses after middle age. The structural change that is responsible is perfectly well known. The sensory cells in the part of the organ of Corti toward the base of the cochlea simply degenerate and vanish, as do the nerve fibers that connect with them (see Figure 4-7). Having said this, we can add little more about the process at the present time, except to speculate as to whether arteriosclerosis of the small blood vessels may be partly responsible and to wonder why the part of the organ sensitive to high tones is almost invariably first involved. Perhaps the very small size of the artery to that part of the cochlea is a factor.

Drugs, allergens, and noise. Two general causes are popularly blamed for many cases of hearing loss or even total deafness. One is drugs, and the other is noise. There is general agreement among physicians that some drugs sometimes cause or contribute to a hearing loss and that sufficiently prolonged exposure to enough noise certainly can do so. Furthermore, if such a toxic or noise-induced hearing loss occurs, it is a sensory-neural hearing loss based on a degeneration of sensory cells and nerve fibers, such as occurs normally with advancing age. The audiograms and all other tests reveal no consistent differences: all three are typical sensory-neural hearing loss. Because of similarity to presbycusis and the large individual differences in susceptibility, the importance and even the reality of toxic and noise-induced

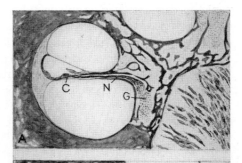

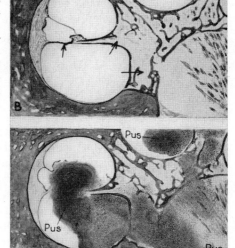

Fig. 4-7. Two types of neural impairment are represented in this figure. Section A represents a normal cochlea. The location of this section in relation to the inner ear as a whole is shown by the rectangle in Fig. 3-6. The organ of Corti C, the fibers of the auditory nerve N and N VIII, and the ganglion cells G are labeled in this section.

Section B shows the lower turn of a cochlea of an aged person with high-tone neural loss. The arrows show where the organ of Corti, the nerve fibers, and the ganglion (nerve) cells have degenerated.

Section C shows the destruction of the organ of Corti, basilar membrane, and nerve by pus, as in meningitis.

hearing loss were in some doubt for many years. Now, however, one drug has emerged as a real danger to hearing and the case against noise is clearly defined.

DRUGS AND POISONS. Tinnitus and sensory-neural hearing losses due to quinine and to salicylates (aspirin) have been known for years, especially in sensitive individuals. Less clear cut are the tinnitus, hearing loss, and vertigo thought by some to be associated with excessive use of tobacco, coffee, or tea. Rare toxic effects from carbon monoxide, arsenic, lead, and other poisons need not be discussed here.

Recently a group of antibiotic drugs, notably dihydrostreptomycin and kanamycin, and to a less extent streptomycin and neomycin, have been found to be definitely ototoxic, especially for certain susceptible individuals. To make matters worse, dihydrostreptomycin, for some unaccountable reason, has been used routinely in various mixtures with penicillin for so-called prophylactic therapy. The hearing loss from dihydrostreptomycin often does not appear for two or more months after the medication has been given. Therefore dihydrostreptomycin was not, for a long time, suspected of causing any trouble. It has now become clear, however, that these particular drugs should never be used unless there is a specific and compelling indication for them.

ALLERGENS. Hypersensitivity of the tissues of the middle ear, the Eustachian tube, and the inner ear to various foreign proteins in the air or blood stream has been described. Perhaps the most common is the sensitivity to bacteria called "bacterial allergy." Occasionally, a patient has tinnitus or a hearing loss whenever he or she eats particular foods, such as wheat, milk, eggs, chocolate, nuts, or citrus fruits. Certainly severe pollen allergies contribute to blockage of the tubes and may make an individual more susceptible to the various types of otitis media.

Noise. MASKING BY NOISE. A background of noise interferes with hearing and may completely submerge or *mask* a sound that we wish to hear. One mechanism of masking is quite simple. Nerve fibers are already being stimulated by the noise, and the more sensitive fibers may be carrying as many impulses per second as they can. Like a country telephone, the line is busy, and the new sound, if it is weaker than the noise, cannot set up enough additional nerve impulses to be recognized or *discriminated* from the background. We cannot hear a whisper in a boiler factory any more than we can see the stars in the daytime. There are other more complicated effects, both in the sense organ and in the nervous system, which are simply part of the normal adjustments of the ear to the general level of sound that is reaching it.

TEMPORARY HEARING LOSS. Quite different from this everyday matter of masking is the "auditory fatigue" or temporary hearing loss that is produced by long exposure to loud sounds. Whoever has worked in a really noisy factory, driven a tractor on a farm, or indulged in much pistol or skeet shooting can recall how his ears rang for hours afterward and voices sounded muffled and indistinct. Loud sounds could be heard as well as ever, but he was temporarily hard of hearing. After a few hours, or by the day following at least, his hearing had recovered. Recovery from this hearing loss is usually so complete that the hearing loss may properly be considered a fatigue rather than an injury. We call this a *temporary threshold shift*.

It is a curious fact that the temporary threshold shift produced by exposure to a loud tone or noise is confined almost entirely to frequencies *higher* than the frequency of the offending tone or noise. *The greatest shift is for tones about half an octave above the exposure tone,* but all of the higher frequencies may be more or less affected.

Hearing for lower tones, on the other hand, remains almost as good as ever. Furthermore, the high tones, in addition to being more annoying (although not more painful), also cause a more rapid shift of threshold. The greater susceptibility of the ear to fatigue by high tones offsets the greater intensity of the low components in most loud noises, both natural and man-made. For most noises, therefore, the temporary effect is usually a partial high-tone loss, *most severe for frequencies above the range essential for speech.* Ears vary so much in their susceptibility, and noises vary so much in their spectra, that isolated numerical statements are not very meaningful, but an example may be given from some wartime experiments. Exposure to a 1000 cps tone at 120 db (about at the threshold of discomfort) for half an hour usually caused a temporary threshold shift of about 35 db over the upper half of the speech range. Hearing was usually normal the next day, but the last part of auditory sensitivity to recover completely was almost always the band *between 3000 and 5000 cps.* This band seems to represent a vulnerable spot in the sense organ of hearing that recovers more slowly, regardless of what tone or noise produces the threshold shift.

PERMANENT INJURY FROM NOISE. Temporary threshold shift may be called "fatigue," but somewhere injury begins. We know that the muzzle blast of a big gun or the explosion of a nearby shell may rupture the drum membrane or cause permanent sensory-neural hearing loss. (Curiously enough, if the membrane *does* rupture, there is likely to be less permanent sensory-neural loss of hearing than if it does not. Blast deafness is rarely total in any case.) In animal experiments it was found that blasts may disorganize the organ of Corti or shake great pieces of it loose into the surrounding fluid. The injured part of the organ does not regenerate but instead is replaced by a layer of simple cells. The same sort of permanent injury is produced by a sufficiently intense noise or pure tone. The intensity required to cause real disintegration depends in part on how long the noise lasts.

ACOUSTIC TRAUMA. Injury to the ear by a single brief exposure to sound, particularly to an explosion or gun blast, is called "acoustic trauma." This term has been, and in European countries still is, used to include loss of hearing from prolonged and repeated exposure to noise. It is useful to distinguish the two conditions, however, particularly for medicolegal reasons. In acoustic trauma, as we use the words, it is easy to identify the actual incident and the time that it happened and usually the responsibility for it. From the audiological point of view the loss of hearing may be very severe at first, but much recovery can be expected and improvement usually continues for several months. This is in sharp contrast to the chronic noise-induced hearing loss among industrial workers in very noisy trades. Their improvement in hearing after the first forty-eight hours off the job is very slight indeed.

Another form of acute injury to hearing is a loss resulting from a blow to the head. A blow on the external ear, the old-fashioned "boxing the ears" of children as a form of punishment, can cause not only severe pain in the middle ear and possible injury to the drum membrane or fracture or dislocation of the ossicles but even permanent injury to the inner ear. The injury is caused by a violent wave of air-conducted "sound." Similar damage to the inner ear may even be caused by a very sharp blow on the skull, such as may occur in an automobile accident. Here the injury is best described as acoustic trauma by bone conduction. This accident is rare, however.

Noise-induced hearing loss is the preferred term for what was once called "boilermakers' deafness" or "industrial hearing loss." It is a loss of hearing that develops gradually over months and years. The loss *almost always begins at 4000 or 6000 cps,* where the recovery from temporary threshold shift is slowest, but this depends somewhat on the spectrum of the noise.

NOISE EXPOSURE.   The ear can tolerate for a few seconds a painfully loud noise that would disrupt the organ of Corti or at least cause degeneration of some of its sensory cells if continued for minutes. In other words, the duration as well as the intensity of the exposure is important. Injury from noise exposure depends on decibels, on frequency, and also on duration measured in seconds, hours, months, or years. The sound levels necessary to produce rapid injury, say 150 db or more, rarely occur as sustained sound except near the exhaust of some jet engines and rockets. Those who work in such situations must take special precautions, and certain areas may be forbidden entirely as too hazardous for hearing. But for the more ordinary, less severe noise exposures, the usual practical question about injury is: "Will the temporary hearing loss produced day after day and week after week ultimately become permanent?" The answer is "Yes," *if* the noise is loud enough and if a long exposure is repeated often enough; but we do not know how loud and how often is "enough." Some ears are more susceptible to temporary threshold shift than are others, and there are probably similar differences in resistance to permanent injury. In the practical situations of the drop-forge worker or the antiaircraft gunner who has suffered a permanent hearing loss, we rarely know how loud the sound was that finally caused the permanent injury. Rules and devices for prevention of noise-induced hearing loss are given in the next chapter.

OTHER POSSIBLE EFFECTS OF NOISE.   We need not fear any mysterious general effects, such as fatigue, headache, neurosis, or sudden death, from any special sounds or combination of sounds. On careful investigation, the persistent rumors about such effects prove to be unfounded. The ears are much more sensitive to noise than is any other part of the body and are always injured first. To be injurious, sounds must be powerful, and usually long lasting or repeated as well. *There is no magic in any strange disharmony or in any high-frequency "ultrasonic death ray" at any practical intensity.* Noise is unpleasant, but in a wartime experiment designed to imitate piloting an airplane, a steady loud noise did not measurably impair the performance of men in any of a large variety of tests of coordination, steadiness, memory, puzzle solving, and the like. Those who *must* work in noise soon learn to disregard it. We may guess that those who dislike their work and are irritable tend to blame noise more than it really deserves for their ills.

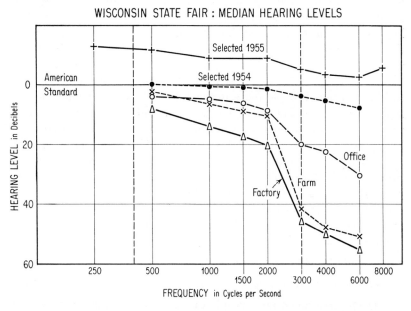

WISCONSIN STATE FAIR : MEDIAN HEARING LEVELS

FREQUENCY in Cycles per Second

Fig. 4-8. Factory and farm workers show more high-tone hearing loss than do office workers. The "selected" groups are young adults who were judged to be otologically normal and with no history of noise exposure or otic pathology. The deviations of their median hearing levels from the American Standard zero level and also the differences between the "selected" levels in 1954 and in 1955 are discussed in Chapter 7. The best estimate of the combined effects of age, noise-exposure, and so on, among office, farm, and factory workers is given by the divergence of their median levels from the selected 1954 levels. (*Data from "1954 Wisconsin State Fair Hearing Survey,*" by A. Glorig, et al., *American Academy of Ophthalmology and Otolaryngology, 1957, and from Glorig, Quiggle, Wheeler, and Grings, Journal of the Acoustical Society of America, 28:1110–1113 [1956].*)

AGGRAVATION OF HEARING LOSS BY NOISE. There is always the uncomfortable possibility that although brief exposure to noise under 120 db over-all will not permanently damage a normal ear it may seriously injure a hard-of-hearing ear. Many have probably been discouraged from using a hearing aid, perhaps on the advice of a physician, lest the loud sound of the instrument accelerate the degenerative process that caused the hearing loss. Such advice may amount to conservative cruelty. In the first place, if the hearing loss is due to a failure of sound to reach the inner ear, the ear is thereby *protected* from any possible injury by the sound. Thirty decibels of conductive hearing loss, the least for which it is worthwhile wearing a hearing aid, represents a protection nearly as great as that offered by the best ear plugs. Thirty decibels of protection will reduce the maximum output of the most powerful instrument below any reasonable danger limit. If, however, the hearing loss is due entirely to degeneration of the nerve or sense organ, the caution is in order: the additional burden of loud noise might accelerate the degeneration. However, in this type of loss the intense sounds actually sound loud to the listener, and he is not likely to need a very high-powered instrument to get the best result that a hearing aid can give him. He is not likely to tolerate anything approaching the danger zone and may need to be encouraged to use more power rather than less. Simply because some users of hearing aids have continued to lose hearing does not mean that the instrument is responsible. A patient may forget how deaf he really is until he takes off his hearing aid, and he may blame the instrument for what he thinks is an increase in his hearing loss. The progressive hearing loss of old age becomes worse whether an instrument is used or not. *Caution is legitimate with sensory-neural hearing loss*, but if, as in "mixed hearing loss," there is also some conductive loss, the protection given by the conductive hearing loss will guard the inner ear against excessive noise either from the instrument or from noisy surroundings.

CONGENITAL DYSACUSIS

In children and young people the most common cause of sensory-neural hearing loss, if we are to accept medical statistics at their face value, is *congenital,* but the meaning of the term as it appears in medical records is not entirely clear. It is a sort of wastebasket classification in which are placed all cases of impaired hearing in children for which no other likely cause can be found. The term "congenital" may be wrongly applied to cases in which the impairment is actually due to scarlet fever, meningitis, or some other disease of childhood which destroyed hearing before the child learned to talk. There is no doubt, however, that babies may sometimes be born deaf and also that there is a hereditary tendency, fortunately very rare, for the sense organ of hearing and the auditory nerve to degenerate at an early age without apparent cause.

Congenital deafness or dysacusis may be caused by almost any severe virus infection of the expectant mother during the early months of pregnancy. The first three months, when important rapid development of the embryonic eye, ear, and central nervous system is going on, are a critical period for such injury by a virus. Some viruses, such as mumps and influenza, are more dangerous than others in this respect. The epidemic of German measles in Australia about 1942 is a well-known example. About 1946, some 16 per cent of the cases listed as congenital in the schools for the deaf in Australia were associated with *German measles (rubella) in the mother during the first three months of her pregnancy.* Similar reports have come from other countries, but fortunately the ordinary strains of measles and German measles do not seem to be as damaging as those responsible for that particular epidemic.

Congenital abnormalities of this type cannot be cured; like all cases of neural hearing loss, they are based on complete degeneration of essential sensory cells and nerve fibers. These cells, once they have degenerated, cannot be restored, nor can their function be taken over by other nerve or sense organs, except indirectly, as in the substitution of sight for hearing. Rubella during the first three months of pregnancy may also cause aphasia or mental retardation as well as abnormalities of the eyes or the ears. *But knowledge of the danger from German measles, mumps, and influenza during pregnancy may lead to preventive measures that will considerably reduce the incidence of congenital deafness in future generations.*

Another threat to normal development is the so-called Rh factor of the bloods of the parents. Specifically, if the mother is Rh-negative, the father Rh-positive, and the unborn child Rh-positive, the mother's system may develop a reaction against the Rh-positive factor as though it were a bacterial toxin or a virus. Thus the mother's own self-protective reaction may injure the developing fetus, with effects similar to those of actual viral infection. The danger period from Rh-incompatibility is just before, during, and after birth. It may cause a toxic condition in the mother and an abnormality of the blood of the infant known as jaundice of the newborn, or icterus neonatorum. Although life may be saved by blood transfusion, there may be permanent damage, sometimes to the ear, more often to the brain, and sometimes elsewhere. It is some comfort to know that abnormalities from the Rh-factor are relatively rare in the first-born child.

HEREDITARY DEAFNESS OR HEARING LOSS

We have mentioned hereditary degeneration of the auditory nerve, but very little is known about this condition. It appears that degeneration may begin at any age and that this atrophy occurs in families. For example, one little girl of eight became hard of hearing in both ears without apparent cause. She developed a hearing level of 30 db at 256 cps and of 80 to 100 db at 1024 cps and above. Her hearing level by bone conduction (at the frequencies at which it could be measured) was almost the same as by air conduction. Her case was clearly a sensory-neural impairment. Her mother was also very hard of hearing and said that her loss of hearing had occurred at the same age and without apparent cause. The hearing losses of all four ears, both the mother's and the daughter's, were of the same type and were nearly identical. More frequently, hereditary deafness is the result of a failure of normal development of the inner ear, with or without abnormalities of the eye or the brain or both. Congenital malformation of the external or of the middle ear may also be hereditary.

The existence of hereditary sensory-neural deafness is well enough established so that those who suffer from it should give serious thought to the question of marriage with others who are similarly afflicted. If *both* parents have true hereditary deafness or dysacusis (not merely a "congenital" impairment resulting from German measles or other infection in infancy or in their mothers), their children will almost certainly be born deaf or soon become deaf. Even marriage of someone who has hereditary deafness into a family in which there are other cases of hereditary deafness, although the intended spouse may actually have normal hearing, is risky. If, however, one prospective parent comes of a family that is free from the hereditary trait, the chances that the children will become deaf are small, and marriage may properly be considered. In case of doubt, a doctor or other counselor who is well acquainted with the laws of heredity should be consulted.

CAUSES OF DEAFNESS IN CHILDREN

In 1928 an extensive study was made of the causes of deafness and severe hearing loss in the children enrolled in public schools for the deaf in nine midwestern states. The figures are based in part on the records of the schools and in part on inquiry and examinations by a group of doctors led by Dr. G. E. Shambaugh, Sr. The results were corroborated by a similar but smaller study in eastern Pennsylvania and New Jersey and are our most authoritative guide as to the relative importance of various causes of severe auditory handicap. These studies are still the largest and most complete that have been carried out, but unfortunately they are seriously out of date. Many of the infectious diseases of childhood, such as scarlet fever, measles, influenza, pneumonia, whooping cough, typhoid fever and diphtheria, which then accounted for about 15 per cent of the entire population of totally deaf or severely hard-of-hearing children, have now been brought under control to such an extent by protective "shots" of antitoxins or vaccines or by the early use of sulfa drugs or antibiotics that they now cause far fewer cases of deafness. Two new causes, maternal infection during pregnancy and Rh-incompatibility, have been identified. Meningitis, a specific infection of the brain, is rapidly coming under medical control, as is typhoid fever. Infections of the middle ear and the mastoid bone are diagnosed earlier and on the average are better treated, whether by surgery or by drugs.

Several studies have been published that give the causes of deafness, as nearly as could be determined, in certain special groups such as the children enrolled in a particular school for the deaf. These figures, valuable as they are for some purposes, do not give a correct picture of either the etiology or the incidence of deafness in the general population. The samples are too small and too highly selected. For this reason we do not cite them here.

If a broad survey of causes of deafness in children were made today it too might well be out of date in another thirty years. It would probably resemble Dr. Shambaugh's survey in one respect, namely, a high percentage of "congenital deafness," either definite or probable. The definitely hereditary group would be a rather small percentage. "Congenital deafness" would now be subdivided to show maternal infection and Rh-factor, and a considerable number would probably be listed as "dysacusis from brain injury," "cerebral palsy," and so on. And if the survey were honest it would certainly show at least 25 per cent as "unknown"!

Meningitis. Meningitis was in 1927 the commonest single cause of acquired total deafness in childhood. Meningitis begins as an infection of the membranes surrounding and protecting the brain. The infected spinal fluid invades the inner ear through the normal connections between the inner ear and the cranial cavity, and, although the patient may recover, the nerve and sensory structures of the inner ear may be completely destroyed. Figure 4-7 illustrates such total destruction. The knowledge of the nature of the injury in meningitis and in other forms of neural deafness allows us to state categorically that *no type of treatment, medication, or stimulation will improve the hearing of anyone whose deafness is due to meningitis or for whom a diagnosis of long-standing neural deafness can be made.*

Other infectious diseases. Sensory-neural deafness or hearing loss occasionally appears as a complication of influenza and some of the common infectious diseases of childhood. In mumps, for example, there sometimes appears to be an infection of the brain which spreads to the inner ear, but there is not, as in meningitis, the extensive destruction of tissues other than the delicate sensory cells. Fortunately, mumps almost always affects only one ear, and a loss of hearing in one ear results in relatively little social or practical handicap. The hearing loss from measles and scarlet fever may be neural, apparently from the absorption of toxins, or it may be a consequence of infection of the middle ears. Unlike mumps, these diseases tend to affect both ears. The middle-ear hearing loss from measles and scarlet fever is, of course, a conductive hearing loss like that caused by any other type of otitis media.

SENSE-ORGAN DYSACUSIS

Much attention has been turned during the last twenty years to what we now recognize as sense-organ dysacusis. The condition is not necessarily a permanent degeneration of sensory cells or nerve fibers, as in presbycusis, noise-induced hearing loss, congenital deafness and toxic degeneration, but faulty function of a sense organ that may still become healthy again. The cause or causes of the abnormality are completely unknown, but it usually involves the nonauditory or vestibular labyrinth, either alone or in addition to the organ of hearing. For this reason the most common as well as the most distressing and disabling condition is *vertigo*, or violent dizziness. The attacks come and go and may begin quite suddenly. When at their worst, the patient cannot walk or stand and may even have difficulty lying quietly in bed. Between attacks there may be little or no vertigo but abnormalities of hearing may now be noticed. One of these is tinnitus. This may be a violent, distressing roar, unlike the mild, high-pitched whistle of nerve degeneration or otosclerosis. It, like the vertigo, is a clear symptom of overactivity of the sensory cells. They are "hyper-irritable" and set off spontaneous discharges of nerve impulses, which in turn create the illusions of sound and of movement. Hearing is less sensitive than normal, but the patient complains chiefly that although he *hears* words they "don't come clear" and he can't make them out. He suffers, as we say, from a loss of discrimination. Both the hearing level for tones and the discrimination for speech may fluctuate considerably, now better, now worse, over periods of days or weeks. The patient may experience one or another form of diplacusis ("double hearing") and often a feeling of fullness in the affected ear.

Sudden attacks of vertigo, tinnitus, and deafness are usually known as *Ménière's disease* in honor of the Frenchman who first described it in 1861. An anatomical abnormality known to be associated with it is a distention of the membranous labyrinth, like a toy balloon, as though the endolymph in it were under increased pressure. This finding in a few cases has suggested the somewhat speculative name *endolymphatic hydrops* for the disease. Dozens of causes for Ménière's disease have been suggested but none have been established as anything more than merely plausible. The most popular theory at the present moment is some kind of spasm or intermittent partial blocking of the circulation of the inner ear. The disease, with its unpredictable ups and downs, is often as puzzling to the otologist as it is distressing to those who suffer from it. It now appears, however, that a strong psychosomatic element underlies Ménière's disease, very much as it does with peptic ulcer and some forms of vascular disease.

Diplacusis. An abnormality of hearing that is not a change of hearing level but depends rather clearly on faulty function of the sense organ is the failure to hear the pitch of sounds correctly. A watery swelling or "hydrops" of the cochlear structures should change their physical properties, such as mass, elasticity, or stiffness, enough to alter the "tuning" of the basilar membrane. A given frequency, say 1000 cps, may now agitate the organ of Corti a little nearer to or farther from the apex. The new position may correspond to the normal position for 950 or 1050 cps, and, according to the principles of the neural specificity of pitch, the pitch that we hear will be that of a 950- (or 1050-) cps tone. The pitch scale will be distorted, and if the two ears are affected unequally, the same frequency will have a different pitch in the two ears. This inequality of pitch—"hearing double" —is known as *diplacusis,* in this case, *diplacusis binauralis.* Careful comparisons show that most people have a little diplacusis for some parts of the frequency scale most of the time; but unless the condition becomes rather considerable or is tested for carefully, they are, fortunately, quite unaware of it. The brain can average out small pitch differences between the ears just as it averages small differences in color vision between the two eyes.

Diplacusis may become an annoying or serious feature of sensory-neural dysacusis. The degeneration of the hair cells and nerve fibers is not necessarily uniform from the high-tone end of the basilar membrane toward the low-tone end. There may be islands of normal cells with rather sharp boundaries and a correspondingly jagged audiogram. We believe that if the frequency of a tone corresponds to a gap where some or all of the cells are missing, the first tone to be heard as the sound is made more intense may be the pitch that belongs to a neighboring patch of normal sensory cells. The vibration always spreads more or less along the basilar membrane because, as has been pointed out, the basilar membrane is a continuous structure; it is merely a matter of which is stimulated first, insensitive cells in the right place or sensitive cells some distance away. If the degeneration is very spotty, or if some of the sensory cells are abnormally irritable, the tone may be impure, noisy, or buzzing, or more than one tone may be heard simultaneously. This is *diplacusis monauralis.* A rough, buzzing, noisy quality instead of a pleasant pure musical tone is often heard by patients with sense-organ dysacusis, as in Ménière's disease. Our most detailed present information on diplacusis, and the interpretation we have given, comes from wartime studies on normal ears that had suffered a temporary threshold shift or auditory fatigue from exposure to a very loud, pure tone. The amount of pitch shift was in some cases nearly an octave, or the tone sounded noisy and impure, or one ear heard two pitches at once. Usually the shift and the buzzing were less for very loud test tones than for those that could only just be heard. In Ménière's disease, however, the abnormal quality of sounds and poor discrimination are present with both loud and faint test sounds. Of course, these distortions of sound, including the diplacusis, reduce the ability to understand speech far below what we would expect from simple pure-tone threshold tests.

Central Dysacusis

By *central dysacusis* we mean an impairment of hearing that cannot be explained by abnormality of sense organ or auditory nerve. The difficulty, whatever it may be, lies somewhere in the central nervous system. The nearly equivalent term *retrolabyrinthine dysacusis* means that the cause lies behind (or beyond) the labyrinth and includes tumors of the auditory (or vestibular) nerve trunk as it passes from the temporal bone to the brain stem. These *acoustic tumors* usually are benign, grow slowly, and cause a hearing loss by the mechanical pressure on the nerve fibers. Symptoms of neural hearing loss, mild tinnitus, and vertigo increase slowly over the years and are difficult to diagnose with assurance until other cranial nerves or the brain stem also begin to suffer from the pressure. Although the tumors are not malignant, they offer a difficult problem to the surgeon because their location inside the skull at the base of the brain makes their removal a serious operation.

Any type of general disease of the brain, such as other brain tumors, arteriosclerosis, cerebral hemorrhage, plugging of cerebral blood vessels (thrombosis or embolism), multiple sclerosis, syphilis or brain abscess, may affect the auditory pathways anywhere along their course from the auditory nerve through the brain stem and up to the outer layers of the temporal lobe of the brain. These same diseases, and also birth injuries, gunshot wounds, skull fractures, and the scars and adhesions from any or all of these may also affect the brain. When understanding the meaning of words is concerned, more of the brain is required than for simple hearing of a sound, but we cannot say just how much or what particular parts of the brain are needed for these complicated tasks. The pure-tone audiometer is here of little use as a measuring tool. Instead, we must center our attention on what kinds of things the person can and cannot do, how rapidly he can do them and under what conditions of fatigue, motivation, and so on.

In this area it is not the otologist but the neurologist, the neuro-surgeon, the psychiatrist, the psychologist, and the educator who are the partners of the audiologist. It is from them that the appropriate concepts must be sought for describing the defects due to old age, disease, and brain injury, for devising tests for assessing performance, and for making diagnosis and prognosis. Some of these will be considered in Chapter 8. In general, however, we have left the area in which anatomical localization, such as "middle ear" or "auditory nerve," and quantitative physical measures, such as decibels and cycles per second, are very helpful. For all of the senses anatomical localization is clearest in the sense organs themselves and next clearest in the peripheral nerves. The deeper (or the "higher") we get in the nervous system the less clear is *any* localization. To be sure, a large part of the gray matter of the cortex of the brain is identified as visual cortex, another area as auditory, another as cutaneous, another as motor, and so on, but these assignments are general and exact boundaries are vague. In animal experiments we must remove *all* of the auditory cortex on *both sides* in order to demonstrate clearly any lasting handicap at all. Following a lesser removal, learned auditory tasks (conditioned reflexes) may be lost, but if even a small bit of auditory cortex remains, relearning is usually possible, and often is faster than the original learning process.

In the study of the cortex it has been hard to devise tests that are difficult enough, that is, complicated enough in the right way, to provide tests that are both valid and reliable. The central nervous system has a way of finding other ways to do a job. A legless animal can no longer run, walk, or even crawl toward its goal but it may nevertheless *roll* in the right direction. The inherent versatility and plasticity of the nervous system with its possibility of "vicarious function," i.e., a region taking over a function that it does not ordinarily perform, is disconcerting for the experimenter, but it is the salvation of the educator who trains a child who has suffered a brain injury at birth, and of those who are concerned with the rehabilitation of wounded veterans.

But plasticity and versatility and vicarious function are limited, and they become more and more limited with advancing age. Also, the tasks performed in the new way may require more attention and higher motivation and may be more fatiguing. One defect of an abnormal brain may be just the inability to "pay attention," so performance may be good one moment and poor the next, or vary greatly from day to day. The most characteristic feature of some abnormal conditions is the variability of behavior, performance, and test results. This is in sharp contrast to the highly reproducible auditory thresholds of a trained normal listener or of a patient with conductive hearing loss or with some types of neural hearing loss.

"Central dysacusis" includes many disorders and must be defined more closely, if possible. Three major types are common enough and clear enough to deserve special description.

VERBAL DYSACUSIS (SENSORY APHASIA)

Verbal dysacusis means a failure to understand the meanings of words even though the sounds are heard quite perfectly and correctly. A popular term for this condition is "word deafness," and the word "aphasia" is being used more and more widely. An ingenious suggestion by Dr. L. Meyerson, which never became popular, however, was to call the primary reception of acoustic signals "hearing" and the understanding of the meaning of the signals "auding." Verbal dysacusis may be caused by injury to parts of the cerebral cortex, the familiar "gray matter," concerned with hearing. Difficulties with speech and reading, in other words, with the whole central process of the meanings of symbols, whether auditory or visual, are frequently associated with verbal dysacusis.

Verbal dysacusis, also called "auditory agnosia" or "central auditory imperception," has long been recognized as a symptom and has been associated in a general way with injuries to the temporal lobe (particularly the left temporal lobe) of the brain. The symptom is clear in an adult who has fractured his skull in an automobile accident. A corresponding injury incurred at birth or in infancy before the child has ever learned the meaning of words is obviously harder to identify. The defect now appears as an inability or difficulty in *learning the meaning of words* or other sounds. This symptom is familiar, although it is not always easy to distinguish such "congenital auditory agnosia" from a peripheral neural deafness because the child may simply pay no attention to sounds. The symptoms and the progress are different in the child from what they are in the adult, partly because word meanings have never been learned by the child and partly because of the greater "plasticity" of the child's brain, but the conditions are fundamentally similar.

The term "sensory aphasia" has been applied to this symptom, although it is less specific than "auditory agnosia" or "verbal dysacusis." Others prefer to speak of "aphasoid" children because "aphasia" means inability to speak and properly should include only those who have lost or have not acquired the power to formulate and articulate speech. These disabilities are sometimes called "expressive aphasia" and "motor aphasia" to distinguish them from sensory or receptive aphasia or verbal dysacusis.

As was pointed out earlier, one basis of the terminology used here is anatomical: (1) external and middle ear (conductive), (2) cochlea (sensory-neural), and (3) retrocochlear (central). The term "central" is used in just this sense, to locate the impairment in the central nervous system without any implication that it is either "organic" or "functional." "Central dysacusis" is not a synonym for "aphasia" but overlaps with it. "Aphasia" refers to cetrain impairments of the function of language. It would be wrong to use "aphasia" too broadly to include all central auditory impairments just as it would be wrong to include the expressive and motor aspects of aphasia under the term "central dysacusis." In the term "central dysacusis" the word "central" says that the impairment is more than faulty function of the ear. The word "dysacusis" implies that the condition is a sensory rather than a motor difficulty and that it may or may not involve what we vaguely call "understanding" or "the language function." It may or may not have a recognizable anatomical basis. We have deliberately avoided the term "aphasia" because its meaning seems to be changing rapidly. It originally meant "absence of the ability to express one's thoughts in speech," but it now seems to include sensory agnosia as well and sometimes the ability to understand the meaning of symbols of any sort. This is a far cry from a simple inability to use words correctly and meaningfully.

Our understanding of the neurological and physiological basis of the aphasias, the agnosias, and the related conditions of cerebral palsy, epilepsy, and the like, is advancing rapidly but we still must approach the practical problems of the clinic on the basis of direct observation and experience and not from neurological or physiological theory.

PHONEMIC REGRESSION AND OLD AGE

The term "phonemic regression" was coined a few years ago by Dr. Raymond Carhart to describe a condition that he noticed fairly often in elderly people who came to his hearing clinic at North-western University. They complained of difficulty in understanding what other people said. By pure-tone audiometry these elderly people showed nearly normal hearing levels, at least up to 2000 cps, provided the tests were carried out carefully, deliberately, and sympathetically, and with adequate rest periods. But with speech audiometry, particu-larly with recorded speech tests, these people had great difficulty. They understood only a few words correctly and soon became discouraged.

It is easy to recognize in this the pattern of old age. The attention span becomes short and the person will not and cannot be hurried. Given time, he may answer correctly, but never quickly. He has much more difficulty with the complicated acoustic patterns of speech than with simple pure tones. That is why Dr. Carhart calls it *phonemic* regression. These people have the high-tone sensory-neural hearing loss of presbycusis but their failure to understand words is far greater than can be explained by this loss alone.

The cause of phonemic regression lies in the brain, not in the ear. Generalized cerebral arteriosclerosis is probably the most common cause. Many individual cells have died throughout the brain and there may be many bits and patches where the loss is more than just a thinning of the cell population. The brain still remembers old ex-periences and habits but it learns or remembers little that is new. Attention is short. Naps become frequent. And even familiar perform-ances, like recognizing the meaning of words or sentences, while often still possible, may require special motivation and plenty of time. For elderly people with phonemic regression a hearing aid is of little help, nor does it help to shout at them. It is more important to speak *clearly, simply,* and, above all, *slowly.*

PSYCHOGENIC DYSACUSIS (FUNCTIONAL DEAFNESS,
NONORGANIC DEAFNESS)

It is not generally recognized that psychological changes in the personality may be the cause of auditory difficulties. In such cases there is a partial or total inability to hear, although there is no structural change in the auditory apparatus itself. The nerve impulses initiated in the ear by sound waves do actually reach the brain, but *they are not consciously heard.* Such deafness is technically called *psychogenic* dysacusis. The person suffering from it is sometimes said to be *functionally deaf.*

Psychogenic dysacusis must not be confused with *malingering.* The malingerer *knows* that he can hear, whereas the functionally deaf do *not know* that their hearing is still normal. The malingerer *pretends* that he is deaf in order to escape unpleasant duties, such as service in the armed forces, for example. The possibility of malingering must be considered, not only in the military situation but in medicolegal situations whenever the person being tested may gain financially if he has a sufficient impairment of hearing. It is not always easy to be sure how much hearing loss is real and permanent and how much is simulated or perhaps just added by always giving one's self the benefit of the doubt and making no effort to pick out rather faint signals. Specific tests for malingering are discussed in Chapter 8.

Laymen in general have been unaware of the existence of psychogenic dysacusis, or functional deafness, and the medical profession has tended to underestimate its importance, in spite of occasional obvious cases of "miraculous" cures at shrines, by faith healers, or for no evident or reasonable cause. The experience of World War II showed, however, that psychological factors may be among the common causes of deafness and hearing loss in military service. Of course, hearing loss is not necessarily *either* organic *or* psychogenic. Very often it is both, in uncertain proportions. The best estimate we can find is based on a careful study of the last five hundred cases admitted to the Hoff General Hospital (United States Army) at the end of World War II for auditory rehabilitation. Fifteen per cent of these men were found to have indications of a psychogenic factor in their hearing loss. For some of them the history of the hearing loss did not coincide with the usual clinical history or with the results of the otological examination. For others the audiogram varied widely from day to day, or the hearing loss for speech was much more or much less than the audiogram suggested it should be. Perhaps a hearing aid gave no improvement at all or else a startlingly great improvement. These 15 per cent, a total of seventy-five men, were treated by appropriate methods (which we shall not attempt to describe) for psychogenic dysacusis. The accuracy of the original estimate was substantiated by the fact that sixty out of the seventy-five, or "12 per cent of all patients admitted, had either a complete return of hearing to normal or a substantial improvement" at the time of separation from the Army.

This figure, high enough to make some otologists incredulous, does not mean that 12 to 15 per cent of the cases of hearing loss were *purely* psychogenic, but it does mean that psychological factors accounted for at least a significant part of the hearing loss in approximately one in eight men whose hearing became inadequate in military service. The special stresses of combat service obviously increased the proportion of cases of psychogenic dysacusis. Psychogenic hearing loss was a prominent factor in the army cases studied, and in all probability it is more prevalent and important in civilian life than has previously been suspected, but the importance and prevalence in civilian life of psychogenic deafness, as distinct from a mild psychogenic overlay, is still an open question.

Hysterical deafness.   The most common type of psychogenic deafness is called *hysterical deafness*. In this type, deep emotional conflicts within the personality structure involve the sense of hearing and manifest themselves in a total loss of hearing. Conflicts of which the individual is unconscious, rather than an impairment of the auditory mechanism, are the real cause. The disturbing emotional problem is converted into an impairment of hearing. Such substitution for the emotional problem is called *conversion,* and the resulting deafness is termed a *conversion hysteria.* Hysteria may involve senses other than hearing. A man may suffer from hysterical blindness or from anesthesia or paralysis of any part of the body without any physical impairment of the eye or nerves or muscles. But in any case of hysterical loss, the individual is unaware of the conflict which has found a substitute solution, or at least he does not understand its true nature.

It is impossible in this chapter to describe the different types of emotional disturbance which find their solution in hysterical symptoms. In every personality there are some emotional conflicts which do not present any problem in the ordinary course of living. In general, however, the more severe the emotional conflict, the less able is the individual to withstand strain of any kind. Actually, 38 per cent of the cases of "blast deafness" (acoustic trauma) admitted to Hoff General Hospital were diagnosed either as purely psychogenic or else as organic hearing loss with a large functional overlay. For example, a soldier exposed at close range to the burst of a large shell or a land mine escaped with his life, but was temporarily deafened by the noise. Later his ears recovered, but his unconscious emotional forces prevented his regained "hearing" from becoming conscious. What was probably a true physiological deafness at first was continued as a psychogenic dysacusis. Some men who regained most of their hearing spontaneously after a temporary blast deafness have reported that their recovery of hearing was quite sudden, or that for a time their hearing fluctuated with their mood or condition. They heard poorly when tired or nervously tense and better than usual when relaxed by a convivial dose of alcohol. These stories clearly suggest a *temporary* psychogenic dysacusis that passed off without recognition or special treatment.

A particular kind of emotional conflict may be the basis of hysterical deafness in time of war. Since hearing serves to create, through language, a structure for the moral code, and since war liberates the basic aggression in human nature, conflict is inevitable. From childhood on, we have been taught not to kill. War reverses that moral prohibition as well as many others. It is not surprising, there-fore, that the conflict present in accepting this reversal should, in some persons, result in the rejection of hearing. To liberate his basic aggres-sion, such a man must say, "I will not hear the voice of conscience." The hearing apparatus through which the moral code was formulated then becomes involved in a basic emotional conflict that is sometimes solved by a complete or partial rejection of the apparatus itself—with consequent deafness. This rejection is, of course, not conscious but takes place at the unconscious level. The soldier is utterly unaware that his deafness is *psychogenic* and was not caused by physical injury to his ears.

When a civilian becomes hysterically deaf (which apparently happens only rarely), we can infer that his inner conflict is correspond-ingly more severe, since the loss of hearing is precipitated by a milder stress. We must also infer that hearing has an unusual importance for such a person. There are, of course, great individual differences in the relative importance of the sense of hearing. In most of us one type of imagery plays a stronger part than do the others; vision, hearing, or the sense of motion may predominate in our relation to the world. When asked to recall the melody of a song, one person may *picture* the printed score, another may *hear* the melody, while a third may *feel the finger positions* required to play it.

In addition to these individual differences, however, auditory images generally affect most of us powerfully in the emotional field. This is particularly true in emotionalized memory. In terrifying situa-tions, it is often the sounds involved in the experience, rather than the sight of it, that convey the horror. If one has witnessed an accident in which a man was hurt, his cries may persist in memory long after the visual image of the experience has faded.

This tendency of auditory imagery to persist in memory is strengthened in the man whose perceptive interests and imaginative capacities are integrated around hearing. If the experience which he is trying to forget is charged with emotional material, as it always is in war, it is possible for repression to blot out hearing and to make him deaf.

As for the civilian who becomes hysterically deaf, previous ex-perience must contain incidents or situations that threaten him as deeply as combat does the soldier. An understanding of these incidents or situations can be gathered only through a careful case study of his development.

Therapy of psychogenic dysacusis. The prevention and the therapy for all other forms of dysacusis, deafness, and hearing loss will be found in the following chapter. It is appropriate, however, to consider the therapy of psychogenic dysacusis here because it illustrates very vividly the nature of the disorder. In fact, the diagnosis of psychogenic dysacusis usually rests almost entirely on the success, at least temporary, of some attempt at therapy.

The most effective treatment of hysterical deafness is based on the *positive suggestion* that the hearing loss is only temporary. To make the patient accept positive suggestion is difficult because in many of the hysterically deaf we see what Charcot, the great French psychiatrist, has called *la belle indifférence* to their conversion symptoms. Since they have achieved even a false resolution of their emotional conflict, they appear placid and quite undisturbed by the fact that they have given up their hearing. When they describe their deafness, they rarely emphasize their own feelings about the loss, but instead point out the objective or practical inconvenience of not being able to hear a car start, for example, or to hear directions. Even these practical difficulties are usually brushed aside by such a remark as, "But that is not important."

It is better to teach the patient how to *listen* than to teach him speechreading, for speechreading may only help to confirm the symptom of deafness and make it less accessible to treatment. By suggestive therapeutic methods the hysterically deaf may be encouraged to regain their hearing. But, unless some relief from the basic emotional conflict is achieved by the therapeutic process, the cause for the conflict remains, and the conversion symptom may merely shift over into another sensory field or take the form of a partial paralysis. A "cure" of psychogenic dyacusis may be only temporary, but this at least demonstrates that part or all of the deafness or hearing loss is functional. It does not mean that the cure is necessarily permanent or that the fundamental problem may not again appear in some other incapacitating symptom. If the hearing losses of the soldiers at Hoff General Hospital were purely the result of combat pressure, release from army service may have been sufficient to make their cure permanent. It is probable that a civilian who becomes functionally deaf from the pressures of living cannot be cured without psychiatric therapy deep enough to change the patient's personal concept of himself and his relationships with others.

Depression deafness. Hysterical deafness does not include all the cases of deafness or dysacusis that should be classified as psychogenic. Dr. D. A. Ramsdell (see Chapter 18) has differentiated a type, which he terms "depression deafness," in a schizophrenic personality structure. Personality tests, case histories, and the presence of recognized schizophrenic symptoms indicate that this type of dysacusis is not due to conversion, as has been previously supposed. (Schizophrenia is a type of mental disorder characterized by a progressive isolation of the individual from reality. Feeling unable to meet the practical demands of his environment, the patient escapes into an unreal world of phantasy.)

An intensive study of depression dysacusis reveals that there is a particular pattern in the case histories of such patients. The patients emphasize the subjective effects of their hearing loss and show definite hypochondriacal symptoms. They speak, not of the objective inconvenience of their impairment as does the hysteric, but of the change in their own feeling state. They are perplexed and frightened, and find the world about them incomprehensible and overwhelming. Failure of the sense of hearing to operate normally in such a patient is not due to conversion as a means of solving a basic conflict. The simulation of hearing loss or deafness acts as a protective defense against the precipitation of a schizophrenic episode. Hearing, more frequently than do the other senses, becomes involved in the schizophrenic's escape from reality.

It is a well-known fact that hearing may be accentuated in early schizophrenia to the point where the patient hears imaginary voices or has "auditory hallucinations." The reverse may also be true, and the patient may become deaf as part of the schizophrenic process. Such a patient is basically suicidal, but since he stops short of an actual biological death, the case may more properly be described as one of partial suicide. By giving up hearing, the patient succeeds in arriving at the state that one individual has described as "being buried alive." The patient restricts himself to a world that lacks the movement and flow so characteristic of the complete world of reality. He severs the auditory coupling, which is the chief link in maintaining an experience of aliveness and of identification with a moving world. In schizophrenic depression, the reward for the deafness, which corresponds to *la belle indifférence* in the hysteric, is the maintenance of only a visual orientation to the world around him.

In any case of psychogenic deafness or hearing loss, careful diagnosis should always be made before therapy is undertaken. Superficially the two types of psychogenic dysacusis appear much alike, but the treatment appropriate for depression deafness is quite different from that indicated in hysteria. For cases of depression deafness, therapy should be as painstaking and as careful as if one were dealing with threatened suicide because the wrong type of therapy may precipitate a psychotic episode.

It would be unwise to attempt here a detailed explanation of the therapy for either type of psychogenic dysacusis. If medical examination and tests of hearing indicate that the hearing loss is not due to impairment of the hearing apparatus, professional psychiatric aid should be obtained.

The variety of types of central dysacusis is illustrated by the experience of one particular clinic. Here 8 per cent of the children referred for communication disorders were eventually diagnosed by psychiatrists as autism or infantile schizophrenia, another 7 per cent had severe emotional disturbances, 14 per cent were mentally retarded, 15 per cent had auditory agnosia or verbal dysacusis, and 19 per cent had one or another type of central dysacusis as well as deafness or a hearing loss.

Suggested Readings

FOWLER, E. P., SR. *Twenty Years of Research in Otosclerosis, and Correlated Problems, 1926–1946.* New York: Central Bureau of Research, American Otological Society, 1946.

FOWLER, E. P., JR. *Nelson Loose-Leaf Medicine of the Ear.* New York: Thomas Nelson & Sons, Inc., 1939.
A textbook of medicine intended for physicians.

———, and M. BASEK. "Causes of Deafness in Young Children," *A.M.A. Archives of Otolaryngology,* 59: 476–484 (1954).

GOODHILL, V. "Pathology, Diagnosis and Therapy of Deafness," in *Handbook of Speech Pathology,* L. E. Travis, ed. New York: Appleton-Century-Crofts, Inc., 1957, Chap. 9.
A fairly detailed exposition of the medical and surgical aspects of deafness.

HOPKINS, L. A., and R. P. GUILDER. "Pedigree Data 1930–1940." Clarke School Studies: Concerning the Heredity of Deafness. Ann Arbor, Mich.: Edwards Brothers, Inc., 1949, Monograph I.

HOPKINS, L. A., and M. T. MACKLIN. "Studies on the Inheritance of Deafness in the Pupils of the Clarke School for the Deaf," *The Laryngoscope,* 56: 570–601 (1946).
One of the most thorough studies of the heredity of deafness in the medical literature.

JORDAN, R. C., moderator. "Deafness in Children–Knowledge and Practice," *Transactions of the American Academy of Ophthalmology and Otolaryngology,* 61: 706–727 (1957).
The subtitles are Evaulation of Hearing in Preschool Children; Problems of Testing and Managing Children with Communication Difficulties; Otosurgical Developments and the Hard of Hearing Child; and Nonmedical Care of Children with Hearing Impairment.

KNAPP, P. H. "Emotional Aspects of Hearing Loss," *Psychosomatic Medicine,* 10: 203–222 (1948).

MARTIN, N. A. "Psychogenic Deafness," *Annals of Otology, Rhinology, and Laryngology,* 55: 81–89 (1946).

PENFIELD, W., and T. RASMUSSEN. *The Cerebral Cortex of Man.* New York: The Macmillan Company, 1950.

PENFIELD, W., and L. ROBERTS. *Speech and Brain-Mechanisms.* Princeton, N.J.: Princeton University Press, 1959.

SENTURIA, B. H. *Diseases of the External Ear.* Springfield, Ill.: Charles C Thomas, 1957.

VAN EGMOND, A. A. J. "Congenital Deafness," *Journal of Laryngology and Otology,* 68: 429–443 (1954).
An excellent survey lecture.

5

THE MEDICAL TREATMENT OF HEARING LOSS AND THE CONSERVATION OF HEARING

Hallowell Davis, M.D., and
Edmund Prince Fowler, Jr., M.D.

This chapter might have been entitled, as it was in the first edition, "Medical Aspects of Hearing Loss." The abnormalities of structure and function and the types and the causes of deafness and hearing loss have, however, already been described separately in Chapter 4, and the remaining "medical aspects" are essentially (1) the medical treatment of some few conditions that are amenable to it, (2) the hygiene of the ear, (3) the various types of prostheses, particularly those that are placed in the middle ear, and (4) conservation of hearing. Actually, medical treatment has rather little to offer to restore lost hearing, but preventive medicine can and does contribute greatly to the conservation of hearing.

In the present chapter we shall first review the possibilities and principles of medical treatment of the conditions described in Chapter 4. We shall then see how these possibilities, coupled with appropriate systematic audiometry, provide conservation of hearing.

Medical Treatment of Hearing Loss

EXTERNAL EAR

The blockage of the external ear canal by impacted wax is rather frequent, particularly in later adult life. When blockage occurs there is little the patient himself can do except visit a doctor, who will remove the impacted wax without injury to the canal or the drumhead. Normally the wax works its way out unnoticed bit by bit; but there are

125

some people whose wax simply does not come out of the canal in this way and every six months or every year they should have the wax removed by a doctor before it "macerates" or otherwise injures the skin of the canal. Hydrogen peroxide is sometimes used to soften the wax, which may then be washed out by irrigation with warm water. If this is done the canal should be thoroughly dried afterward. Actually, if the ears are kept clean, the average person does not develop impacted wax. The constant insertion of the earmold of a hearing aid or of matchsticks or hairpins often pushes the wax so deep into the canal that it must be removed by a doctor. Impacted wax sometimes makes, by reflex, an annoying dry cough. Persons fearing tuberculosis have even had X rays taken when their only trouble was impacted wax.

EXTERNAL OTITIS

The skin of the external canal is in some areas very closely attached to the underlying cartilage and bone, so that any infection of it is very painful. It is unwise, as a rule, to open a limited external otitis with a knife, as is often done with similar abscesses elsewhere in the body, to let out the pus. Incision, and other types of manipulation as well, will often spread the infection and produce a diffuse external otitis.

The physician can now treat external otitis quite effectively with the newer drugs, such as sulfonamides or neomycin with hydrocortisone. The old-fashioned eardrops of alcohol and boric acid are sometimes effective, but often painful. For the patient, the important thing is to keep water out of the canal. Water softens the skin and spreads the infection more widely. If the canal has been wetted, either from essential washing away of dead skin or wax, or inadvertently, from ill-advised use of any watery medication, such as hydrogen peroxide, the canal should be dried out out with 95 per cent ethyl alcohol. The alcohol will sting for a few minutes, but the ultimate benefits justify the temporary discomfort.

Another variety of external otitis (the "eczematoid" type) is a chronic scaling of the skin that is very difficult to treat successfully. Fortunately, this type rarely causes deafness, unless the canal is neglected and allowed to fill with wax and the cast-off scales of skin.

AERO-OTITIS MEDIA

Aero-otitis media depends entirely on failure to ventilate the middle ear through the Eustachian tube while descending from a high to a low altitude. *The best way to avoid aero-otitis is not to fly while suffering with a cold.* Colds inflame the tissue at the mouth of the Eustachian tube and prevent its proper function. Continual swallowing on descent will, with partially blocked tubes, help to equalize the pressure. This is helped by chewing gum which produces enough saliva to allow for sufficient swallowing to open the tubes and equalize the pressure while making a normal descent. Airline pilots are instructed to descend or to depressurize a cabin at a rate of not more than 300 feet a minute. Occasional swallowing during such a slow descent will suffice for most people. Passengers in sleeper planes should be awakened during descent, and children and others who constantly have trouble with their Eustachian tubes during flight should be given water to drink.

Professional aviators and commercial travelers who must do a great deal of flying and who have recurrent aero-otitis should have their Eustachian tubes treated medically if they wish to continue flying without developing some permanent loss of hearing. In a similar category are submarine crews, deep-sea divers, skin divers, and caisson workers. If the tubes do not open with swallowing, yawning, or moving the jaws about, an attempt should be made to open the Eustachian tube by strong blowing of the nose. If this does not work, a doctor may employ a drug like ephedrine to shrink the mucous lining of the nose temporarily, or he may have to inflate the tube with various blowing or swallowing maneuvers (Valsalva or Politzer), or with a catheter passed through the nose (Figure 5-1). In rare instances of severe aero-otitis, incision of the drum may be necessary to remove the fluid.

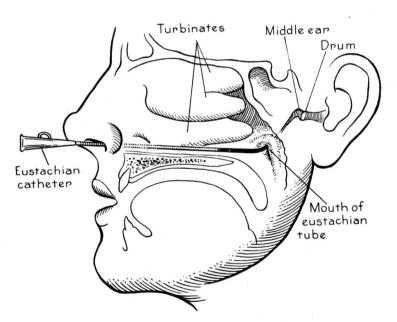

Fig. 5-1. A catheter can be introduced through the nostril and inserted into the opening of the Eustachian tube.

ACUTE AND CHRONIC OTITIS MEDIA

Chronic otitis media, particularly if it is recurrent or frequently reactivated, forms adhesions that impede the transmission of sound and may destroy the eardrum membrane, the ossicles, and other structures. It is a common and important cause of hearing loss. Of course, the first concern of an otologist confronted with a case of otitis media is with the general health and safety of the patient. If some loss of hearing must be risked or even deliberately produced by removal of the ossicles together with the pus and diseased tissue in order to be sure to check the infection, the otologist does not hesitate to do so (see Chapter 6). Where possible, of course, he spares the hearing, but his first concerns are life and health. Treatment of otitis media by drugs may help restore or save hearing, but unless the infection is very mild, it is best to provide drainage for it. Drainage is nature's most effective way of getting rid of infection and the products of infection. The surgeon easily provides drainage by incising the lower back portion of the drum, where the incision has been found to cause no loss of hearing. If the drum is not opened, it will usually rupture spontaneously sooner or later. It has been found that more hearing loss and more mastoiditis requiring surgical attention occur after spontaneous rupture of the drum than after surgical incision.

The bacteria that usually cause acute infection of the middle ear can be killed by sulfa drugs or by various antibiotics, notably penicillin. There are physicians who treat all otitis media with these drugs without surgery. This, however, is not good practice, because subacute, or chronic, otitis media is likely to recur in certain cases if drainage is not provided in addition to drug therapy. *Acute otitis media should not be treated by patients themselves or by druggists.* The tendency is to stop the drug as soon as the pain or the discharge subsides, and this is too soon. On the other hand, prolonged use of the drugs without medical supervision is dangerous. Inadequate dosage only extends the disease and makes the bacteria less susceptible to the drug being used. It is the recurrent, subacute, or chronic types of otitis media that cause hearing loss, and it is in these conditions, as a rule, that complications develop.

Prostheses. Occasionally the hearing in an ear with a perforated drumhead from chronic otitis media can be helped by closing the perforation with an artificial substance. This can be a piece of cellophane, cigarette paper, a plastic tube (Pohlman prosthesis), a piece of cotton wool soaked in mineral oil, or a bland ointment. The latter is preferable if infection is still present because it can be medicated. Success with such prostheses indicates that tympanoplasty may be successful (see Chapter 6). Some patients prefer to continue to use the prosthetic substances for years; indeed, this is sometimes safer than surgery.

Prevention of otitis media by surgery and radiation. Also aimed at the prevention of recurrent and chronic otitis media are the *surgical removal of the adenoids* that block the Eustachian tubes and the *treatment of nasal infection.* Blockage of a tube and nasal infection both predispose to infection of the Eustachian tube and therefore to otitis media.

If surgical removal of the adenoids does not enable the Eustachian tubes to open readily (and it often does not), the remaining adenoid tissue about the mouth of the tubes may be treated with *radium* or *X ray.* The lymphoid tissue that makes up the adenoid is extremely sensitive to radiation, and a very small dosage will often shrink the offending tissue, restore proper function of the tubes, and so prevent further otitis media and the development of hearing loss. Radiation is especially useful to submarine personnel and to aviators who must have perfectly functioning Eustachian tubes. Of course, radiation should not be used for neural deafness, otosclerosis, or other diseases where blockage of the tube is not a factor in the causation of the disease.

Blowing out the ear. *Inflation,* whether performed by an instrument fitted to the nostril or by a silver catheter passed through the nose to the pharyngeal orifice of the tube, will improve the hearing, temporarily at least, if there is a plug of mucus blocking the tube. Often inflation is the only effective relief for temporary middle-ear hearing loss, but the method can be abused and is useless in cases of otosclerosis or of neural hearing loss. An old theory has been proved false: that wiggling the ossicles back and forth by blowing air up the Eustachian tubes will loosen them and improve the hearing. Inflation through a catheter is now reserved for diagnostic purposes and for patients who have a temporary blocking of the tubes by excessively thick secretions. Many people can clear their own tubes by yawning or blowing the nose. The self-inflation maneuver of Valsalva is familiar, i.e., blowing while holding the nose. If this does not work, the Politzer maneuver may succeed. The otologist places the olive-shaped tip of an air-filled "Politzer bag" in the patient's nostril and squeezes the bag as the patient swallows. Too much strong inflation may produce a loose, floppy drumhead, however, and there is always the danger, too, of forcing infected material up the tube from the back of the nose.

TREATMENT OF SENSORY-NEURAL HEARING LOSS

Physicians are on sure ground in objecting to the theories of those who say that manipulation, injections, or stimulation by sound can improve a hearing loss that has been clearly established as neural. If sensory cells or nerve fibers have once degenerated, they *cannot* be restored. Of course, the conductive component of a mixed hearing loss might be improved by surgery, but not the neural component. Whatever effects may have been obtained in particular cases either must have resulted from the training that the patients received that enabled them better to understand speech with whatever residual hearing they may have had, or must have been pure self-delusion. Of course, nearly all deafened patients want to believe that their hearing is being improved by whatever is being done for them, and the therapist wants to believe that he is helping the patient. The powerful suggestion acting on both of them too often gives rise to a false belief that the new form of therapy, whatever it may be, has actually improved the hearing. Moreover, "nerve stimulants" cannot restore the missing fibers or cause degenerated sensory cells to resume their function. Nevertheless, patients are continually being dosed with vitamins, antihistamines, and many other types of medication, with the expectation that the function of their long-defunct auditory nerves will be improved. The suggestion that hearing may be restored by stimulation by sound is, of course, utterly fantastic. The only possible beneficial effects of drugs are the arrest of the disease process and perhaps, in some cases, the relief of tinnitus.

Incidentally, the cessation of a severe tinnitus not only eliminates a very distressing symptom but may improve the hearing to a certain extent by removing an interfering masking noise. The improvement, however, is never more than ten or fifteen decibels. Unfortunately, the relief of tinnitus by any direct treatment is so rare that one wonders whether the disappearance is not always spontaneous when it does occur. Tinnitus, it must be remembered, is a subjective symptom and as such is susceptible to suggestion. Many a patient has been taught by a sympathetic and understanding physician to minimize his head noises.

MÉNIÈRE'S DISEASE AND
SUDDEN HEARING LOSSES OF VASCULAR ORIGIN

There are two types of sensory-neural hearing loss which are sometimes amenable to medical treatment: Ménière's disease, i.e., the sudden attacks of vertigo, deafness, and tinnitus described in Chapter 4; and certain sudden, severe hearing losses, with or without vertigo, which are presumably of vascular origin. Both conditions often have a strong psychogenic component in that they seem to occur most often in highly energetic, driving perfectionists when life stresses become excessive. Often the symptoms occur after a distressing, frustrating, emotionally disturbing event rather than during it. Also, the ear symptoms frequently occur in patients who have developed other recognized psychosomatic diseases, such as high blood pressure or gastric ulcer.

Essentially, the treatments for Ménière's disease and sudden vascular hearing losses are very similar, from the medical standpoint, to those used for other vascular diseases elsewhere in the body. If the disease is entirely in the ear, the otologist is likely to prescribe some vasodilator drug, such as nicotinic acid or injections of histamine. In the sudden catastrophic types of severe hearing loss, often designated as "sudden deafness," he may, in addition, prescribe anticoagulation drugs, such as those used for apoplexy, for venous thromboses, or for heart attacks. This treatment should be carried out in a hospital under the supervision of a man skilled in the use of anticoagulants. Some physicians also recommend procaine, given intravenously, again in a hospital under rigid supervision. The procaine increases the blood flow through the small blood vessels but it increases the work that the heart must do, and the heart must be in good condition to take on this added load. These various treatments must be started at once to be effective, and unless they are accompanied by careful study of the patient's stress situations and the possibility of alleviating them, the hearing losses are likely to recur; each time they do recur they are more likely to remain permanent.

Apart from prompt treatment directed toward the vascular system and proper attention to the patient's emotional stresses, there is no really satisfactory medical treatment for Ménière's disease. Many drugs, special diets, and several bizarre forms of treatment have been tried and encouraging results have been reported with some of them. The drug or regimen chosen depends on the theory of the cause of the disease that is favored by the physician, or it may be on a purely empirical basis. Nicotinic acid, to cause dilation of the small blood vessels, is a favorite drug; methantheline and propantheline are also popular. A full list would include atropine, histamine, Diamox, a salt-free diet, and many others.

In some patients some of these drugs have had clear favorable effects. The symptoms have improved while the drug was being taken regularly, but became worse when the dosage was reduced or stopped. Other patients have shown little or no consistent benefit. It is very difficult, however, to establish a firm case for any drug or any theory: one of the major characteristics of Ménière's disease is the fluctuation of symptoms—the spontaneous remissions and the return of "attacks" without obvious cause. The only sure relief from the symptoms of Ménière's disease is the surgical destruction of the labyrinth described in Chapter 6. The advantages of medical treatment are that it does no harm, it gives opportunity for spontaneous improvement, and it is of benefit in many cases.

PREVENTION OF NEURAL HEARING LOSS AND DYSACUSIS

As mentioned in Chapter 4, several drugs are specifically toxic for the inner ear. The most important of these are kanamycin, neomycin, and, especially, dihydrostreptomycin. These should be avoided unless essential for preservation of life. Certainly, they should never be used prophylactically. Large doses of other less toxic drugs, such as straight streptomycin, aspirin and other salicylates, and quinine and quinidine should be used with caution. Some individuals, especially those with poor kidney function, are very susceptible to these drugs. The onset of tinnitus or of slight vertigo will often herald the occurrence of an ototoxic reaction to them.

Some of the severe congenital hearing losses of childhood can be prevented by improved methods of resuscitation at birth and the more careful anesthetizing and medication of mothers in labor. Substitution transfusions in babies with Rh and AO incompatible blood may save some, but many of these measures, especially the saving of tiny, premature babies, probably increase the number of children in the population who survive with communication disorders.

Conservation of Hearing

The movement for conservation of hearing really began with the preventive measures and screening audiometry in schools more than thirty years ago. The part played by the American Hearing Society is mentioned in Chapter 20. The development of the group screening audiometer by the Bell Telephone Laboratories (the Western Electric 4C audiometer) was an epochal event for conservation of hearing, not only in children but, as we shall see, in adults also.

Another organization that has continued actively to promote conservation of hearing, particularly from the point of view of preventive medicine, has been the Committee on Conservation of Hearing of the American Academy of Ophthalmology and Otolaryngology. This committee, composed of leading otologists who are interested in problems of hearing and a few nonmedical consultants, encouraged the establishment of conservation of hearing programs, particularly in schools. Later, through its Subcommittee on Noise in Industry (now known simply as the Subcommittee on Noise), it extended its efforts to this wider field. Still more recently it has established additional subcommittees on hearing in children, hearing in adults, audiometers, research in otolaryngology, and the like.

The problems and programs of conservation of hearing divide naturally into the three age groups: children, adults, and elderly people. Surgical treatment of hearing loss is described in the following chapter, and the methods and programs of special education and training and of auditory rehabilitation are covered in later chapters.

CHILDREN

The basic threat to the hearing of children is from infection in the middle ear; that is, from unrecognized or untreated chronic otitis media or from recurrent attacks of acute otitis media. Therefore, the program for conservation of hearing in children is primarily a program for (1) the detection of chronic otitis media, "glue ears," and the like; (2) the detection and treatment of conditions leading to blocked Eustachian tubes and to frequent head colds; and (3) the provision of adequate and effective medical and surgical treatment for the children found to have these conditions.

Adequate numbers of otologists, pediatricians, and general practitioners, as well as enough hospitals and other facilities, are now available in most communities to care for these children. An important part of the job, however, is to inform and persuade parents of the importance of doing something about the conditions when they are found. We will leave aside the problems of medical economics: the "who pays" and the how and when. The part of the job in which we are interested in this chapter is the detection of the cases that need attention.

Screening audiometry. It is often not easy to identify an ear with chronic otitis media unless the ear is actually discharging pus. Even a fully trained otologist looking at the eardrum membrane with his otoscope may see nothing clearly abnormal. The only effective means of picking out the children who may need attention is to test their hearing. Tests of hearing, including pure-tone audiometry, are described in Chapter 7, but it is obvious immediately that it would be both time consuming and wasteful to test every ear at all frequencies when most ears are perfectly normal. The answer is "screening audiometry." All of the children in a school are tested briefly and quickly to identify or screen out, as by a sieve, those who may possibly have something wrong. Those who are thus screened out are then given a full, careful audiometric test and otologic examination. Of course, a good many of them turn out on the full test to be normal or very nearly so. The screening test is planned to screen out the borderline cases so as not to let any really abnormal cases go undetected.

Two general forms of screening audiometry were developed specifically for use in schools. One is *group speech audiometry,* developed by the Bell Telephone Laboratories. It screens a whole roomful of children at once. The youngsters write down on prepared blanks the numbers that they hear spoken at successively lower and lower levels. These test words are played from a phonographic disc. The other form is "sweep-frequency audiometry," carried out individually with a pure-tone air conduction audiometer. The very high and the very low frequencies may be omitted and only one intensity or "screening level" is used. If these few test tones are heard, the child's hearing is within normal limits.

There is no great difference in the over-all time per child between the two methods. Individual screening is likely to be further shortened by the omission of some of the test frequencies, but it is not yet clear just which frequencies must be retained.

The important point here is not the technique of screening or the criteria employed but *the concept of screening audiometry as part of an annual physical checkup.* This is the approach made by preventive medicine.

We note in passing that the emphasis that was placed for many years on hearing for the very high frequencies—8192, 11,584, and 16,000 cps—has now evaporated. It was originally thought that these very high tones were particularly sensitive indicators of middle-ear disease or of beginning neural hearing loss. It now appears that, for purely physical and anatomical reasons, audiometry above 6000 cps is unreliable. No individual will give the same answers when tested on successive days. For one thing, small differences in the application of the earphone can cause large differences in standing wave patterns in the ear canal. Nor is the test valid. Even if high threshold levels for very high frequencies are confirmed on repeated tests, they do not now appear, as the result of a recent careful, long-term follow-up study, to give real and useful warning signs. For screening audiometry, 6000 cps is high enough.

ADULTS

Otitis media continues to be a threat to hearing throughout life, but adults are more aware of trouble with their ears and their hearing and are in a position to do something about it. Not so many adult ears suffer from sheer neglect. It is much easier to drain an effusion from the ear of an adult than from the ear of a child because the adult does not require a general anesthetic. Otosclerosis strikes the ears of young adults, but there are no preventive measures against this disease. The problems of otosclerosis are the problems of surgery or of a hearing aid. The particular subtle danger to the hearing of adults against which precautions can be taken is noise.

Hazardous noise-exposure. Noise hazards for hearing have for many years been associated with certain industries, notably boiler-making and weaving. The growth of heavy industry has increased the noise levels and also the number of workers exposed to them. The aircraft industry, particularly since the development of jet engines, has added new problems. Moreover, quite recently it has become clear that gunfire, including skeet shooting as well as artillery, machine guns, and small arms, and even the tractor on the farm are significant hazards to hearing. But noise-induced hearing loss develops slowly. Noises that are not painful or even really uncomfortable after the first week or two may gradually impair hearing.

For many years a sort of tacit conspiracy of silence kept the problem of noise-induced hearing loss from public view. Workers in very noisy places were pleased with their relatively high wages, and industry feared litigation, insurance problems, and compensation payments. (The problem of handicap and compensation is discussed in Chapter 9.) "Noise control" has now become practical and popular, thanks to technical advances in acoustical engineering, to community concern about aircraft noise, and to a variety of military problems, including communication in noise. Court decisions in the states of New York and Wisconsin have recognized noise-induced hearing loss as compensable under workmen's compensation laws. Industry now cooperates with the Research Center of the Subcommittee on Noise of the American Academy of Ophthalmology and Otolaryngology to gather more information so that we will be able eventually to state clearly just what is a hazardous noise-exposure.

Now that it is common knowledge that hazardous noise-exposures actually do exist, a major objective in the conservation of hearing of adults is to do something about the hazard, both in industry and in military situations. There are several approaches to the problem: to reduce the noise, either at the source or in the transmission; to remove all personnel from noise areas; to use protective devices such as ear-plugs or ear muffs; to identify noise-susceptible persons and remove them from noisy situations; and to institute "monitoring audiometry" to identify the persons who are actually beginning to develop a noise-induced hearing loss before they develop enough permanent threshold shift to constitute any practical handicap.

Monitoring audiometry was first formally defined and named in a symposium of the Armed Forces–National Research Council Committee on Hearing and Bio-Acoustics on "Problems in Military Audiometry." The concept is very much the same as that of screening audiometry for children. We watch or "monitor" the hearing of all those who have a hazard of noise-exposure and find which ones require special attention. That attention may be ear muffs or it may be removal from the noise. Monitoring audiometry is regarded as part of a routine periodic health examination or physical checkup. The audiometry required is more elaborate than that for screening school children but less elaborate than what the otologist requires for diagnostic purposes.

"A GUIDE FOR CONSERVATION OF HEARING IN NOISE"

For the benefit of industry, in 1957 the Subcommittee on Noise (in Industry) revised its "Guide for Conservation of Hearing in Noise." This authoritative, carefully considered, and carefully worded statement reviews the fundamentals of hearing loss and noise-exposure and then outlines a hearing conservation program. We cannot do better than to reproduce its section on general information in full.

BASIC INFORMATION ABOUT HEARING LOSS AND NOISE-EXPOSURE

Although there is still much to be learned about the relations of hearing loss to noise-exposure, we have accumulated enough information through experience and research to enable us to organize and conduct hearing conservation programs. This basic information is, in brief:

1. **Many noise-exposures can produce a permanent hearing loss that may affect communication by speech.**

2. Noise-induced hearing loss may be transient, permanent, or a combination of transient and permanent.

3. Permanent noise-induced hearing loss is due to destruction of certain inner ear structures which cannot be replaced.

4. The amount of hearing loss produced by a given noise-exposure varies from person to person.

5. **Noise-induced hearing loss first affects man's hearing of sounds higher in frequency than those necessary for communication by speech. Therefore most early noise-induced hearing losses pass unnoticed unless they are detected by suitable hearing tests.**

6. **Four major factors characterize noise-exposure:**
   (a) **overall noise level**
   (b) **composition of the noise**
   (c) **duration and distribution of exposure during a typical workday**
   (d) **total time of exposure during a work-life.**

7. Man's hearing ability and noise-exposure can be measured reliably by competent, properly qualified personnel. (The measurement and evaluation of impact noises, which are produced by drop hammers, riveting guns, etc., present special problems.)

8. **To be effective a hearing conservation program should include:**
   (a) **a noise-exposure analysis**
   (b) **provision for control of noise-exposure**
   (c) **measurements of hearing.**

INDICATIONS OF THE NEED FOR A HEARING CONSERVATION PROGRAM

The initiation of a hearing conservation program should be considered whenever persons have

1. **Difficulty communicating by speech while they are in the noise, or**
2. **Head noises or ringing in their ears after working in the noise for several hours, or**
3. **A loss of hearing that has the effect of muffling speech and certain other sounds after several hours of exposure to the noise. (This hearing loss is transient and usually disappears in a few hours.)**

• • •

Absence of pain should not be construed to mean absence of hearing loss. Pain is produced in the ear when noise levels are of the order of 130 db: noise-induced hearing loss, however, may be produced at considerably lower noise levels. Pain and annoyance are not reliable indicators of a potential noise-induced hearing loss. The decision to initiate a hearing conservation program should not be influenced by the presence or absence of these symptoms.

Ultimately, the analysis of noise-exposure is the only completely satisfactory way of establishing the need for hearing conservation.

OUTLINE OF A HEARING CONSERVATION PROGRAM

A hearing conservation program consists of three parts.

1. Analysis of Noise-Exposure

Noise-exposures are analyzed in terms of:
   (a) overall level
   (b) composition of the noise

(c) duration and distribution of exposure during a typical work-day
(d) total exposure time during a work-life.

Measurement of *each* of these four factors of noise-exposure is important for hearing conservation. Even though two different noises have the same overall level, their compositions may differ considerably (to such an extent, in fact, that one may produce a permanent hearing loss while the other may not). Also, the auditory effects of continuous noise-exposure are different from the effects of intermittent exposure to the same noise.

2. *Control of Noise-Exposure*

Noise-exposure may be reduced by:
  (a) Environmental control
    (1) reducing the amount of noise produced by the source
    (2) reducing the amount of noise transmitted through air or building structures
    (3) revising operational procedures
  (b) personal protection

The most satisfactory method of environmental control of noise-exposure is to control the noise at the source. Unfortunately, this is not always possible. When the amount of noise produced by the source can not be sufficiently reduced a combination of control methods may be required to conserve hearing.

3. *Measurement of Hearing*

A hearing conservation program should include
  (a) preplacement hearing tests, and
  (b) routine periodic follow-up tests.

These tests of hearing are the most important part of a hearing conservation program. They provide a record of the initial status of an employee's hearing and make it possible to follow any subsequent changes in hearing ability. Preplacement and follow-up tests help to identify persons who may be highly susceptible to noise-induced hearing loss. Test results will show whether the conservation program is effective or not.

Even when noise-exposures are not severe enough to warrant a hearing conservation program, it is desirable to test hearing systematically as part of routine physical examinations.

RESPONSIBILITY FOR CONSERVATION OF HEARING

Medical Responsibility

The conservation of any human function is primarily a medical responsibility. Hearing conservation is no exception. Prevention, diagnosis and treatment of hearing loss; validation and approval of audiometric records; and the final assessment of measurements of hearing are medical responsibilities. **Any hearing conservation program without medical supervision must be considered inadequate.**

Direct medical supervision of a hearing conservation program is highly desirable. Here a physician is responsible for the organization and administration of the testing program as well as for checking and evaluating audiometric records. The physician himself does not perform all the operations necessary to the conduct of the program: he delegates responsibility for many of the technical activities to members of his staff, setting up standards or limits within which they can operate semiautonomously. Whenever medical records show that control of noise-exposures may be inadequate, the physician in charge so reports. The responsibility for making necessary noise measurements and for effecting further environmental noise-exposure controls then devolves on the industrial hygienist, members of the engineering or safety departments or other persons assigned to the task. Although the actual operations of measurement and protection are performed by both medical and non-medical personnel, the physician ultimately is responsible for the health of the employee.

Medical supervision must be available if a hearing conservation program is to serve its dual purpose of preventing hearing loss and providing valid records for compensation claims. Many companies do not have a full time medical department and cannot provide direct medical supervision for a conservation program. These companies can, however, satisfy the general requirement of medical supervision by employing medical consultants.

General Co-operation

The success of hearing conservation depends on the complete co-operation of employer and employee alike. All groups stand to benefit equally from a hearing conservation program, and all groups should give the program their active support. Supervisory personnel should initiate noise measurements, make the environmental changes that are necessary for noise-exposure control, furnish any required ear protection and make it readily available to all employees, acquaint all employees with the benefits to be derived from hearing conservation, and, by example, promote attitudes that will benefit the program. Each employee should make proper use of the personal protection that is provided, obey environmental regulations, and participate willingly in the hearing testing program.

In the Guide there follows a section on technical information. Much of this material has been covered in Chapters 2, 3, and 4 of this book, but the following statements on Hearing Conservation and Noise-Exposure are new.

3. Hearing Conservation and Noise-exposure

Two things must be considered before we can set a limit beyond which noise-exposures are judged to be severe enough to warrant an organized program of hearing conservation. First, can a realistic hearing conservation program provide complete protection for all ears; and second, what do we know about the effectiveness of the different components of noise-exposure in producing hearing loss.

(a) Limitations of a Practical Hearing Conservation Program

The aim of hearing conservation is to prevent loss of hearing for all persons exposed to noise, but unfortunately complete protection cannot always be realized. Sometimes practical programs can achieve only a limited goal. For example:

(1) Prevention of hearing loss at all audible frequencies may not prove possible. Particular efforts should then be made to protect hearing at the frequencies most important to communication by speech (500, 1000, and 2000 cps).

(2) Prevention of hearing loss in every person who is exposed to noise may not be possible. Some few ears are highly susceptible to noise-induced hearing loss. As yet, there is no predictive test that will enable us to identify persons with highly susceptible ears. No practical general rule of protection is equally effective for all persons exposed to noise: the protective measures that prevent loss of hearing in normally-susceptible ears are not effective for highly susceptible ears.

(b) Noise-Exposure and Hearing Loss

Noise-induced hearing loss depends upon noise levels and exposure time. Any attempt to assess the need for hearing conservation must take account of both.

The effects of continuous exposure to steady noise may depend on the way the sound energy is distributed in the noise. Early noise-induced hearing losses are usually confined to the frequencies around

4000 cycles per second. As the exposure lengthens the losses spread to lower frequencies, whose audibility is more directly involved in the understanding of speech. Data on noise-induced hearing loss, both temporary and permanent, indicate that the losses occur at frequencies above those that characterize the exposure sounds. Since the most important frequencies to be protected are in the range 500 to 2000 cps inclusive, it follows that the 300-600 and 600-1200 cps bands deserve our major attention if we are trying to protect man's hearing for speech.

At the present time our knowledge of the relations of noise-exposure to hearing loss is much too limited for us to propose "safe" amounts of noise-exposure. We can however, point to certain noise levels that indicate when it is advisable to initiate hearing conservation programs. These levels will not be general because a different level is needed for different types of noise and different schedules of exposure. The hearing conservation level that we now specify tentatively applies only to years of exposure to broad-band steady noises with relatively flat spectra. **It does not apply to short exposures, and above all, it does not apply to impact noises or narrow band noises.** This tentative hearing conservation level is stated as follows:

> **If the sound energy of the noise is distributed more or less evenly throughout the eight octave bands, and if a person is to be exposed to this noise regularly for many hours a day, five days a week for many years, then: if the noise level in either the 300-600 cycle band or the 600-1200 cycle band is 85 db, the initiation of noise-exposure control and tests of hearing is advisable. The more the octave band levels exceed 85 db the more urgent is the need for hearing conservation.**

The 85 db is *not an overall* sound pressure level: it refers to two particular *octave bands*. The overall level of noise is always higher than the level in any one octave band; in typical industrial steady noises it may be as much as 20 db higher.

Overall and octave band levels measured in three typical industrial noises are reported in Table I. For all three of these noises the overall level exceeds the level in the 300-600 or the 600-1200 octave bands by at least 10 db and for one noise by 16 db.

The section of the Guide on ear protectors is also worth quoting:

2. *Use of Personal Protection*

Ear protectors in effect reduce noise levels at the inner ear. Ear protection is particularly important when noise-exposures cannot be controlled adequately by environmental changes.

(a) Types of Ear Protector

Ear protectors may be
(1) Ear plugs, or
(2) Ear muffs

Ear plugs are designed to occlude the ear canal. They may be made of rubber, neoprene, plastic, or cotton impregnated with wax. Contrary to popular opinion, dry cotton affords **no** protection. Material and shape have little to do with the effectiveness of commercially available plugs except as they affect acceptance by users.

Ear muffs are designed to cover the external ear. At frequencies above 1000 cps muffs provide about the same protection as plugs. At frequencies below 1000 cps only certain recently designed muffs provide as much protection as plugs. (See Table II for some typical attenuation figures.)

Whether to wear plugs or muffs or both depends in part on the work situation. Will the employee's head be confined to a work space so small there is no room for muffs? Must he wear a hard hat in addition to ear protection? And so forth. There are advantages and disadvantages to the use of either plugs or muffs, and before a choice is made between the two, all the circumstances of a particular job should be considered.

(b) Fitting and Indoctrination

An employee's ears should be examined and his hearing tested at the time he is fitted with ear protectors. Plugs should be fitted individually for each ear: if the ear canals are not the same size or shape they may require plugs of different size. To promote the acceptance of ear plugs an employee should be allowed to choose from three or four different makes at the time he is fitted.

As with other kinds of personal protection (hard hats, safety glasses, safety shoes or respirators) it may be difficult to convince employees that they should wear ear protectors. Successful personal protection programs are based on thorough indoctrination of personnel. An employee *must* be impressed with the importance of ear protection and the benefits to be gained from its consistent use. He should be told

(1) Good protection depends on a good seal between the surface of the skin and the surface of the ear protector. A very small leak can destroy the effectiveness of the protection. Protectors have a tendency to work loose as a result of talking, chewing, etc., and they must be reseated from time to time during the work day.

(2) A good seal cannot be obtained without some initial discomfort.

(3) There will be no untoward reactions as a result of the use of ear protectors if they are kept reasonably clean. (Skin irritations, injured ear drums, or other harmful reactions are exceedingly rare. A properly designed, well fitted and clean ear protector will cause no more difficulty than a pair of safety goggles).

(4) The use of ear protection will not make it more difficult to understand speech or to hear warning signals.

Most of the available ear protectors, when correctly fitted, provide about the same amount of protection. The best ear protector, therefore, is the one that is worn properly. Properly fitted protectors can be worn continuously by most persons and will provide adequate protection against most industrial noise-exposures.

Ear plugs do not provide the same amount of attenuation in the field as in the laboratory, probably because of incorrect fitting and failure to maintain a good seal even with properly fitted plugs. Limited research data indicate that in the field ear plugs provide on the average about 5 db less attenuation than in laboratory tests.

A list of the manufacturers of ear protectors is available on request.[1]

CONSERVATION OF HEARING IN ELDERLY PEOPLE

For elderly people the problem of hazardous noise-exposure becomes less and less important and the maintenance of reasonable hygiene of the ear becomes more and more routine. There are fewer and fewer risks, as people grow older, from dirt and water or even from the common cold. The characteristic hearing loss of old age (presbycusis) is neural, but we have no idea about how to protect against it. Neither can we protect against cerebral arteriosclerosis and the other conditions that we lump together as "senile changes." They are the province of the new branch of medicine known as *geriatrics*.

Something can be done, however, to *protect communication by speech*. As hearing begins to deteriorate in elderly persons they can begin to use hearing aids. They can also take lessons in speechreading, and if their hearing losses become severe they can even learn how to keep their own voices pleasant and intelligible. These suggestions

[1] These extracts from the "Guide for Conservation of Hearing in Noise" are reprinted by permission of the Subcommittee on Noise of the Committee on Conservation of Hearing, American Academy of Ophthalmology and Otolaryngology.

sound very simple and obvious, but the people who could benefit from them find them difficult to carry out, even if they can be persuaded to try. The problem is to *start soon enough* while the elderly man or woman is still adaptable, able to learn, and willing to make the necessary effort. As will be explained in other chapters, the person who becomes hard of hearing, particularly the elderly person, often does not recognize or admit his incapacity. He may blame others for not speaking up or for mumbling their words. By the time his hearing loss has become an obvious handicap it may be too late to "teach the old dog new tricks" and to alter his habits of a lifetime. To overcome such individual inertia and to create a healthy, constructive social point of view toward these and other problems of aging are the objectives of conservation of speech communication in elderly people.

Suggested Readings

American Standards Association. "The Relations of Hearing Loss to Noise Exposure." Report of Exploratory Subcommittee Z-24-X-2. American Standards Association, Inc., 70 East 45th Street, New York 17.

COX, J. R., JR. "Industrial Noise and Conservation of Hearing," in *Industrial Hygiene and Toxicology*, F. Patty, ed., 2d ed. New York: Interscience Publishers, 1958, Vol. I, Chap. 18.

FOWLER, E. P., JR. *Nelson Loose-Leaf Medicine of the Ear*. New York: Thomas Nelson & Sons, Inc., 1939.
    A textbook of medicine intended for physicians.

GOODHILL, V. "Pathology, Diagnosis and Therapy of Deafness," in *Handbook of Speech Pathology*, L. E. Travis, ed. New York: Appleton-Century-Crofts, Inc., 1957, Chap. 9.
    A fairly detailed exposition of the medical and surgical aspects of deafness.

HARRIS, C. M., ed. *Handbook of Noise Control*. New York: McGraw-Hill Book Company, 1957, Chaps. 4, 7.

ROSENBLITH, W. A., and K. N. STEVENS. *Handbook of Acoustic Noise Control*. Vol. II, *Noise and Man*, Wright Air Development Center, Technical Report 52-204, 1953.

6

THE SURGICAL TREATMENT
OF HEARING LOSS

T. E. Walsh, M.R.C.S., L.R.C.P.

As described in previous chapters, the ability to hear requires an intact nerve of hearing to convey to the brain the nerve impulses set up by sound waves. For normal sensitivity of hearing there must also be an efficient apparatus to convey sounds from the outside world to the sense organ in the inner ear. This conduction apparatus consists of the external ear and canal for the collection of sound waves and the drum and ossicles of the middle ear. At the present time we are unable to restore any tissue that may have degenerated in the brain, the auditory nerve, or the inner ear. The surgical treatment of hearing loss is, therefore, aimed at correcting abnormalities of the conduction apparatus.

Surgical Treatment of the Middle Ear
and the Mastoid

The function of the Eustachian tube in equalizing the pressure of air in the middle ear with that outside the eardrum has already been described. The tube normally opens only momentarily when we swallow or yawn. If any obstruction is present, so that the tube cannot open when it should, the air contained in the middle ear is partly absorbed and the drumhead is pushed in by the air pressure outside. When the drum membrane is thus "retracted," its free motion is limited and its efficiency as a conducting mechanism is reduced. The result is a temporary, partial loss of hearing.

In addition to allowing the passage of air between the back of the nose and the middle ear, the Eustachian tube offers a pathway up which infections of the nose and throat can easily extend into the middle ear. Such infection is more likely to occur when the mouth of the Eustachian tube is surrounded by lymphoid tissue (adenoids), which easily becomes infected in colds or sinusitis.

The adenoids, tonsils, and sinuses are therefore doubly important as indirect causes of hearing loss. They may prevent ventilation of the middle ear, and they may favor infection. Enlarged tonsils and adenoids should therefore be removed surgically. If there is a tendency to recurrence of adenoid tissue, the radiation treatments mentioned in the previous chapter may prove helpful.

The spread of infection up the Eustachian tube is frequently helped by the improper forcible blowing of the nose, which is so commonly practiced. Children in particular should be instructed to blow the nose gently with both nostrils open so that the pressure does not force infected material from the nose up the Eustachian tube to the middle ear.

The condition of *serous* or *mucous otitis media* has been described in Chapter 5 and the necessity for removal of the fluid to restore hearing and to prevent the formation of adhesions has been pointed out. Often a simple incision of the drumhead or puncture by a needle with suction will clear up a serous effusion. Occasionally the condition can be relieved by inflating the middle ear by way of the Eustachian tube. Sometimes, however, adequate drainage cannot be obtained through the Eustachian tube or perhaps the opening in the drumhead heals too quickly. In this situation the hole in the drumhead can often be kept open with a small piece of plastic tubing. In adults the puncture of the drumhead is usually done without anesthesia, but in children this procedure is not an easy one, especially if a plastic tube is to be inserted.

If the exudate in the middle ear is thick and the disease is of long standing, elimination of the large surface of the mastoid cells may be necessary. This requires the operation known as *mastoidectomy*, which will be described below.

Of course, if the accumulation of fluid is due to blockage at the nasopharyngeal end of the Eustachian tube, it may be relieved or recurrence prevented by removal of enlarged adenoids or by treatment of the overgrown lymphoid tissue by radiation. These measures are not likely to be effective, however, if the fluid is thick and mucoid.

The symptoms of inflammation of the middle ear, or *otitis media,* and its medical treatment by sulfonamides and penicillin were discussed in Chapter 5 as part of the medical treatment of the ear. If, however, the inflammation is not recognized early and is not promptly and efficiently treated, pus will form in the middle ear. This condition is technically known as *suppurative otitis media* and popularly as a "rising," a "bealing," or a "gathering" in the ear. If the drumhead is not incised promptly to relieve the pressure within, it may rupture spontaneously. Unless the infection is very mild, the drum should be opened *promptly,* if it has not done so of itself, and the pus within it allowed to drain out. Following a spontaneous rupture, the perforation does not always heal; but, if the drumhead is incised by the surgeon early in the course of the infection and the pus behind it is able to drain, the incision usually heals well with no residual loss of hearing. If, however, the infection is neglected, mastoiditis, with its attendant danger of further complications, may occur and the hearing be permanently impaired. *Prompt attention to infection of the middle ear will do much to prevent the loss of hearing that frequently accompanies perforation of the drumhead and chronic diseases of the middle ear.* Contrary to popular belief, the hearing loss which sometimes persists after mastoid surgery or incision of the drum membrane is due to the disease and not to the surgery.

Chronic otitis media may follow acute otitis media if the acute otitis is not properly treated. The hearing then becomes further impaired because, as a result of the infection, the ossicles become bound together with scar tissue or may actually be eaten away by the disease process. There is also the further danger that in certain cases the infection may spread into the skull and lead to meningitis and brain abscess. Operation for chronic otitis media is indicated to ensure the safety of the patient, to check the formation of scar tissue, and also to restore the hearing as far as it can be restored.

MASTOIDECTOMY

The operation of mastoidectomy for chronic otitis media has been considered a terrible and dangerous procedure by most laymen. It is usually, however, a lifesaving operation, and in the hands of a competent otologic surgeon it is not dangerous.

There are several kinds of mastoidectomy. The "simple" or "complete" mastoidectomy, performed for acute mastoiditis, aims to remove the diseased tissue in the mastoid bone and to establish free drainage of pus from the mastoid and the middle ear. "Radical" mastoidectomy is performed in chronic cases when the disease is not only in the air cells of the mastoid bone but in the middle ear as well. Its object is to remove all diseased tissues from both cavities and to create a single cavity that will eventually become lined with skin and cause no further trouble. "Simple" mastoidectomy, performed for acute infection of the mastoid air cells, causes no appreciable hearing loss if there are no other complications. The hearing may be expected to stay within normal limits. "Radical" mastoidectomy, on the other hand, performed most frequently for chronic running ears, usually leaves a hearing level

of about 35 to 40 db because the middle ear is destroyed in the operation, even if it has not already been destroyed by the infection. The
final level actually represents an improvement of hearing in about one
third of all cases over the conductive loss which existed before operation while the middle ear was plugged with pus. For another one third
there is no significant over-all change in hearing, and for the remaining third the hearing is worse after the operation than it was before. Of
course, if, as is frequently the case, there is also some sensory-neural
hearing loss, the impairment due to it will remain and will be added
to the 35 or 40 db of conductive impairment produced by the operation.
It should be clearly understood that *radical mastoidectomy is a lifesaving operation or is performed to prevent further deterioration of
the inner ear and not for the sake of any possible improvement of
hearing.*

Surgical Alleviation of Conductive Hearing Loss

The two major diseases of the middle ear, otitis media and
otosclerosis, have been discussed in some detail in previous chapters.
The surgical treatment of acute otitis media is an important surgical
procedure, but there are now also surgical operations that aim at
combating a disease process as well as at improving the conduction of
sound to the inner ear. One of these is *myringoplasty,* or repair of a
persistent perforation of the drum membrane. Closely allied to this
operation is the use of a "prosthesis," which is a mechanical substitute
of some sort for a missing ossicle. The other two operations, aimed to
relieve or circumvent the fixation of the stapes by otosclerosis, are
stapes mobilization and *fenestration.*

We shall merely mention here in passing that surgery may be
done to overcome congenital malformations of the external or the
middle ear. If the external canal is closed (atresia) it may be opened
by surgical procedures. Frequently, the benefit from such an operation
is limited from the point of view of hearing because of malformations
of the ossicles or other parts of the middle ear as well as of the external
canal. Surgery is also often undertaken to improve the appearance of a
malformed or missing external ear (pinna). This is usually done by a
plastic surgeon rather than by an otologic surgeon.

TYMPANOPLASTY AND MYRINGOPLASTY

There are many cases of chronic otitis media in which the disease
is not sufficiently severe to warrant a radical mastoidectomy. However,
the hearing in such cases is decreased because of the scarlike adhesions
and perhaps because of other anatomical changes that have taken place

in the middle ear and perhaps also because of perforation of the tympanic membrane. For many years plastic operations have been performed in such cases either to re-form the middle ear or perhaps only to close the hole in the drum membrane. The more extensive operation was formerly known as "modified radical mastoidectomy," but it has recently been improved and popularized under the name "tympanoplasty." Here we should remember that "tympano-" refers to the entire middle ear, and not merely to the drum membrane. For the simpler operation, directed to closure of a hole in the membrane and nothing more, we use the term "myringoplasty."

Myringoplasty. In many cases the tympanic membrane has been perforated as the result of an old healed otitis media. The ear is perfectly dry. There is no discharge, but the patient's hearing is depressed because of the hole in the drumhead. Such holes can sometimes be closed by cauterizing, cutting or scraping the edge of the perforation, and then providing some sort of scaffolding, such as cigarette paper or cotton, to assist the epithelium to grow across and thus heal the perforation. Some surgeons have had considerable success with these procedures but others have not. A recent approach to the closure of perforations is to separate the epithelium from the fibrous portion of the drum membrane for a distance of about 2 or 3 mm from the edge of the perforation. A skin graft, which is then placed over the raw surface that has been exposed, receives its blood supply from it. In many instances the skin graft will "take" and close the perforation. Such operations may improve the hearing from levels between 20 and 30 db to a level of 15 db or better, i.e., within normal limits.

Tympanoplasty. When disease is still present in the upper part of the middle ear (the attic) a more extensive operation is required. The objective now is to remove the diseased tissue, particularly from the upper part of the middle ear, as well as to re-form a middle ear so that sound may be conducted to the oval window through any remnants of the ossicles which may be present. At the same time the round window is walled off from the oval window by what remains of the drum membrane. The reduced middle-ear cavity is still connected with the Eustachian tube, as in the fenestration operation (Figure 6-2). In this situation the sound waves reach the oval window, exposed directly to the external canal, and the round window, protected by the drum membrane, with somewhat different intensities and perhaps also with significant phase differences. The situation is very similar to the end result of the fenestration operation except that it has not been necessary to create a new fenestra because the stapes is still mobile in the oval window.

OTIC PROSTHESIS

In some cases in which there is a perforation through the drum membrane or in which most of the drumhead has been destroyed by disease it is possible to improve hearing by means of some material, such as cotton soaked in an oily ointment, or perhaps a piece of artificial membrane or tissue of some sort. Sometimes, but not often, such a piece of flexible membrane placed over the perforation in the drum membrane is effective. More frequently, the cotton or an emulsified ointment is used to isolate the round window from the oval window and thereby produce a difference in acoustic pressure between them. Of course, a prosthesis of this sort has to be changed from time to time when it becomes dry or if it moves from its original position.

Another type of prosthesis is known as the *Pohlman prosthesis.* This is a small bristle of nylon attached to an artificial membrane of paper or plastic. It is so placed that the bristle actually makes contact with the head of the stapes. In some suitable cases this type of prosthesis may give very good hearing as long as it remains properly in place, and it may remain in place for a number of days. Obviously, however, it must be put in place by an otologist, and it is often difficult for him, even with all his special instruments, illumination, and knowledge of anatomy, to make contact with the "hot spot" that gives the desired improvement of hearing. Eventually the device gets out of place; in any case, it must occasionally be renewed or cleaned. Some patients are able to learn to replace it themselves, but there is always the danger of infection in the cavity if they do so. Furthermore, only a very small minority of the hard of hearing have the particular abnormality of the middle ear that is suitable for an otic prosthesis.

STAPES MOBILIZATION

The concept of forcibly breaking loose a fixed stapes and thus restoring its function is as old as it is simple. It was attempted many times during the last quarter of the nineteenth century and in the early nineteen hundreds, but without much lasting success, and the operation was finally abandoned. Recently, the more complicated fenestration operation has been proved to be practical, lasting in its benefits, with high probability of success but limited in the hearing level that it can yield. A few years ago Dr. Samuel Rosen of New York revived the simple stapes mobilization, and this operation is now at about the stage of development that the fenestration operation had reached in 1945.

In the stapes mobilization operation the middle ear is approached by way of the external canal. The skin is cut near the attachment of the drum membrane and the membrane is freed from its attachment for about half its circumference and laid to one side. The head of the stapes is not readily visible from the ear canal, but, by careful grinding with fine drills under a powerful dissecting microscope, enough bone is removed to obtain a good view. The surgeon has several very fine knives, hooks, probes, chisels, all specially made for this purpose, with which he carefully manipulates the head and the footplate of the stapes in various ways. His objective is to break the footplate free as a whole or else to fracture it in such a way that part of it, attached to one crus or to both crura, can move. Sometimes the crura break before the footplate comes free. It is a very delicate maneuver and some surgeons seem to be rather more successful at it than others. There also seems to be a considerable element of luck as to just how favorably a particular stapes will break. Once the stapes has been either fractured or broken loose nothing needs to be done except put the drum back in place and allow it to heal. The entire operation is brief and the aftereffects are those of a minor rather than of a major surgical operation.

The two great points in favor of the stapes mobilization operation are, first, the relatively minor character of the operation and its freedom from uncomfortable aftereffects and, second, the very good hearing level that is sometimes obtained. In a few cases the level for speech returns very nearly to zero. This is possible because the operation leaves the ear with a normal drum membrane and a good set of ossicles, even though the stapes may be a bit broken and chipped. If it is mobile and part of a chain, a piece of stapes works nearly as well as a whole normal one.

The drawback to the operation is the uncertainty of the result. At the time of this writing, no guarantee can be given beforehand, and the patient must accept his fortune, good or bad. The proportion of successes varies from one surgeon to another, with odds from about two to one in favor to about two to one against; of course, many of these are partial successes or near misses, depending on the definition of success.

Mobilization has the added advantage, in the minds of many surgeons, that in case of failure it is usually possible to resort to the more elaborate, somewhat more limited, but much more predictable fenestration operation. It has been stated that it is more difficult to do a good fenestration operation after an attempted mobilization on account of the scar formation, but the consensus now seems to be that the added difficulty is not great enough to affect materially the chances of success.

The stapes, once mobilized, often stays mobile. This cannot be guaranteed, but the percentage is encouraging. The chances of immediate refixation seem to be lower than was predicted by the skeptics of a few years ago. If early fixation occurs, it usually takes place within the first three months after the operation. It is still too early to make any statement about the probability of late fixation, i.e., more than a year after the operation.

FENESTRATION

The following historical account of the development of the fenestration operation, retained (with some small changes) from the first edition of our book, is of some interest in illustrating the step by step advance on an international basis. Such a development is characteristic of most advances in medicine and surgery. As long ago as 1876, Kessel, in Germany, suggested removal of the immobile stapes. The removal, of course, left the oval window open. The opening was allowed to close with scar tissue, and Kessel hoped that the scar would be flexible enough to enable sound to enter the inner ear. His attempts were not successful because of the difficulty in removing the footplate of the stapes and because infection entered the inner ear from the middle-ear cavity.

In 1897, Passow, another German, tried a different approach. He made an opening into the basal turn of the cochlea and covered the opening with periosteum, the membrane which normally covers bone. Immediately after the operation his patient experienced a marked improvement in hearing, which, however, lasted only a few days. The danger of infection was a bugbear of this operation, and, because of it and the consequent danger to life and the fleeting nature of the hearing improvement, the procedure was not generally adopted.

In 1910, Bárány, the great Swedish otolaryngologist (a native of Austria), suggested making an opening into the posterior vertical semicircular canal to reduce the danger of infection of the labyrinth. The surgical approach to the posterior vertical canal is made through the mastoid bone under aseptic conditions, and there is, therefore, little chance of infection. He performed this operation, and the immediate improvement in hearing was marked, but it lasted only two weeks.

In 1914, Jenkins, in England, opened the horizontal semicircular canal in two patients. In one case he covered the opening with a skin graft and in the other with a flap of skin taken from the posterior wall of the external auditory canal. The hearing improved markedly in both cases immediately following the operation, but it fell below the preoperative level in one case and was lost completely in the other shortly afterward.

Holmgren (1920), in Sweden, and Sourdille (1924), in France, continued working on this problem and gradually evolved improvements in approach and technique. It was Sourdille who evolved the flap of skin from the wall of the canal, which will be described in the next section, and left it attached to the drum. Some of his cases were successful, but in a large percentage of them the "fenestra" (from the Latin word meaning "window") closed, and the gain in hearing was lost.

Finally, since 1930, in America, Julius Lempert has further improved the technique of the operation. Whereas Sourdille performed his operation in two stages, Lempert devised a one-stage procedure. By attention to minute details of technique, Lempert improved his results. He, too, was disturbed, however, at the frequency with which the newly created fenestra closed and, in searching for a reason, argued that the window, made as it was in the limb of the horizontal canal, was so narrow that bone could easily bridge the gap. He therefore devised a new technique in which he placed the fenestra farther forward over the wider ampullated end of the horizontal canal and over the vestibule. He was now able to create a window a full millimeter in width. This added size alone made it less likely that the window would close, and now Lempert and his disciples seem to have finally solved the problem of how to reliably prevent the bone from healing over and closing the new fenestra. Close attention is given to removal of all bone dust and chips. The bone from the center of the opening is removed all in one piece. The edges of the fenestra are ground down thin and smooth and the skin flap from the wall of the ear canal is pressed firmly down over the fenestra. The object is to bring the flap in contact with the membranous semicircular canal and with the edges of the cut endosteum that lines the bony canal on the inside. If the canal and the endosteum heal to the skin flap the bone cannot grow over the opening. With present technique not more than about 3 per cent of fenestras close again. Those that do close do so within the first six months.

The principle of the operation, as developed by Sourdille, is illustrated in Figures 6-1 and 6-2. In Figure 6-1, which is a diagram of the correct anatomical relationships as described in Chapter 3, the normal path of sound across the middle ear and into the inner ear by way of the stapes and oval window is indicated by arrows. Figure 6-2, another diagram, is intended to show (1) the fixation of the stapes by otosclerosis; (2) the degeneration of some of the sensory cells of the cochlea, which so frequently occurs in the later stages of otosclerosis; (3) the opening of a fenestra through the bony wall of the middle ear into the horizontal semicircular canal; (4) the skin flap from the ear canal covering the fenestra; and (5) the displacement of the ear-drum and removal of the incus and most of the malleus. The new path of the sound waves is indicated, for simplicity, as entering the inner ear through the fenestra. Of course, both windows must be mobile and both are affected by the sound pressure outside. The movement inside occurs because of the *difference* in pressure on the two windows at each instant. The pressure is probably greater on the average on the new fenestra than on the round window, which lies behind what is left of the drum membrane. The pressure wave at the round window may also be a little earlier or a little later than at the fenestra ("out of phase," as we say), and this phase difference may increase the differ-ence in instantaneous pressure. It does not matter much which way the fluid in the cochlea moves during the compression phase of a sound wave in the canal. What is important is *how much* it moves; and as a matter of experience the drum membrane over the round window niche is an important factor in getting a good differential between the two windows.

Description of the operation. The present fenestration operation in the hands of a well-trained and competent otologic surgeon is not dangerous to life. The danger that is present, other than that of any operation in which an anesthetic is used, is that the hearing may be entirely lost in the operated ear. This can occur from difficulties at operation or may follow a postoperative inflammation of the delicate structures within the labyrinth. There have also been a few instances

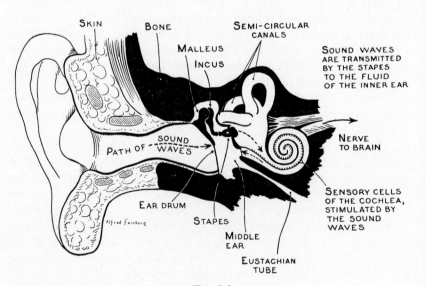

Fig. 6-1.

of facial-nerve paralysis. This condition, however, is only temporary, and recovery is spontaneous. In no case, in the care of a skilled surgeon, should there be danger of permanent injury to the facial nerve.

The operation may be performed under any type of anesthetic. A skin incision is made in the ear canal and the mastoid bone is exposed and entered. The spongy interior, composed of the partitions between the mastoid air cells, is removed sufficiently to allow approach to the enlarged ampullated end of the horizontal canal and to the middle ear. Great care is taken to control all bleeding, as the fenestra cannot be successfully made in the presence of any blood. The posterior superior bony wall of the external auditory canal is gradually removed until the joint between the malleus and the incus is exposed. This procedure is done with care so that the skin of the external auditory canal and the drum are not injured. Then the incus is removed, and the head and neck of the malleus are amputated. The skin of the external canal is now separated from the bone of the posterior and superior walls, but its attachment to the drum is left intact. Thus, a flap of skin is formed which can be laid down over the fenestra. This flap of skin is carefully inspected for any particles of bone that might stick to it, and these are removed. All bleeding is again controlled. The fenestra is now made in the ampullated end of the horizontal canal by carefully burring through the bony capsule (Figure 6-3). The skin

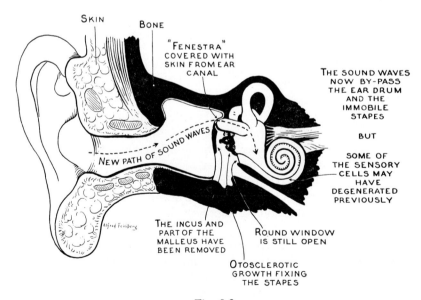

Fig. 6-2.

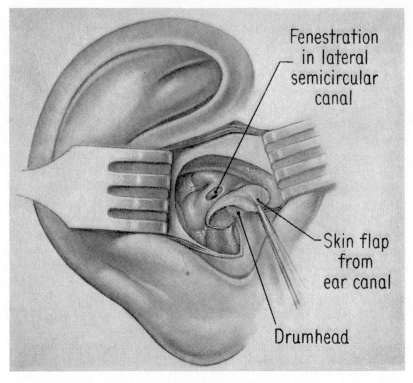

Fenestration
in lateral
semicircular
canal

Skin flap
from
ear canal

Drumhead

Fig. 6-3. (*This figure is reproduced through the courtesy of Dr. Julius Lempert, New York, and the Archives of Otolaryngology.*)

flap is then laid over the fenestra. The cavity is packed and a dressing is applied over the ear.

Course of events after the operation. The average length of stay in the hospital is from five to seven days. Immediately after the operation, and even on the operating table if the operation is done under local anesthesia, hearing may return dramatically, and the patient, very hard of hearing before operation, may be able to hear the softest-spoken word. This degree of improvement may be diminished for the first few days after the operation because of some inflammatory change due to the surgery. It gradually improves after a period of two or three weeks.

After the operation the patient is somewhat dizzy for the first twenty-four hours. With the new techniques and the use of isotonic fluid for irrigation during the operation there is very little postoperative labyrinthitis and most of the dizziness can be very easily controlled, so that we expect the patient to be out of bed the day after the operation, although he may be somewhat unsteady. Of course, certain movements of the head cause dizziness and the patient must be careful to take things easy for a few days. It is unusual nowadays if the patient is not sitting up and eating full meals within forty-eight hours of the operation. The patient is urged to be up and walking about as soon as he is able after the operation, usually the second or third day. On the fifth or sixth day the dressing is done and all packing is removed from the ear. Only some sterile cotton is left to close the canal. The patient is allowed to go home the day that the dressing is done.

The first dressing is seldom uncomfortable and should never be painful. The ear must be treated at intervals until it is completely healed. These intervals are usually two to three weeks, depending on the techniques that the surgeon prefers. Healing is usually obtained in four to nine weeks.

When the patient leaves the hospital, there are precautions that must be taken for his safety. It must be remembered that the labyrinth has been disturbed and that sudden movements of the head may give rise to dizziness. Such sudden movements must therefore be avoided. For instance, when he is about to cross a street in traffic, the movement of looking each way should be a slow and deliberate one.

Because the horizontal semicircular canal has been exposed (except for its covering of skin) and is now quite accessible to the outside, it can easily be stimulated by changes in temperature. On cold days and when it is windy, cotton should be worn in the ear. The result of stimulation by the cold air is dizziness. It follows, of course, that swimming must be forbidden. It would be extremely dangerous to allow cold water to enter the ear canal following fenestration.

After complete healing has taken place, it is very important to have the cavity cleaned about every six months. Normally, the outer layers of skin all over the body shed dead cells. Elsewhere on the body surface these cells fall off unnoticed. In a cavity such as that left after fenestration, the dead cells may accumulate and must be removed.

Until healing is complete, superficial infections with parasitic fungi are rather common and may cause a delay in healing. It is important that the aftercare demanded by the surgeon be carefully followed.

The cosmetic effect of the operation is of minor importance, but it is well to know that in most cases no change in appearance from the normal can be noted when healing is complete.

EVALUATION

The fenestration operation and stapes mobilization must be judged by the answers to four major questions:

For what kinds of deafness is it suitable?
What are the discomforts and dangers?
What are the chances of success?
How permanent are the benefits?

The first and second of these questions we have already answered. Both operations are theoretically suitable for conductive but not for neural hearing loss. Fenestration causes some temporary discomfort. Stapes mobilization causes far less discomfort from vertigo, and the like, after the operation and does not require any periodic aftercare. The danger of losing the hearing of the operated ear entirely is about the same for the two operations. The danger to life is practically negligible for both of them.

The chances of success of both operations depend, of course, upon whether the operation is confined to suitable cases or whether it is tried on patients who have a good deal of neural loss in addition to their conductive loss. We must also set up some definition of "success."

The objective of the fenestration operation and of stapes mobilization is to restore the patient to a satisfactory hearing level for everyday speech. By this is meant that he should, if the operation is successful, be able to hear ordinary conversation without a hearing aid. He should be able to hear adequately in most theaters, movies, and churches. A final hearing level for speech of 30 db, which in the context of workmen's compensation laws corresponds to less than 25 per cent handicap in the hearing of everyday speech (see Chapter 9), is generally accepted as the borderline of success, i.e., a reasonably adequate level for practical everyday communication.

The fenestration operation is now so well standardized that if it is performed by an otologist who specializes in this operation its outcome can be predicted within a very few decibels with considerable confidence. The reason for the consistency in the results is that the operation completely by-passes the fixed stapes and produces a new sound-conducting system. The new system, illustrated in Figure 6-2, is not as efficient as the normal ear with its complete drum membrane and its chain of ossicles, but it is simple and its performance is therefore predictable. It makes no difference how much conductive loss there was before operation. After the operation the efficiency of transmission for speech is reduced by about 23 db. For the "ideal" cases of purely conductive hearing loss it has been the uniform experience over a period of more than ten years for most of the leading otologic surgeons in this country that half of their cases show a final hearing level of 23 db or better. The variability from case to case is such that half of the cases fall in the range from 21 to 30 db inclusive.

Of course, if the patient has any sensory-neural loss the number of decibels estimated to be due to this cause must be added to the 23 db that must be expected as the residual conductive impairment. The assessment of a small sensory-neural loss in the presence of a large conductive loss is not very easy because of the "Carhart notch" in the bone-conduction audiogram, as explained in Chapter 4.

The other sources of uncertainty about the result of the fenestration operation are the possibility of accidental injury to the inner ear during the operation (less than 1 in 100) and the possibility of closure of the fenestra (about 1 in 30). There are also a very few additional unexplained failures.

In summary, then, for cases which show no evidence of sensory-neural loss, the over-all chance of a final hearing level for speech of 30 db or better is about 80 out of 100. The chances are even for a final level of 23 db or better. The chance of a final level of 20 db or better is about 28 out of 100.

The result of stapes mobilization is less predictable. We have already pointed out that there is a considerable element of luck in just how the stapes breaks. It is theoretically possible for hearing to be restored to the zero hearing level, and this sometimes happens. Surgeons differ from one another more with respect to success in stapes mobilization than with respect to the success of fenestration. Perhaps during the next few years a way will be found to make the stapes mobilize reliably the way we want it to. If this can be done, stapes mobilization should become the operation of choice. At present it is the "sporting proposition": a better pay-off if you win, but only fifty-fifty odds for substantial improvement.

Ten years ago there was still much discussion as to whether the fenestration operation tends to protect the ear against nerve degeneration. To a physiologist the possibility always seemed very remote, and since that time no evidence has appeared to support such a theory. The theory of conservation or protection of cochlear function is not much of an argument in favor of having an operation as opposed to simply using a hearing aid. The practical decision should be made on other grounds than this.

Surgical Treatment of Ménière's Disease

Surgery can improve a sensory-neural hearing loss of one but only one variety. If the loss is due to pressure on the auditory nerve or the cochlear artery from a tumor of the auditory nerve, removal of the tumor may restore some or all of the lost hearing. Improvement is more likely if the hearing loss came on rather rapidly and the operation is performed promptly than it will be if the tumor grew slowly. In this case the nerve cells and hair cells are likely to be injured or starved beyond hope of recovery. The operation for removal of the tumor is not undertaken to restore hearing, however. It is undertaken to protect life, because further growth may cause pressure on vital centers in the lower brain stem.

Surgery may be employed in severe cases of Ménière's disease, not to cure the disease but to give the patient relief from a disabling vertigo or an intolerable tinnitus. The "Day operation" or the "Cawthorne operation" is performed something like a fenestration operation but the surgeon deliberately enters the inner ear and destroys the membranous labyrinth. The operations differ chiefly in surgical details of the means used to inactivate or destroy the labyrinth. Still another method (Arslan) employs high-intensity ultrasound, applied locally to the labyrinth, for this purpose. Such operations are justified because the brain compensates very well for the loss of the nonauditory labyrinth, although the vertigo from irritation and spontaneous discharge of this sense organ can be completely disabling. The only question is how long to wait for a spontaneous improvement or how severe must the symptoms be before operating.

At one time an effort was made to spare the hearing when the nonauditory labyrinth was destroyed. One method was to cut the vestibular nerve but spare the cochlear nerve. It soon appeared, however, that the hearing of the affected ear was so badly impaired by the same disease process, whatever it is, that speech could not be understood usefully and there was often a very loud and annoying tinnitus. If there is reasonably good hearing in the remaining ear the patient usually prefers unilateral deafness to the tinnitus and diplacusis; and he may get it whether he wants it or not as a result of the operation if the utricle, saccule, and semicircular canals are really thoroughly destroyed.

The Day, the Cawthorne, and the Arslan operations represent a type of operation that is now fairly common in neurosurgery. The neurosurgery does not restore a normal state, but distressing, undesirable symptoms are relieved by deliberate, well-placed, controlled destruction of a certain bit of tissue that is acting abnormally. A loss of function is often far preferable to faulty abnormal overactivity.

Suggested Readings

BILGER, R. C., A. C. GOODMAN, and T. E. WALSH. "The Fenestration Operation: A Perspective in Time," *The Laryngoscope,* 69: 141–163 (1959).

DAVIS, H., and T. E. WALSH. "The Limits of Improvement of Hearing Following the Fenestration Operation," *The Laryngoscope,* 60: 273–295 (1950).

FOWLER, E. P., SR. *Twenty Years of Research in Otosclerosis, and Correlated Problems, 1926–1946.* New York: Central Bureau of Research, American Otological Society, 1946.
A summary written by an otologist for otologists.
GOODHILL, V. "Pathology, Diagnosis and Therapy of Deafness," in *Handbook of Speech Pathology,* L. E. Travis, ed. New York: Appleton-Century-Crofts, Inc., 1957, Chap. 9.
A fairly detailed exposition of the medical and surgical aspects of deafness.
KOPETZKY, J. S. Nelson Loose-Leaf Surgery of the Ear. New York: Thomas Nelson & Sons, Inc.
This is a textbook of surgery intended for otolaryngologists.
LEMPERT, J. "Fenestra nov-ovalis with mobile stopple," *Archives of Otolaryngology,* 41: 1–41 (1945).
ROSEN, S. "Simple Method for Restoring Hearing in Otosclerosis: Mobilization of Stapes," *Acta Oto-Laryngologica,* 44: 78–88 (1954).
SHAMBAUGH, G. E., JR. "Correlation of the Predicted with the Actual Result of Fenestration in 164 Consecutive Cases," *The Laryngoscope,* 62: 461–474 (1952).

PART 3

AUDITORY TESTS AND HEARING AIDS

7

AUDIOMETRY

Hallowell Davis, M.D.

Audiometry means the measuring of hearing. There are many tests of hearing: some old and many new, some crude and some very refined and elaborate, some intended for screening and others designed for medical diagnosis. We shall make a rapid survey of these tests and name and classify or characterize most of those that are in current use in hearing clinics. We shall, however, be content to point out the principles that are involved and the kind of information that each test yields. We shall not discuss the details of technique and precautions. This is not a "cookbook of audiometry." Neither do we go far into controversial questions of theory or the "last word" from experimental psychophysics. Other authors and the current journals provide adequate treatment of these various topics. We are writing only a guide for the beginning student or the interested worker in a related field.

Types of Hearing Tests

In Chapter 2, "Physics and Psychology of Hearing," it was pointed out that there are several different aspects of hearing. We may be interested in testing any or all of them, and different types of test are appropriate for each one. First and most obvious is *sensitivity*. How weak a sound can be heard? Then there is the *recognition of pitch*. Do pure tones sound pure and musical, and is the ear "in tune," so to speak? There is also auditory *discrimination*. How small a difference in pitch or in loudness can a person detect? Can he recognize difficult words? Can he pick out speech from a background of noise or of many voices as well as he should? And finally there is *tolerance*. At what intensity does a sound become uncomfortable or painful?

165

Originally the interest in audiometry lay almost entirely in sensitivity. From the medical point of view the object was to determine whether the fault lay in the sound-conducting mechanism of the middle ear or in the neural mechanism of the inner ear. More recently, however, the importance of tolerance, of correct recognition of pitch, and of auditory discrimination has been recognized, and tests for these .other aspects of hearing have been developed. The otologist now wants to distinguish impairments of the sense organ from those of the auditory nerve or brain stem, and both such conditions from what we now call central dysacusis.

CRUDE TESTS OF SENSITIVITY

To bring the study of hearing out of the realm of guesswork and to guide the medical treatment of its problems, we need tests and, above all, *measurements* of hearing. When someone is totally deaf in both ears, there is usually no doubt about it, but to devise a simple and reliable test to determine whether a man's hearing is good enough for him to enter military service or bad enough to entitle him to compensation for injury is a very different matter. It is not easy or simple to measure the sensitivity of hearing accurately, partly because it requires complicated apparatus to deliver sounds of known intensity to the ear and partly because physical sound has two major dimensions—frequency and intensity—and the loss of hearing for some frequencies may be much greater than for others. The difficulties are overcome by the electric audiometer; but the instrument is expensive, and the quiet surroundings required for accurate measurements of hearing may be difficult and even more expensive to provide. For rapid and approximate testing, therefore, the crude but time-honored methods—the *conversational voice*, the *whisper*, the *coin click*, and the *watch tick*—will still be used.

These four simple tests solve in different ways the problem of which frequencies to test. The voice and the whisper represent two kinds of sound that are most important for a man to hear, and if he can hear (and understand) the human voice, we do not much care whether or not he can hear the cricket's chirp. The frequencies most important for good understanding of speech extend from about 400 to about 3000 cps, and the voice test therefore gives some idea of the usefulness of hearing over this range. The watch tick and the click of coins, on the other hand, are high-frequency sounds, mostly above the range that is really needed to understand speech. They are useful because loss of hearing often begins with a loss of sensitivity for high frequencies and the defect can be detected much earlier by the coin or the watch than by the voice or the whisper. In a very general way the hearing for speech is impaired most by conductive hearing losses, which affect all frequencies. Sensory-neural loss is most often a high-tone hearing loss, which almost always begins and is most severe above 2000 cps. The spoken voice and the watch tick or coin click supplement one another in just this way, and *to the extent that they can be standardized*, they are useful tools for rough-and-ready testing.

Two major difficulties with all simple tests, in addition to the necessity of providing a quiet test room with walls that do not reflect the test sounds, are standardizing the sounds and measuring their intensity. We have to assume that one man's voice is as easy to understand as another's, that watch ticks are alike, and that any two coins struck together in various ways will give off the same sound. Of course, many efforts to standardize these tests have been made. For example, certain key words, usually numbers such as "sixty-six," "ninety-nine," are regularly used in the voice test. Those who do much testing of this sort try to speak always with the same loudness and distinctness; but we need not be concerned here with details.

The whisper test has the advantage over the conversational voice that it is relatively easy to standardize the loudness of a whisper by whispering only at the end of an expiration. Incidentally, the whisper represents at fairly even intensity the frequency range needed for good understanding of speech. In ordinary conversational voice the low frequencies are much more powerful than most of the high frequencies.

The intensity with which the sound of the voice, watch, or coin reaches the ear is varied by the tester coming closer and closer to the subject. This is theoretically a reasonable method because the intensity of sound varies inversely as the square of the distance it travels. (Twice as far away, one fourth the intensity at the ear; three times as far, one ninth; and so on.) In practice this rule almost always breaks down badly because of echoes from the walls of the room. Only in specially sound-absorbent rooms does the rule mean much for distances of more than six feet or so.

When we test the sensitivity of the ear, we do not merely want to know that someone can hear our voice at twenty feet and our watch at five, or that he can detect a tone of 1000 cps at one ten-thousandth of a dyne per square centimeter. We want to know whether or not he is "normal"; that is, how he compares with his fellow men. We therefore establish the performance of a large number of "presumably normal" men and women and then express the performance of the man with poor hearing as a ratio with respect to the normal. Thus, we may say that someone's hearing by the whisper test is 5/20 ("five over twenty"), meaning that he can just understand at five feet a whisper that the average man understands at twenty feet. Hearing level is given in decibels and is precisely what we want, namely the ratio (or, more exactly, the logarithm of the ratio) of the subject's threshold of hearing to that of a standard "normal" man.

TUNING FORKS

The first step in refinement of auditory tests was to use a series of pure tones of known frequency and thereby map the threshold of hearing up and down the frequency range. This is the principle of the modern electric audiometer; but before the development of the science of electroacoustics the sounds could be generated only by whistles, tuning forks, or modified musical instruments. Tuning forks are still dear to the otologist and serve him well for preliminary orientation, for an approximate cross check on any more elaborate audiometry, and for several special diagnostic tests. The octave frequencies of 64, 128, 256, 512, . . . cps were chosen for the standard sets of tuning forks. The otologist often uses his own ear as a standard of comparison. When the patient says he can no longer hear the tone the otologist quickly moves the fork into position close to his own ear. If he cannot hear it himself or if it sounds very faint the patient must have normal or nearly normal hearing for that frequency. At least he does if the room is quiet enough and the otologist himself has normal hearing. And if the patient cannot hear the fork at its loudest, his hearing for that frequency is abnormal to a real and practically significant degree. No exact measurements are possible, even though the striking of the fork may be quite well standardized by practice, but very useful practical information is obtained rapidly.

The most common diagnostic tests carried out with tuning forks are the Schwabach, the Rinne, and the Weber tests.

The *Schwabach test* is a test of bone conduction. Instead of holding the vibrating fork close beside the entrance to the ear canal the otologist places the tip of its hilt gently but firmly against the mastoid process of the skull behind and below the patient's ear. He then notes by how many seconds the hearing of the fork is shortened or prolonged relative to a normal ear, usually his own, in the same environment. "Schwabach shortened" or "bone conduction decreased" means that the patient's bone conduction is not as good as the average. This will be the situation if the patient has a sensory-neural hearing loss. If bone conduction is "lengthened" or "increased," a conductive hearing loss is suggested. The patient's hearing by bone conduction may actually be better than the examiner's because a conductive loss protects the bone-conducted tone against masking by air-conducted background noise, and it also prevents the radiation of acoustic energy out from the ear canal after it has reached the inner ear by bone conduction.

The *Rinne test* compares the patient's hearing by bone conduction with the patient's own hearing by air conduction. Like the Schwabach test, it is really a test of how much the ambient noise masks air-conducted as opposed to bone-conducted sound. The hilt of the tuning fork is applied to the mastoid, as in the Schwabach test, but when the patient no longer hears the sound, the fork is held close to the patient's ear instead of near the otologist's ear. If the patient again hears the tone he is said to have a "positive Rinne." It is normal to hear about twice as long by air as by bone conduction with the usual initial standard blow. If the patient does not hear the tone by air it is a "negative Rinne." The presumption in this case is a conductive hearing loss in that ear.

The *Weber test* compares the hearing by bone conduction in the patient's two ears. This test also depends on differences in masking by the ambient room noise. The hilt of the vibrating fork is applied to the center of the patient's forehead and he is asked *where* he hears the tone. If both ears are normal they will be equally stimulated and equally masked, and the sound will be heard as if it is in the center of the head. If there is conductive loss on one side the sound is heard better by that ear (by bone conduction, of course). Thus the sound is heard in the abnormal ear, which is less masked. The Weber is said to be "lateralized" to the right or the left, as the case may be. If, however, one ear is normal and the other has a *neural* loss, the Weber is lateralized to the normal side. If the two ears are both abnormal but symmetrically so, the Weber will not be consistently lateralized to either side.

Many other tuning fork tests have been suggested but most of them are variations on these same themes. All of them, including those described, have their pitfalls and difficulties, but their value for initial orientation and for final confirmation should not be overlooked by the electronically oriented audiologist.

THE ELECTRIC AUDIOMETER

In a pure-tone audiometer an alternating current of the desired frequency is generated by an electronic oscillator circuit. Nearly all models now provide a series of fixed frequencies in octaves based on 1000 cps. The number and choice of frequencies depend on the particular use for which the instrument is designed, as will be explained below. Formerly, instruments with continuous adjustment of frequency, such as the Peters, the Sonotone, and the Western Electric model 6B, were also popular, but the use of fixed frequencies has now become standard practice. The intensity of the sound output is regulated by means of a dial graduated, according to the American Standards for Audiometers, in 5 db steps. The electric current produces sound in a receiver or an earphone held by a spring headband snugly against the subject's ear. Usually two receivers, carefully matched to one another, are provided, with a switch on the instrument so that the sound can be delivered to either ear at the choice of the operator. Sometimes one of the earphones is a dummy, provided simply to exclude distracting sounds from the ear not under test. The receiver is provided with a rather firm sponge-rubber cushion that makes a good, but comfortable, acoustic seal against the side of the subject's head. A wide range of intensities, as much as 110 or 120 db at some frequencies, is available for the test tones so that any useful remnant of hearing can be detected.

An additional 10 db of intensity is provided in some special instruments in use in schools for the deaf, but it is questionable whether the sense of hearing or the sense of feeling is being tested at these very high intensities. A remnant of hearing at such a high level is not very useful even with modern hearing aids. For ordinary testing the range of 110 or 120 db is quite sufficient; moreover, the additional step is a

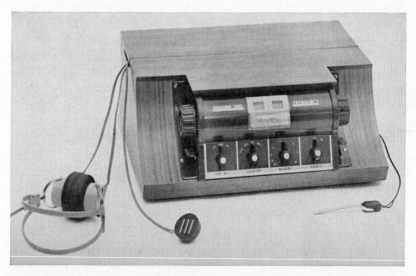

Fig. 7-1. An electric audiometer for general diagnostic purposes has both air-conduction and bone-conduction receivers. A microphone is provided to facilitate giving instructions to the patient. The frequency is selected by the large knob at the right and the intensity by the large knob at the left. The interrupter controls are just below these knobs. The other switches control the input (tone or speech), the receiver used (right, left or bone), the masking noise (by air conduction) and the power. (*Maico Electronics, Inc.*)

difficult task for the engineer who designs an attenuator that must cover the greater range.

The test tone is turned on and off by the operator. A special switching circuit is provided to cause the current to fade in and out gradually enough to avoid any audible click that might be produced by a sudden start or stop. On the other hand, the rise time is not more than half a second so that it is quite practical for the operator to use very brief pulses of tone as test signals if he wishes. In earlier models the test tone faded in and out very gradually and was normally on unless the operator interrupted it by means of the switch. Most modern audiometers can be operated with the tone normally on or normally off. The thresholds obtained with the earlier models are practically identical with those obtained with more rapid interruptions or pulses, but the subject can usually make up his mind more rapidly and with less effort with the briefer signals. The net result of using rather brief pulses is a saving of time on the over-all test.

Sometimes a signal circuit is provided whereby the subject holds down a push button as long as he hears the tone and releases it when he ceases to hear. Most audiometrists now prefer, however, to have the subject raise his finger when he hears the tone rather than press a button. The speed and promptness with which the finger is raised give an observant operator much additional information as to the certainty with which the subject feels that he hears the tone.

Another accessory is a "masking circuit" that generates a buzz to be delivered to the ear opposite to the one being tested. This may be

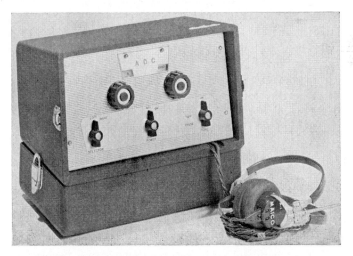

Fig. 7-2. This audiometer has only air-conduction receivers. It is suitable for monitoring audiometry and can be carried easily by hand. (*Audiometer Sales Corp.*)

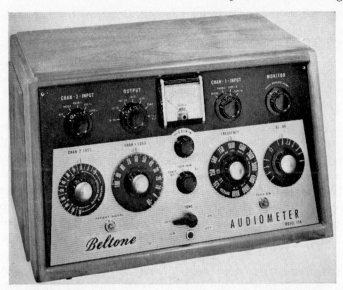

Fig. 7-3. For certain tests, such as loudness balance, an audiometer requires two channels. This instrument also has a VU meter with which to monitor speech. An accessory turntable (Fig. 7-7) and a microphone make it a complete speech audiometer. (*Beltone Hearing Aid Co.*)

necessary if the ear being tested is quite hard of hearing and the opposite ear hears well by bone conduction. In this situation, unless a masking noise is used, the good ear may hear the vibrations carried across through the skull before the threshold of the poorer ear is reached. Still another accessory is a *bone-conduction vibrator* that delivers vibrations to the mastoid process of the temporal bone instead of generating sound waves in an earphone. The same electrical circuits are employed with no change except in the scale on which the amount of hearing loss is read.

The more elaborate electric audiometers intended for diagnostic purposes may have still other features that allow the operator to perform tests such as loudness balancing or measurement of the difference limen for loudness in addition to determining hearing levels by air conduction and bone conduction. Some of these additional tests will be described briefly below.

STANDARDS FOR AUDIOMETERS

When electric audiometers were first introduced each company designed its own model with features that seemed best according to the judgment of its engineers and consultants. This situation led to some confusion and uncertainty, particularly with respect to just what values were taken as the reference level on the intensity scale to represent normal hearing. There was also some concern that the purchasers of audiometers should have assurance as to the accuracy of the frequency scale, stability of output with varying line voltages, and so on. In 1951, however, the American Standards Association issued a standard for audiometers for diagnostic purposes and in 1952 another for screening audiometers.

The American Standards Association is a voluntary association of manufacturers and consumers which has written standards for many branches of American industry. These standards are a convenience for all concerned and are regularly made the basis of specifications or procurement both by government and by industry. In the field of acoustics, for example, there is not only an American Standard Terminology but standard specifications for such items as the sound level meter, octave band filters, microphones, meters, and methods of sound measurement. The American Standards are revised from time to time to keep pace with technical progress and the state of the art, and at the present writing (1959) the standards for all audiometers are being reviewed and will presumably soon be combined into a single new American Standard.

The American Standards for Audiometers specify such features as the frequencies that are to be provided and the permissible limits of deviation. They require that certain features, such as a clickless interrupter switch, the headband, appropriate cushions for the receiver, be provided. They specify the variation in output that is permitted as the line voltage varies over considerable limits and they set limits of tolerance for the accuracy of the attenuator. Finally, they specify the sound pressure that must be produced at each frequency, measured in a standard "coupler," when the intensity dial of the audiometer is set to zero. Limits of tolerance for the pressure calibration are given also.

Another organization that assisted in the development of standards and specifications for audiometers was the Council on Physical Medicine of the American Medical Association through its Consultants on Audiometers and Hearing Aids. The consultants set forth certain minimal requirements and also certain additional recommendations for both audiometers and hearing aids and maintained for many years a program of so-called acceptance of instruments that met these requirements. Audiometers were accepted only after a sample of the model in question had been examined by an independent anonymous laboratory and certified as having met the published requirements. The requirements conformed in general to those of the American

Standards Association but were revised more frequently and therefore tended to represent a more advanced stage of thinking and practice than did the American Standards. By their recommendations the Consultants on Audiometers and Hearing Aids gave semiofficial guidance to the manufacturers as to the needs and desires of medically oriented users of their instruments.

The program of acceptance of audiometers and hearing aids by the Council on Physical Medicine is no longer in force. Its minimum requirements and recommendations are matters of record but they give no assurance that any particular model meets the requirements. Very recently, however, the Committee on Conservation of Hearing of the American Academy of Ophthalmology and Otolaryngology has established a Subcommittee on Audiometers. This committee announced in 1958 that it would "list" models of audiometers that were found by test, in independent but well-qualified laboratories, to meet the American Standards for Audiometers. This listing does not, of course, assure the purchaser that *every instrument* of that model necessarily meets all of the specifications quantitatively, but it assures him that the company in question has been able to produce such an instrument. The company at least has the necessary technical "know-how." This, after all, was the essence of acceptance by the Council on Physical Medicine, although the Council was also concerned with advertising claims. The listing by the Committee on Conservation of Hearing will amount substantially to a stamp of technical approval of the manufacturer. It should give useful backing to the voluntary cooperative effort represented by the American Standards Association.

The National Bureau of Standards has also cooperated in the development of the American Standard and it preserves the instruments on which the definition of the American zero level for audiometry rests. It serves as the final arbiter in any questions that may arise concerning the accuracy of calibration of new instruments in this country.

THE ZERO HEARING LEVEL

The pure-tone audiometer measures the deviation in decibels of a subject's threshold of hearing from an arbitrary standard chosen to represent "normal hearing" (see Chapter 2). The problem of intensity calibration of pure-tone audiometers is threefold. First, how is normal to be defined; second, what particular set of actual measurements or calculated figures should be chosen to represent the desired "normal hearing level"; and, third, how are manufacturers of audiometers in all countries to know what the values are, in engineering terms, to which their instruments should conform?

At the time this chapter is being written (1959) all of these questions are under discussion. An effort is being made to arrive at a set of *international zero reference levels for audiometry.* The desirability of an International Standard is as obvious as the desirability of a common system of weights and measures and a common language of scientific terminology, but that does not mean that an International Standard automatically comes into being. Most research laboratories in the United States use the metric system, but in everyday life the same scientists talk and think in terms of miles per hour, pounds per square inch, degrees Fahrenheit, and so on. And unfortunately, although American manufacturers and otologists agreed some years ago on an American Standard for Audiometers which includes a set of zero reference levels, the British have adopted a different set of levels; and European sentiment clearly favors the British rather than the American as the basis for the desired International Standard. The Japanese, on the other hand, have adopted a standard that is very close (within 3 db at all frequencies) to the American Standard.

The American Standard is based on data obtained in 1935–1936 in a field health survey conducted by the United States Public Health Service. The British Standard is based on tests conducted under laboratory conditions. Each type of data has been reproduced in corresponding studies carried out under similar conditions. The difference seems to depend on the rather casual approach that is usual in a clinical test versus a laboratory atmosphere with its higher motivation of the subjects. This whole problem of reference levels is discussed more fully in an addendum at the end of this chapter.

There are still minor international differences to be clarified that seem to depend on differences between the British and the American standard acoustic couplers and others that involve attempts to measure acoustic pressures under an earphone actually applied to the human ear, but the basic situation is that for twenty years America has been committed to a perfectly valid "clinical" standard while Great Britain, and perhaps by now other European countries as well, has adopted a very logical and highly reliable "laboratory" standard. It is not a matter of right or wrong or of error in measurement: it is a difference in point of view. And in the opinion of many it would be far better for everyone to adopt either one or the other or some arbitrary compromise between the two as an International Standard, in spite of the inconvenience of a period of change and readjustment, rather than to have two standards, according to which, for example, a hearing level of 20 db means a perfectly normal level in one country but a definitely abnormal level in another!

THE RANGE OF NORMAL LEVELS

Very few persons have audiograms that fall exactly on the zero line at all frequencies. Each person's audiogram has minor ups and downs that may be quite constant from test to test. Also, people differ in auditory sensitivity just as they do in height and weight. We have explained how the zero reference level was determined experimentally as the median or as the mode of a group of values. The individual thresholds scatter over a range of many decibels. In Figure 2-4 this range was illustrated by the indefinite shaded boundary of the auditory area.

The concept of a "range of normal" is very familiar to the physician but less so to the layman or even to the lawyer. Nevertheless, the physician's definition of "abnormal" is likely to be rather fuzzy and he hesitates to draw a sharp line at any one level and say, "Here is the limit. Anything beyond this is abnormal," because to him "abnormal" implies that something has gone wrong. It implies disease. The statistician, however, finds another way out. From the number and scatter of the original measurements that determine the zero level he can calculate the limits within which any given percentage of new cases can be expected to fall. One common convention is arbitrarily to take two "standard deviations" as the range of normal, which practically means that we agree to call the most deviant 2 per cent "abnormal" (without inquiring into cause) and to consider the other 98 per cent as "within normal limits." The situation is a little more complicated than here stated when, as with hearing, the deviations from the center of the group are greater in the direction of poorer hearing than of better hearing and "abnormality" lies only on the poorer side of center, but the principle should be clear, nevertheless. On this basis, hearing levels of 10 db (American Standard) for frequencies up to and including 2000 cps and of 15 db at 4000 cps and higher are definitely within normal limits. We shall return to these questions in Chapter 9. (See especially Figures 9-1 and 9-2.)

Incidentally, it was in very nearly this way that the limits of normal for the 4C Group Hearing Test, described below, were established. A small but definite percentage lay beyond the arbitrary cutoff point and these were therefore automatically considered "abnormal." It later came as a shock to some people to learn that calculations from the results of the test applied to New York school children showed that there must have been 3,000,000 hard-of-hearing children of school age in the United States. This result had been built into the test by statistical definition at the start.

The heart of the audiometer, from the engineer's point of view, is not the generator that determines frequency or the "attenuator" that varies the intensity, since these are now routine in the electronic art; it is the receiver, which converts the electrical into acoustical energy. It is not easy to design and construct an earphone that is reasonably efficient for all of the frequencies we wish to test and that will maintain its original efficiency year after year. And the operator is at the mercy of the earphone. If the earphone is put out of adjustment by accidentally falling on the floor, its loss of efficiency in generating the sound will be interpreted as a lack of efficiency of the ear in detecting the sound. The scale on the instrument does not actually measure the sound but only the electric current that generates it. The careful operator therefore periodically tests his own ear, and if the instrument says that his ear is losing its sensitivity, he tests other presumably normal ears. If most of them show the loss of sensitivity, it is fairly certain that the "calibration" of the audiometer is no longer correct.

CALIBRATION FOR BONE CONDUCTION

The bone-conduction receiver is more difficult to standardize than the air-conduction receiver, and bone-conduction tests are more difficult to carry out properly. Skulls and skin differ to an annoying degree in their ability to conduct sound, and the force with which the bone-conduction receiver is applied to the mastoid is important. Some audiologists prefer to apply it to the forehead instead. The ear not under test must be "masked" by noise delivered through an air-conduction receiver. The ear under test must be open to the room. This makes it more vulnerable to masking by room noise than an ear that is snugly covered by an air-conduction receiver. No satisfactory "artificial mastoid" corresponding to the National Bureau of Standards' "artificial ear" (the NBS-9A coupler) has been developed. There is no American Standard for zero hearing level by bone conduction. Each diagnostic audiometer has bone-conduction values painted on its dial, but the careful audiometrist should verify them with his own group of young adult normals just as his predecessors did in the 1920's and 1930's with the Western Electric 2A audiometer.

Figures 7-4 and 7-5 illustrate air-condition and bone-conduction audiograms, the limits of normal discussed above, and also the limits of measurement of an audiometer that just meets the American Standard for Audiometers for Diagnostic Purposes.

NOISE LEVELS IN AUDIOMETRIC BOOTHS

In all audiometric work it is assumed that the tests are carried out in a room which is quiet enough so that the background noise does not

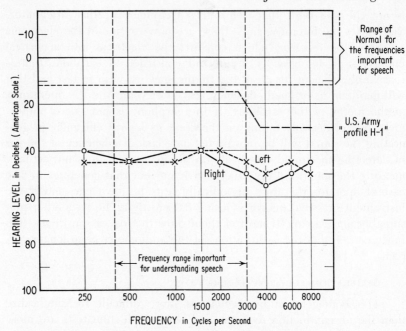

Fig. 7-4. This kind of "flat" audiogram may be produced by otitis media. Hearing by bone conduction (not shown) is presumably normal. The range of normal threshold levels for the frequencies 500 to 3000 cps extends from the lowest output on an audiometer nearly to the 15 db hearing level. The horizontal dashed line indicates approximately the limits of the United States Army "profile H-1" (see Chap. 9) defined as "15 db for average of 500, 1000, and 2000 cps, and 30 db at 4000 and 8000 cps." The range of normal is not sharply limited and is particularly vague below 500 cps and above 2000 cps.

interfere with the test. This is not a very difficult condition to meet if the patients are all very hard of hearing, as they are in a school for the deaf. If, however, we wish to measure normal or nearly normal hearing, special sound treatment for both the exclusion and the absorption of unwanted background noise is necessary. Prefabricated audiometric booths are now available commercially, and in general have proved more satisfactory than reconstruction of a room in an existing building. In a new building, however, acoustic engineers can design satisfactorily quiet rooms for audiometry at reasonable cost if they are consulted early enough in the planning. Sometimes the problem is very difficult for the acoustic engineer, as it is when the audiometric rooms must be located near washrooms, elevators, ventilating fans, or other machinery. The low frequencies are the most difficult and the most expensive to exclude.

The expense of a satisfactory booth will also depend critically on

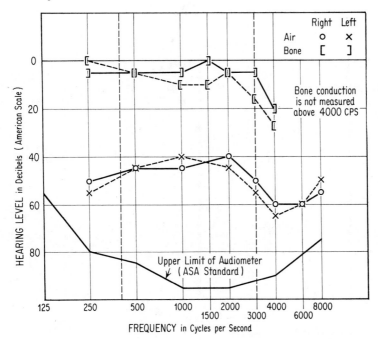

Fig. 7-5. These audiograms show the hearing levels in a hypothetical case of conductive hearing loss with a slight additional sensory-neural loss at 4000 cps. The upper lines show bone-conduction hearing levels within or close to normal limits. Middle lines show abnormal air-conduction hearing levels. Lowest line shows the minimum range of "pure-tone audiometers for diagnostic purposes," as specified in American Standard Z24.5-1951. The vertical dashed lines indicate the band of frequencies most important for understanding speech. The symbols for air and bone conduction are those of the International Code. In American usage, however, the brackets to the right and left (for bone conduction) are often reversed. Arrow heads (< and >) are often used instead of brackets. Universally, however, if color is used, red = right.

just what kind of audiometry is to be done in it. Are we content with measuring thresholds down to (but not below) the American Standard zero? Will an earphone always be over the ear under test or will we want to measure bone-conduction thresholds with an open ear canal? Do we want to measure thresholds at 125 and 250 cps for diagnostic purposes, or will we be content to start at 500 cps, as in monitoring audiometry, or will we only do single-frequency screening at 4000 cps?

Of course, the amount of sound treatment needed depends on the sound levels expected outside as well as on the permissible levels inside. The outside levels depend on local conditions, but for the guid-

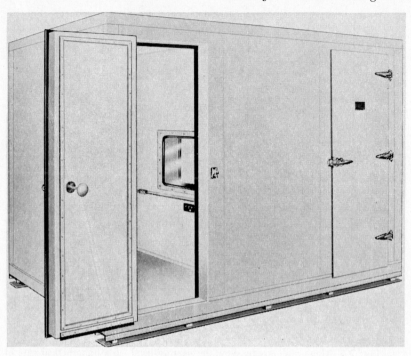

Fig. 7-6. Prefabricated sound-treated booths provide the quiet that is needed for accurate determination of auditory thresholds. The subject sits in a separate compartment from the tester. Both compartments are ventilated, but without raising the ambient noise level above the specifications of the American Standards Association. (*Industrial Acoustics Company, Inc.*)

ance of acoustic engineers an American Standard is now being prepared to tell what octave band sound levels are permissible in an audiometric booth if we are to measure zero hearing levels (American) using properly fitted earphones.

"PERCENTAGE OF HEARING"

The audiogram is an accurate and adequate description of our sensitivity of hearing, but for some purposes it is too analytical and gives us *too much* information. What we would like if we could get it, for purposes like the estimation of practical handicap, is a *single* measure of hearing. It would be very convenient if we could calculate, or measure directly, a "percentage of hearing" that a person has, just to be able to tell him how good his hearing is. Actually, a rule for this was proposed when the electric audiometer was first introduced. It amounted in principle to calculating what percentage of the normal speech area, shown in Figure 2-5, a person has. The hearing levels for 500, 1000, and 2000 cps were averaged. Then, because the total dynamic range of the speech area was 120 db (the range of the audiometer) and what was wanted was a *percentage,* the average level was multiplied by the fraction 100/120 or 5/6. Later this factor was simplified further to the decimal fraction 0.8. This is now the famous Fletcher "point eight" rule for calculating percentage of hearing or percentage of hearing loss. A modification of this rule still (1959) persists in the New York rule for calculating the compensation due for industrial hearing loss.

The phrase "percentage of hearing" is very confusing and should be dropped entirely. We should speak of either the "percentage of handicap" or else simply the "hearing level for speech." The rule for calculating the hearing level for speech from the hearing levels for the three pure tones is still a very good and useful rule. It is the "point eight" part and the concept of "percentage of hearing" that have proved unsatisfactory.

SPEECH AUDIOMETRY

The Fletcher "point eight" rule for the percentage of hearing was simple but arbitrary, and other rules giving different weights to various frequencies have been proposed. The differences of opinion concerning these rules stimulated the development of *speech audiometry* to measure the threshold for speech directly. The principle of speech audiometry was established by the success of the 4C group audiometers for screening school children, and during World War II a rather similar auditory test, using two-syllable words, was developed to provide quick screening for military purposes. The advantages of the single, quick speech test were several. For one thing, the test appeared obviously valid: it measured directly what people wanted to measure. This directness appealed alike to testers and to candidates for military service and to patients. They all *like* speech tests. And, in spite of the fluctuating and elusive physical character of speech, the speech tests for auditory threshold have proved to be very reliable. The test is quick. Above all, the result is a single number.

The principle of a *speech audiometer* is very simple. The test material is speech. Words or sentences may be spoken into a microphone ("live voice testing") or, better, they may be recorded in advance in standard form and at known levels on either magnetic tape or phonograph disc. In either case the speech signal becomes an alternating electric current. Its strength is varied by a calibrated attenuator. The listener may wear earphones or, sometimes, listen with both ears to a loud-speaker. The listener determines, not when he can just hear the voice sounds, but when he can *identify the words.* He may repeat the test words aloud, or check them on a multiple-choice list, or write them down, or perhaps, if the speech material is a set of questions, he may answer the questions. Usually we take the "50 per cent correct" level as the threshold. Or the subject may simply listen to the reading of some simple text and himself set the volume control so that he can just get the gist of what is being said. Of course, each form of test and each sample of speech material must be calibrated separately; that is, we must find the median (or modal) threshold for a reasonably large group of presumably normal listeners.

There are several difficulties with speech audiometry, some of which were immediately apparent while others were not. An obvious one is the problem of physical measurement of the intensity of the speech signal; others concern the choice of words or sentences, others the voice of the talker, and others the purpose of the test.

The problem of physical measurement has been adequately solved, even though measurement of speech is never as precise as measurement of pure tones, because the intensity of the sound-pattern of speech is continually changing. The usual convention is to take a sort of running average of the largest of the excursions of the meter as it swings in response to the syllables of the words. A particular kind of meter, the VU ("vee-you") meter, or "volume indicator," is used for this purpose. The term "volume" in electrical engineering is used to mean exactly this kind of measurement of electrical speech signals, and the dial on a radio or a hearing aid that controls the intensity (loudness) of the output is therefore known as the "volume control." If the talker has the meter in sight himself, he can adjust, or *monitor*, his speech to a chosen standard level. A practiced talker can hold such a general level of conversation, or repeat a given word, within a couple of decibels, which is quite sufficient for our purpose.

More disturbing is the realization that all words, spoken naturally and in sequence, do not have the same physical power. Here we adopt the convention that all the words are to be spoken with the same *effort*, and the monitoring is done only on the strongest syllables. If single words are used, they are introduced by the same carrier phrase or word, such as, "Say the word ———," or "Would you write ——— now." The talker monitors on the carrier and lets the test word come naturally without any extra emphasis. The carrier also serves to warn the listener that the test word is coming so that he is at attention.

But now the choice of material becomes important because all words are not equally intelligible even when carefully monitored. Some can be understood even when barely audible, whereas others must be at a much higher level before even a practiced listener can identify them correctly. Familiar words are more intelligible than the unfamiliar; words of many syllables are easier than monosyllables; and words with weak vowels and many high-pitched consonants, such as "thin" and "sift," are particularly difficult. A word is easier to identify if we know in advance that it is one of a limited list or is a certain kind of word than if it is just "any word."

Of course, it is much easier to recognize a word in context in a sentence than when it is heard alone. Everyone knows the difficulty there is with unfamiliar names or even with numbers when a telephone connection is poor. Therefore *word tests* and *sentence tests* must be standardized separately.

SPEECH THRESHOLD TESTS

If the test is intended to be simply a threshold test to measure the hearing level for speech the choice of the test material and the voice and inflections of the talker are not very important as long as they do not impose any great and unsual difficulty for the listener. A vocabulary beyond his level of education, a foreign language or a very unfamiliar dialect, or sentences so long that he can't remember all the words: obviously, these should be avoided. The absolute values in dynes per square centimeter will vary with the test chosen, but the hearing level of an individual, which is his deviation from the expected normal performance on that particular test, is very constant.

The threshold for speech or *speech reception threshold level* (SRT) may be measured with either words or sentences. Unless a patient is suffering from some form of sense-organ or central deafness or has a very high threshold for speech and a low threshold of tolerance for discomfort, he understands all the items correctly if the intensity is great enough. *If the listener does not understand all of the items correctly at the highest intensity, the test material is not suitable for him or else a threshold test may not be the proper kind of test to apply for the disorder that he has.* Most listeners hear correctly if the intensity is high enough, but as the intensity is reduced, mistakes begin. The level at which half of the items are correctly understood is usually taken as the end point, or "threshold." A rapid but reasonably accurate method is to adjust the volume of continuous speech, such as a simple text read from a book, until the listener can just easily follow the sense of what is being read. Such a continuous, even sample of simple, unemotional text is known in some laboratories as "cold running speech."

Probably most popular recorded threshold tests for speech are the word tests known as W-1 and W-2, prepared by Central Institute for the Deaf. They are direct developments from Auditory Test No. 9, standardized by the Psycho-Acoustic Laboratory of Harvard University for wartime use at the Army and Navy Aural Rehabilitation

Centers. The words are all familiar words of two syllables with equal stress on each syllable (*spondees*) such as "railroad" (see the Appendix). The very similar earlier test, used by the Western Electric Company in its 4C group audiometer, is a series of two-digit numbers, as, for example, "six four," "two three." Both lists have been recorded on phonograph discs, with the words in groups and each group weaker by a known number of decibels than the preceding group. Both lists have been carefully standardized, and the performance of normal ears for each of them is known. With either list properly administered, the *hearing level for speech* may be measured with at least the same precision and reliability that we attain with the pure-tone test of a clinical audiometer. This accuracy is possible because, as their volume is reduced, the words pass quite abruptly from intelligible words to a mere trace of speech sound. The words were selected for their uniform intelligibility by a laborious series of experiments. The use of several words in each group minimizes any errors introduced by a lucky guess or momentary inattention.

Slightly less but still satisfactory accuracy can be obtained by a trained talker reading the words into a microphone. Of course, he has his monitoring meter before him, and he adjusts the attenuator until the listener repeats half of the words correctly. Each talker must "calibrate" his own voice as well as the earphones (or loud-speaker and test room) by measuring the threshold of many normal listeners. The

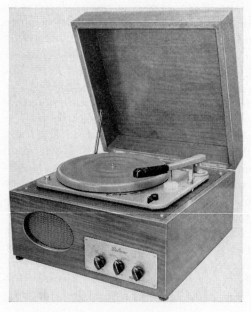

Fig. 7-7. A turntable is needed for recorded speech tests. (*Beltone Hearing Aid Co.*)

calibration cancels out the effects of the talker's particular voice and tricks of pronunciation.

Many *lists of sentences* as well as lists of words have been compiled for auditory tests of this sort. The most extensive and best known are the lists of the Bell Telephone Laboratories. They are framed as questions or directions to tell or explain something, and the listener either answers the question or repeats the sense of it. Sample sentences include the following:

> "What are some of the personal characteristics of the people of Japan?"
> "Is the Hudson River salt or fresh water?"
> "What punishment is inflicted upon a murderer in this state?"
> "Explain how Jersey milk is obtained in Ohio."

Many more of the Bell Telephone Laboratories' sentences as well as sentences and words of the other tests that will be mentioned are given in the Appendix. Long lists are necessary because the same sentence cannot be used twice with one listener. His memory makes it much easier for him to recognize a sentence again even from a single key word. Sentence tests are therefore not so suitable for phonographic recording, but they have the advantage of being more interesting to the listener.

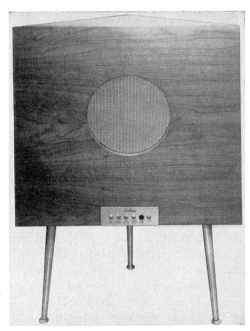

Fig. 7-8. A loud-speaker is used for free field tests and for the assessment of hearing aids. (*Beltone Hearing Aid Co.*)

The Bell Telephone Laboratories' sentences have been found to be too difficult in vocabulary and also to require too much local knowledge of New York City to be entirely satisfactory for general use elsewhere; other lists based on more limited vocabularies and special interests—the military, for example—have been used to good advantage. Some sentences from a simplified Psycho-Acoustic Laboratory list (see the Appendix), designed as questions to be answered by a single word, are

"Which is larger, a man or a mouse?"
"Can you burn your mouth with ice cream?"
"Does a cow have kittens or horns?"
"What month comes after February?"

In an effort to obtain more accurate scoring, still another list was developed in which each sentence contains five key words. The subject repeats the entire sentence, but only errors in the key words are counted. This is a special sort of "word in context" intelligibility, useful for research work. A few samples, with key words italicized, are

"*Clams* are *small, round, soft* and *tasty.*"
"*Sport* is *fun,* but *we need money.*"
"The *boat tipped* and the *fat lady screamed.*"
"It is a *shameful act* to *wipe* your *mouth* on a *sleeve.*"
"*Plug* the *leaky pipe* with a *wad* of *gum.*"

The hearing level for speech turns out to be the same whether it is measured with "cold running speech" or by simple sentences that are repeated back or by simple questions that are answered by a single word, or by repeating back the spondee words of tests W-1 and W-2, or by writing down the numbers of test 4C. It is the same for live voice and for recorded threshold tests. Evidently *these tests all measure the same thing:* if all have been correctly calibrated on similar normal populations, the hearing levels that they measure are all the same. At worst there will be a systematic difference of a very few decibels if the calibrations are not quite equivalent, but the results obtained with one test correlate very nearly as highly with those obtained with another as the results on one test correlate with repetitions of the same test.

The results of any of these tests of the threshold for speech are also very nearly the same as the values we obtain by taking the average of the hearing levels for 500, 1000, and 2000 cps. Only in cases of very irregular audiograms, such as an abrupt high-tone loss beginning near 2000 cycles, or in cases of sense-organ or central deafness do we find serious exceptions to this rule. Other rules, such as averaging the two lowest levels out of these three or giving different weights to the levels for different frequencies, have been proposed again and again, but the simple three-frequency rule first stated by Fletcher in 1929 is still as good a rule as any, and a very good rule, too.

The purpose of a threshold test of speech is fundamentally the same as that of the pure-tone audiogram. It differs in that it practically disregards frequencies below 400 and above 3000 cps and gives a single number for the hearing level of the band between. A speech test may be quicker and may hold the attention better than pure-tone tests. It is sometimes better adapted to group testing. It has special value as a supplement to and cross check on pure-tone testing. Inconsistencies between speech tests and pure-tone tests reveal errors in testing or strongly suggest psychological factors or certain types of sensory-neural loss. And it is very important practically to know that an elderly person, for example, *can* understand speech well at a tolerable level.

SPEECH DISCRIMINATION TESTS AND "ARTICULATION SCORES"

The two-syllable word test and the 4C two-digit test both measure a threshold for the hearing of speech, but the English language is not composed entirely of the easy words that are used in these two tests. The words in these tests were selected precisely because they are easy, and equally easy to understand. A reliable single index of hearing is obtained in this way, but the index does not give a comprehensive view of the way in which someone with impaired hearing understands langauge as a whole.

All the words in the English language are correctly heard by people with normal hearing in ordinary face-to-face conversation; otherwise, the words would not have crept into the language in the first place. But some speech sounds, and therefore the words in which they are used, have a much wider margin of safety than others; that is, some of them can be understood at a much lower volume than are others. (It will be recalled that by *volume* is meant the running average of the intensity of the strongest syllables in speech, and it is assumed that the weaker words and syllables are spoken with the same effort that is used in producing the stronger ones.) If we take a generous sample of English words and speak them one at a time in a "carrier phrase" that offers no context to help the listener to identify the word, we find that some words, which we may call the "difficult" words, require a volume of 25 db or more above the volume at which the first "easy" words are understood. By contrast, the lists of spondee words matched experimentally to be equally intelligible, go from first-word-intelligible to all-words-intelligible in a range of about 6 db.

It is not always realized that the intelligibility of various word lists is a matter of the way the talker utters the words quite as much as it is of the "phonemic composition" of the words. Of course, some sounds—the weak fricatives, such as "th," "f," and "v," for example— depend for recognition on high frequencies in speech, and in speech the high frequencies generally carry less energy than do the low frequencies. In the construction of many word lists much attention was given to including all the sounds (*phonemes*) of the English language and to including them in proper proportion. Actually the voice and enunciation (or "articulation") of the talker are just as important. To be sure, an ear with severe high-tone hearing loss will not hear the high frequencies in speech; but the careless talker may fail to put them in in the first place.

Actually, in ordinary conversation we probably fail to hear correctly and completely many of the difficult words, but we do not realize that we have missed them because we hear part of the word and the context gives us the rest. The context guides us in our choice among several possible words, any one of which we might have heard, just as it tells us which of several meanings of the same word, such as "run," "turn," "meat (meet)," or "so (sew)," is intended. Only when we come to unfamiliar proper names or something out of context do we realize that the speech to which we are listening is something less than 100 per cent intelligible.

We can describe someone's ability to hear speech by means of an *articulation curve*. This tells us what percentage of a specified list of words the listener can identify as the words are spoken to him louder and louder. Of course, we should keep the talker constant from test to test—and the only way to do this practically is to use recorded word lists. The basic idea of describing the understanding of speech by means of a curve instead of by a single index is no more complicated or subtle for the articulation curve than it is for the audiogram, although quantities that are related to one another (that is, the percentage of words correctly understood and their intensity) are different from the intensity and frequency that enter into the audiogram. And once we have a man's articulation curve, we can compare it with an average or normal articulation curve for that particular recording.

The term "articulation" has been used to designate tests in which the listener tells what syllable, word, or sentence he has heard. This use of the term was introduced by communication engineers who were primarily interested in telephone or radio transmission between a talker and a listener. In a later chapter the term "articulation" will be used in its original sense (as it is employed in phonetics) to indicate how well a talker forms his words. In forming the consonants and fricatives, the tongue, lips, teeth, and other parts of our vocal apparatus fit together, or "articulate," with one another like the bones in our joints. The meaning has become extended, however, because the engineers speak of the "good articulation" of a telephone circuit when they mean that it effectively transmits to the listener the articulation of the talker. The tests by which engineers measured the articulation of telephones were called "articulation tests," and now, when the same kinds of tests are used to study the defects of someone's hearing, they are still called "articulation tests." The usage makes sense if we think of the word as meaning *the listener's ability to benefit by someone else's articulation* of the words to which he is listening.

The best-known lists of words used for articulation tests are probably the *PB-50 Word Lists*. These are lists, fifty words each, of reasonably familiar monosyllables and were developed at the Psycho-Acoustic Laboratory at Harvard for wartime research on equipment for communication. Several complete lists are given in the Appendix. The abbreviation "PB" stands for "phonetically balanced." This means that nearly all the phonemes of the English language are represented in every list of fifty words. If only the initial consonants and the vowels are considered, the frequency of occurrence of the various sounds is fairly representative of English speech as a whole.

A rather similar set of fifty-word lists, using a somewhat smaller and more familiar vocabulary, was prepared at Central Institute for the Deaf. Two recordings of the CID lists have been made with different talkers. It so happened that one talker is highly intelligible, so intelligible in fact that the test has many of the properties of the spondee lists and does not give us much new information. The other talker clips his words so badly that some sounds are entirely missing by physical analysis and even the best listener makes a perfect score only with the help of some fortunate guesswork. This recording is too "difficult" to constitute a good standard.

We are still without a proper standard articulation test with normal values established for it. The administration of PB word lists by "live voice" is not satisfactory because talkers are not interchangeable. And even with the same talker the percentage of words correctly repeated at a given intensity level varies 5 or 10 per cent from trial to trial even if the full fifty-word lists are employed.

Nevertheless, certain generalizations can be made that are useful, assuming an "average talker." If a PB list (or any other list) is read too faintly, none of the words can be understood. As the voice becomes louder, more and more of the words are recognized, but even a normal listener does not make a score of 99 or 100 per cent on a PB list until the intensity is at least 25 db above the intensity at which he just recognizes one or two words. If lists are read at several different

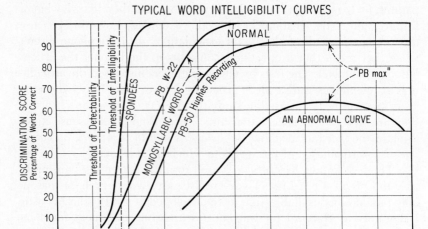

Fig. 7-9. The sound pressure level for speech tests is defined relative to 0.0002 dyne/cm² for the calibration tone (1000 cps) usually recorded on each disc. This meter reading for the calibration tone should match approximately the peaks reached by the VU meter during the carrier phrase.

The articulation curve for spondees rises more steeply than for monosyllables and is fairly constant from one talker or recording to another. The threshold of intelligibility is the sound pressure level at which 50 per cent of spondees are correctly repeated. The threshold of intelligibility for simple sentences and for connected discourse is practically the same as for spondees. This threshold is often called the "threshold for speech." For monosyllables, however, the steepness and position of the curve vary from one talker to another. For some talkers, even normal listeners do not show perfect discrimination scores. For some abnormal ears the articulation curve goes through a maximum and falls again at high speech levels. The plateau or maximum is called the "PB max."

intensities, say 10 db apart, the scores can be plotted, and an *articulation curve,* such as the one in Figure 7-9, can be drawn through the points. We know from thousands of experiments that the articulation curve is in general a smooth S-shaped curve that is steepest at or a little below its middle, and that at the upper end it levels off rather gradually to a plateau.

For normal ears under good listening conditions, the plateau of the articulation curve is at 100 per cent of words correctly understood; but if the words are heard through a communication system that does not transmit all the speech frequencies (or otherwise distorts the sounds), such as an inferior public-address installation, the curve may level off at some lower value, such as 70 or 80 per cent. This means that with such an inferior communication system some words are never correctly understood, no matter how loud the speaker talks or how much amplification is introduced in the system. Just so, *a man with severe high-tone nerve deafness will always fail to hear certain sounds and will never make a perfect articulation score.* On the other hand, the same man may hear *some* words, the easy low-frequency words, as well as anyone else does. He may have a normal *threshold* for speech.

It is a very convenient, although accidental, property of the PB lists that the volume at which 50 per cent of the PB words is correctly understood is a little above the level at which we can easily understand ordinary connected speech. It may seem remarkable that speech is readily understood when only about 50 per cent of isolated monosyllables can be identified separately; but that is the experimental result, both for normal and for hard-of-hearing listeners. In fact, if the connected speech is simple and deals with familiar material, it may be intelligible if the listener really pays attention at a level at which only about 15 per cent of the PB words can be correctly understood.

Practically, the most important thing we want to know about someone's hearing is whether or not he can follow ordinary conversation. Is his hearing *socially adequate?* If not, the position of the 50 per cent point on his PB articulation curve tells us how loud speech must be made (by a hearing aid) in order to make him socially adequate. (Of course, instead of using the PB lists, we can measure directly his threshold for "cold running speech," but the approximate equivalence of the threshold of intelligibility for ordinary connected speech with the 50 per cent score on the PB lists makes it unnecessary to perform the second test if we have already determined a PB articulation curve for other purposes.)

We have described the articulation curve in general and the PB lists in particular because they show us the fundamental relationship between the *intensity* of speech and its *intelligibility.* The position of an articulation curve on the intensity scale is primarily a measure of *auditory sensitivity,* a threshold. The height of the plateau that can be reached is a measure of *auditory discrimination,* that is, of how well difficult words are heard. For some abnormal ears the articulation curve not only reaches a plateau but actually goes through a maximum. Very loud speech is *less* intelligible than speech 10 or 15 db less intense.

The important concept here is that there are two independent properties of speech and hearing. One is intensity. Usually this dominates the situation, and the intensity determines completely (for a given recorded test and a given listener) what the score will be, and if we know the threshold for speech we can predict the rest. But this is not always true. Ears with the same threshold for speech may differ in the maximum percentage of test words they can hear correctly. To test this maximum, the words are given well above threshold. It is the maximum or the height of the plateau that is determined. This is sometimes called the *PB maximum.* A common cause for a PB maximum less than 95 per cent is high-tone hearing loss. Another is sense-organ hearing loss. Another is poor enunciation by the talker. Another is distortion of the speech signal by a poor hearing aid.

DIAGNOSTIC USE OF SPEECH TESTS

One purpose of speech tests of hearing is to verify pure-tone audiometry and detect errors and inconsistencies. The inconsistencies often show that the subject has *impairment of hearing that cannot be measured simply in decibels.* Psychogenic deafness, for example, may take the form of not hearing the human voice but accepting other sounds, or the voice may be heard but the "medical test" of pure tones may be rejected. The senile patient with phonemic regression does fairly well with tones but poorly with speech, and so does the patient with Ménière's disease. Aspects of hearing other than pure sensitivity are sampled by almost any speech test. The important common feature is that a person may have a difficulty in understanding words that is not explained by the faintness of the sounds. It is a mistake to try to measure this kind of difficulty by finding the threshold for one or another speech test. This would imply that there is some constant trading rule whereby the difficulty in question may be met by giving more decibels, but the point is that this is just what cannot be done. The patient hears but he may not understand, even when one shouts at him.

Sometimes the difficulty can be pinpointed a little more closely, and by varying the speech test—or, better, by varying his own voice—a good tester can find whether the difficulty is that the patient simply cannot keep pace with ordinary speech, or that his vocabulary is limited, or that his attention span or his memory span is defective, and so on.

The PB word lists have sometimes been used to assist in the diagnosis of sensory-neural high-tone hearing loss. This form of hearing loss make the hearing of some consonants difficult and the "PB maximum" score is depressed. Unfortunately, however, the words must be rather poorly spoken to make the test difficult enough for this purpose. For example, the Rush Hughes version of the CID recordings of the PB lists seems to be difficult enough for this purpose but the Hirsh recording of the same words is too easy. Here, as in many other situations, a task must be found which the normal person can only just accomplish if it is to separate out those who are slightly but only slightly abnormal.

SOCIAL ADEQUACY OF HEARING

Speech tests may be used to find out how well a person gets along in a practical way with hearing that is not entirely normal. Does he "get by" on the average in everyday situations or does he have some practical handicap? This is the concept of *social adequacy of hearing*. We do not really need all the hearing that a healthy young person has. Speech is perfectly intelligible even when all frequencies above 5000 cps have been filtered out, and it requires careful testing to show that it is less intelligible with only frequencies below 3000 cps remaining. (Ordinary words are not difficult enough to demonstrate the contribution of 4000 cps. The difference shows up much better with nonsense syllables, such as have been used by the Bell Telephone Laboratories in their study of the design requirements of a good telephone.) Also, we can do without frequencies below 400 cps perfectly well. Of course, music now sounds as if it were being played on an old hand-wound phonograph that does not have a big bass or a hi-fi treble; but speech is still good telephone speech. And we don't need all our sensitivity of hearing. Rarely do we listen at threshold. Usually when we don't hear something it is not because the sound is too faint but because some louder sound masks it out.

Otologists have been well aware of the concept of "social hearing." They know that a high-tone hearing loss at 4000 cps and above does not really impair listening except for hi-fi music; and there is so much noise in everyday living that a hearing level for speech of 20 db is considered perfectly adequate and an excellent result for a fenestration operation. Even up to 30 db hearing level for speech a person can "get by," most but not all the time, and then only with some difficulty. Above the 30 db hearing level for speech he definitely needs help, enough to have an operation or put on a hearing aid.

We shall return to this subject in Chapter 9. The point being made here is that although the broad idea of social adequacy of hearing is quite apparent, we do not have a clear measure of it. The best we can do is to say that everyday conditions of living and of listening vary from person to person and from hour to hour. On the average we hear speech at about 65 to 70 db *SPL* (sound pressure level) over all, but sometimes it is down to 45 db and sometimes, as in a noisy subway or at a cocktail party, it is as high as 90 db at our ears. A man with a conductive hearing loss who has a hearing level for speech of 35 db does beautifully at the cocktail party but may hear nothing at a lecture or in church. With effort, he might be able to "get by" with everyday conversation about half of the time. If his hearing level is up to 45 db he probably will hear only in noisy places or when people really speak up for him, perhaps a third or a quarter of the time. People begin to leave him out of the conversation, or he must rely on speech-reading. His hearing is now about at the threshold of social adequacy.

Speech tests are rather convenient for getting the hearing level for speech and for verifying whether a person really can understand loud speech when he hears it. An effort was made to extend the idea of social adequacy of hearing and make it more precise by measuring the threshold for speech and also by obtaining the best articulation score the person could get on a PB word list (the PB maximum score). The two scores determined a "social adequacy index for hearing." Failure of either sensitivity (high threshold) or discrimination (low articulation score) reduced the index below the threshold of social adequacy.

Actually, the idea has not worked out very well. One reason is that the PB recordings never have been standardized well enough to measure a man's discrimination with anything like the accuracy that we measure his threshold level. Also, we do not yet seem to know quite enough about the relation of the hearing and understanding of connected speech in words and sentences to its component frequencies, phonemes, and syllables. Speech is a very dynamic, variable affair and we can define it only in broad statistical terms or in terms of word- and sound-patterns that have not yet been standardized. But this brief discussion of the "social adequacy index of hearing" brings out the point that hearing for speech has at least two independent dimensions: sensitivity (threshold measurement) and discrimination (maximum articulation score). Probably another dimension related to the possible *speed* of understanding should be added, and perhaps still others. The dimension of sensitivity we understand fairly well. This is the dimension in which the hearing aid assists us. The other dimensions are more obscure.

In summary, speech tests have three possible clinical uses that require different forms of test. One is to measure a threshold for speech. For this the spondee word lists were developed and they have proved very satisfactory. Another use is to measure discriminaton, for diagnostic purposes. Here speech is merely a particular kind of auditory stimulus whose necessary properties we are not yet able to specify. The third use is the direct assessment of social adequacy of hearing. Here speech is used in its practical everyday aspect as a means of communication, and both threshold and discrimination are involved. The particular tests of the ability to receive auditory communication still need to be validated in the field.

TESTS OF HEARING FOR LOUD SOUNDS

The upper part of an articulation curve, where the words are heard at high intensities, lies in the upper part of the "auditory area" (Figure

2-5) that is not explored by the audiometer. The audiometer, it has been aptly said, only tells us what we *cannot* hear. More and more, the newer auditory tests have been directed toward discovering *how well we hear at intensities well above threshold* in the middle and upper parts of the auditory area that we customarily use. It is possible to explore the area with pure tones as well as by speech. One pure tone can be matched with another for equal *loudness* or for equal *pitch*. The equal-loudness curves shown in Figures 2-3 and 2-4 represent the results of this sort of matching for loudness. And in Chapter 3 it was pointed out that in nerve deafness the equal-loudness curves in the upper part of the auditory area remain relatively normal, even when the threshold and the lower contours are considerably elevated.

A phenomenon known as *recruitment* has attracted much attention in recent years, partly because it promises to distinguish sense-organ deafness from neural deafness. Many audiologists go so far as to equate recruitment with impairment of the sense organ instead of reserving the term, as one should, for a particular anomaly in the way the ear hears loud sounds.

In Figure 7-10 are represented the auditory area and the speech area for a pure conductive hearing loss, as discussed in previous sections. Figure 7-11 shows the same areas as they might be in a case of sensory-neural hearing loss. An important difference is that in conductive loss the entire auditory area is elevated, except perhaps for the threshold of pain and tickle. (These *may* be elevated also.) For sensory-neural loss the thresholds of pain and tickle and also the threshold of discomfort and the topmost equal-loudness contours all remain normal. Very strong sounds may be as loud and as uncomfortable in such an ear as in a normal ear. If the hearing loss is only in one ear it is easy to make direct comparisons and to plot the "loudness balance" between the two ears at different frequencies and at different sound levels. Of course, at a given level near threshold a sound will be very faint in the abnormal ear but fairly loud in the normal ear. However, as shown in Figures 8-1 and 8-2, the loudness increases more in the abnormal ear for each 10 db increase in level until the two ears hear the *same* loudness at 100 or perhaps 120 db. This abnormally rapid increase in loudness is *recruitment*. The term should mean this and nothing more.

Actually the test for recruitment by loudness balance is now a routine test in diagnostic audiometry, but it is difficult to carry out if both ears are abnormal! For this reason many other tests have been suggested to detect the abnormality of the sense organ that is responsible for it.

The *difference limen for loudness* is one such "test for recruitment." For many years it was assumed on a theoretical basis that if

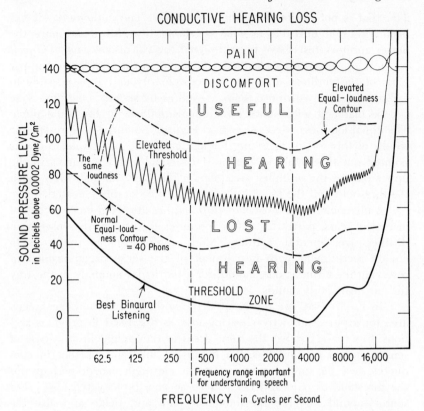

CONDUCTIVE HEARING LOSS

FREQUENCY in Cycles per Second

Fig. 7-10. **Reduced auditory area in pure conductive hearing loss.** The normal threshold zone and threshold for pain are shown as in Fig. 2-4. The threshold for pain is uncertain above 4000 cps. The elevated threshold represents a hearing loss of about 60 db at all frequencies, a so-called "flat" loss, produced by a severe but purely conductive lesion such as otosclerosis. This is the greatest possible purely conductive loss. The case is theoretical, because a conductive hearing loss is rarely perfectly flat, and usually there is some high-tone sensory-neural loss associated with it. The equal-loudness contours are raised without distortion. Nothing sounds very loud. The high equal-loudness contours have been elevated above the threshold of pain. The threshold of pain is not elevated, although the zone of discomfort may rise somewhat. The elevated threshold is a monaural free-field threshold. It is represented as a zigzag line that can be interpreted as showing the individual variability in successive measurements or else as the tracing that might be shown on a recording patient-controlled (Békésy) audiometer as in Fig. 7-12.

there is more increase of loudness per decibel, then the ear should be able to detect a smaller change in intensity than normal. Unfortunately, however, this does not seem to be the case. The "loudness limen" test is not very successful.

More abrupt crossing of threshold, resulting in very precise, confident, and reliable judgments of threshold, seems at first glance to be merely a special case of the loudness limen, distinguishing in this instance the first step in loudness. This test works much better, however, and it is carried out automatically if one uses a recording audiometer of the Békésy type.

Failure of auditory discrimination for words is a common symptom of sense-organ and sometimes neural impairment. This causes very low articulation (PB maximum) scores, perhaps 10 per cent correct as opposed to 75 per cent or more in simple neural high-tone hearing loss. This failure to recognize words is likely to be associated with diplacusis, or false sense of pitch, which was described in Chapter 3.

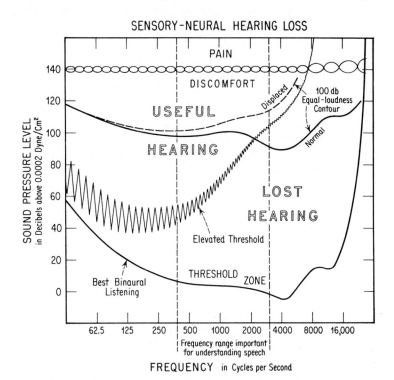

Fig. 7-11. **Reduced auditory area in a hypothetical case of sensory-neural hearing loss.** The normal free field, binaural threshold zone, and the threshold for pain are shown as in Fig. 2-4. The threshold for pain is uncertain above 4000 cps. The hearing loss is of the "gradual" high-tone type and is accompanied by strong "recruitment." The 100 db equal-loudness contour is distorted but is only slightly displaced upward. High-level sounds are nearly as loud as for a normal ear. The threshold of discomfort is unchanged. The zigzag line, representing the elevated threshold as it might be shown by a patient-controlled (Békésy) type of automatic audiometer, covers a wide zone of uncertainty at low frequencies but a very narrow zone where the hearing levels are elevated and recruitment is present.

There may be an abnormal noisy quality heard instead of the pure musical tone. The patient is likely to complain of these effects, but no quantitative tests for them have been systematized. It may be more accurate to speak of these abnormalities of hearing as "symptoms" rather than "signs" or "tests." We shall return to the subject of recruitment in Chapter 8.

AUDITORY DISCRIMINATION IN NOISE

The measurement of auditory thresholds by the audiometer is a measure of simple sensitivity of the ear. The listener merely reports that he hears something. He does not try to distinguish the test tone from any other tone or noise. But nearly all of our actual everyday listening is to much louder sounds, and we are usually interested in recognizing a particular sound or set of sounds against a background of many others. This is called "auditory discrimination." The simplest form of auditory discrimination is the detection of a difference in the pitch or in the loudness of two sounds heard one after the other. We must distinguish between the mere ability to *detect* a faint sound, and the ability to *discriminate* between two sounds that may be quite loud. There is no necessary relation between the two abilities. A man with very keen, sensitive ears may discriminate poorly. He may be a poor listener on a submarine detecting device, for example, where the task is to *recognize* the various underwater sounds. Quite dramatic, on the other hand, is the occurrence of outstanding ability to discriminate in a man who is so hard of hearing that he needs a hearing aid in everyday life. Such a man may perfectly understand speech over the radio or the intercommunicating system of a noisy airplane. Here, where both the noise and the speech that he discriminates from the noise are very loud, his lack of sensitivity is no handicap. His native ability in discrimination, reinforced perhaps by his experience in listening carefully and in making the most of the small differences in what he actually does hear, comes into full play.

Men differ in their native ability to discriminate sounds just as they differ in height, in steadiness of hand, or in visual acuity. For special military assignments, such as radio communication in aircraft or sonar listening, it is sometimes important to recognize ability to hear well in noise. The differences are not wiped out by training. The point is that *in order to measure differences in the ability to understand speech in the presence of noise or to recognize sonar signals, we must test that ability directly with an appropriate test and not with a test that is irrelevant,* like audiometry. A proper kind of test for discrimination is one in which a standard background noise is kept at a constant intensity while speech, heard along with the noise, is varied in intensity. A good measure of discrimination is the maximum score that can be obtained with the PB words, that is, the plateau of the articulation curve, either with or without a standard background of noise.

AUDITORY TRAINING

In the course of auditory training given to new users of hearing aids (described in Chapter 10), practice in auditory discrimination plays a very important part. Some of this training consists of listening to speech in the presence of noise, and some in discriminating between words that sound almost, but not quite, alike. Many lists of paired words were prepared at the Army and Navy Aural Rehabilitation Centers and were used both for drill and for test purposes. The following sample, from the Auricular Training Department of the Deshon General Hospital, is designed for practice on the difference between *m* and *n*. One word of each pair is read by the instructor, and the student checks off the word he thinks he heard:

mine-nine	dime-dine
mew-knew	dumb-done
time-tine	loam-loan

Tests of this sort have been employed in the selection of hearing aids, and they have a certain degree of merit. We must not, however, fall into the error of thinking that there is some special magic in the particular words or sounds that are used and forget about their loudness. *Unless the loudness is controlled, such a test of discrimination is worthless as a test, however useful it may still be for practice.*

The use of pairs of words for on-the-spot trial of hearing aids brings us around the complete circle back to the spoken voice and the whispered voice tests mentioned at the beginning of this chapter. All such voice tests are good in their place as crude tests. They are better than no test at all, but they are accurate only to the degree that they are standardized, to the degree that the loudness of the voice is controlled, or monitored, and to the degree that undesired noise and echo are eliminated from the surroundings.

TESTS OF TOLERANCE

The sensations of discomfort, of tickling in the ear, and of pain that are produced by very loud sounds have already been mentioned in Chapter 2 in the description of the auditory area. Here again, individuals differ as to the intensities of sound that merely cause discomfort, tickle, and pain. There seem to be tough ears and tender ears, or, rather, tough men and tender men. (Women, by the way, seem to be just as tough as men in this respect.) The man with one tough ear usually has another tough ear on the other side of his head. This toughness can be increased by simply listening to loud sounds for a while, even if the sounds are never made so loud as to tickle or become definitely uncomfortable. The increase in tolerance is likely to be greatest if the ear is unusually tender to begin with.

A test for tolerance is very simple in principle. It is like an audiometer or a speech test except that very loud sounds are used. Special apparatus may be required to make the sounds loud enough without distortion. The intensity is increased gradually until the listener indicates that he has had enough. Such tests are very useful in deciding how powerful a hearing aid a man should wear, for, as we shall see, there are definite advantages in using a hearing aid whose output can come close to, but which never quite reaches, the threshold of real discomfort. Any such test, however, must be conducted with care, particularly on anyone with impaired hearing who has not yet become once more accustomed to hearing loud sounds. He may be startled, antagonized, or even frightened if the sound is made too loud too rapidly.

It was surprising to learn through a series of wartime experiments conducted at the Central Institute for the Deaf that the tolerance thresholds of the hard of hearing are on the average the same as those of normal ears. The hard of hearing may scatter a little more widely above and below the average, with some ears more tender and some tougher than the usual run of normal ears, but the differences are much smaller than had been expected.

Types of Audiometry

There are several types and varieties of audiometry that depend on differences in the type of test employed, the purpose for which it is done, the number of subjects tested at once, and so on. We have actually mentioned many of these distinctions but it is useful to list them systematically.

NATURE OF INSTRUMENT AND TEST MATERIAL

The important distinction here is between *pure-tone audiometry* and *speech audiometry*. These are both carried out with standardized electric audiometers. (The spoken voice test, the whispered voice test, and the coin click test are usually spoken of as special "tests" rather than as "audiometry." It would be perfectly proper to speak of "tuning fork audiometry," but in common usage "audiometry" implies an electric audiometer.)

GROUP VS. INDIVIDUAL AUDIOMETRY

Most audiometry is done with one subject at a time. This is *individual audiometry.* The Western Electric 4C audiometer, however, was designed for use in schoolrooms and could test as many as forty children at once. Group audiometers have also been tried experimentally in several military laboratories. Group audiometers offer certain obvious advantages for screening audiometry, which undertakes to screen out only those few who need more elaborate testing.

In the Western Electric 4C audiometer a magnetic phonograph pickup (without amplifier) delivers its output to a set of as many as forty calibrated headphones. The words, actually two-digit numbers, are recorded on the disc in groups at successively lower intensity, and no adjustments are needed. The children write the numbers they hear on previously prepared blanks, which simplify the scoring. The practical problems of administration of the test and the results of its use will be considered in Chapter 17 on hard-of-hearing children.

Any test that requires much writing, even of single words, such as "railroad" or "blackboard," may become a test of the ability to write rapidly or to spell adequately, rather than a test of hearing. In a group test, if the pace is set slow enough for the laggards, the quick ones may become bored and inattentive while waiting for the next word. To meet some of these difficulties the Psycho-Acoustic Laboratory prepared charts with a series of letters or simple diagrams. The test sentences were in the form of instructions to the subject, such as "Draw a circle around the small *a*" or "Cross out the right-hand number." Because the execution and the scoring of the performance are quick and easy, this form of test offers attractive possibilities for group testing with sentences.

Of course, there is no reason why pure tones cannot be recorded like words on a phonograph disc at successively lower intensities and used in a group audiometer for screening purposes. The test tones may be recorded as a series of one to five brief "beeps" or "pips," and the subject may indicate that he has heard them by simply noting on his prepared blank how many "beeps" he hears each time. Such a pure-tone group audiometer was developed and tried for screening audiometry in Armed Forces examining stations. It incorporated several interesting features, such as testing both ears at once, with the signal sometimes appearing in the right and sometimes in the left earphone. The principles involved were approved by a CHABA working group, but the particular instrument has not been generally adopted.

AUTOMATIC AUDIOMETRY

Probably the first automatic audiometer was the instrument developed by Békésy in 1947. This instrument introduced the novel feature of control of intensity by the subject, combined with graphic recording of his adjustments. The frequency of the test tone is automatically increased, slowly and steadily, as the audiogram chart advances under the recording pen. The patient presses a button when he hears the tone. The intensity of the signal is gradually reduced as long as the button is held down. When the subject no longer hears the tone he releases the button. The signal becomes stronger and

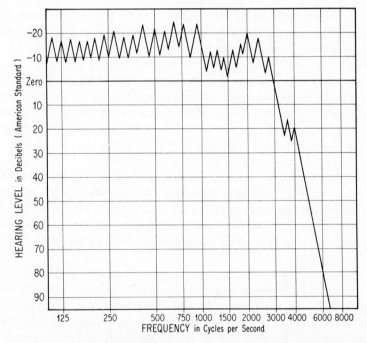

Fig. 7-12. **Audiogram produced by an automatic patient-controlled (Békésy type) audiometer (Grason-Stadler Co., Type E-800).** The instrument traces a red line for the right ear, a blue line for the left ear. The chart moved steadily to the left as the frequency of the test tone changed continuously. The pen moved up or down at a rate of 5 db per second. The direction of movement of the pen was upward (less intense) as long as the patient held his switch closed ("I hear the tone") but was downward (more intense) when the switch was open ("Don't hear the tone"). The subject for this test has an abrupt high-frequency sensory-neural hearing loss beginning just below 3000 cps. He hears nothing at 6000 cps or above. There was a small but significant amount of ambient noise below about 300 cps during this test.

stronger until the subject presses the button again. Thus the pen zig-zags up and down across the chart, reversing its direction each time the button is pressed or released. Usually there is an interval of five to ten decibels between the pressing (hears) and release (does not hear) of the button, but, as we have mentioned above, this range becomes very narrow in an ear that shows loudness recruitment.

The Békésy audiometer has been put to use in many research laboratories and in a number of hearing centers. It has yielded a vast amount of new experimental information on such topics as masking and auditory fatigue. Its accuracy is comparable with clinical pure-tone audiometry. Automatic and semiautomatic audiometers will probably be recognized in the next American Standard for Audiometers, which is now (1959) in preparation.

The military requirements for testing the hearing of many men, whether at induction or at discharge or in monitoring programs for conservation of hearing, have led to the development of several types of group audiometer and also of several automatic and semiautomatic audiometers, both group and individual. The various accomplishments of the different types of audiometer have become somewhat confusing. The problems of military audiometry, among others, were discussed at the annual meeting of the Armed Forces–National Research Council

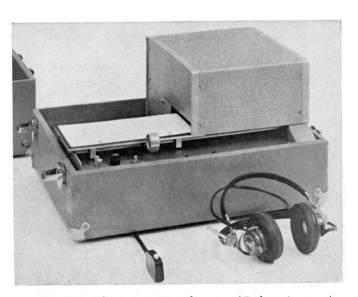

Fig. 7-13. This automatic audiometer (*Rudmose*) uses the patient-control principle to test hearing at six frequencies in each ear. It does not require an operator except to start the machine. (*Maico Electronics, Inc.*)

Committee on Hearing and Bio-Acoustics (CHABA) in 1955. The summary there presented of automatic audiometry is still valid, and we quote it herewith:

> There seems to be some danger that the term automatic audiometry will come to be identified solely with one particular type of automatic audiometer. This is the type in which the subject, by his own responses, controls the intensity of the machine's output. Such an identification should not be allowed to occur, for there are many types of automatic audiometers.
>
> Among the automatic audiometers now in operation are the following:
>
> 1. *The Békésy audiometer.* This has been in operation for several years in many laboratories and clinics. It is the typical "patient-control-of-intensity" instrument. A graph of the crossing and re-crossing of the subject's threshold is drawn by the machine as the frequency is slowly but gradually increased. This graph has the disadvantage that it does not yield numbers directly, but must be interpreted.
>
> 2. *The Rudmose audiometer.* This is a patient-controlled machine, as [is] the Békésy, which employs six discrete frequencies instead of continuously increasing frequency.
>
> 3. *The Brogan audiometer.* This patient-controlled machine, developed at the Air Force School of Aviation Medicine, is one in which the program and patient response is the same as the conventional clinical audiometer. The audiogram is typed on a sheet or punched on an IBM card.
>
> 4. *The Licklider audiometer.* This is a patient-controlled instrument in which the subject identifies in which half of a period of time the test tone was present.
>
> 5. *The Ward audiometer.* This is a pulsing-tone type of group audiometer developed at the Naval School of Aviation Medicine and the Central Institute for the Deaf. Ten men are tested at a time by the method of single descent, using a single attenuator.
>
> 6. *The Glorig audiometer.* Developed at the Speech and Audiology Center at Forest Glen under the combined auspices of the Army and the Veterans Administration, this machine presents tone pulses in groups, part of the pulses to one ear and part to the other. The subject must count the number of pulses in each group.
>
> 7. *Navy audiometers.* Three of these have been developed, all more or less automatic, at the Submarine School in New London, the U.S. Navy Electronics Laboratory in San Diego and the Philadelphia Naval Hospital. In the first two, emphasis was on the group-test aspect and in the latter, automatic administration was the goal.

The audiometer that gives the lowest thresholds is not necessarily the best. Of greater importance is the reliability of the method, i.e., its ability to give the same value on successive trials. The relation between the test values and the audiometric zero given in the American Standard can always be determined experimentally. A second important feature is the amount of maintenance or "down time." The original cost of the machine may also be a determining factor. A final, important consideration is how easily a malingerer can "beat the game" with the machine.

After the objective of the audiometric testing has been determined and carefully specified, a selection should be made between group testing in a large, semipartitioned room and testing in separate booths. In designing the machine, the subjects to be tested must be considered from the point of view of human engineering. In order to get the full cooperation of the subjects, the machine must be quite easy to operate. It must also be sufficiently reliable to remain in calibration and operate with a minimum of technical servicing.

If more than 40 men are to be tested at a time, group tests with scored sheets are probably the method of choice. For between 10 and 40, some other type of group audiometer, possibly the Ward type modified to print the results on a sheet or tape, may prove to be the best compromise. For 10 subjects or less, successive testing with individual instruments such as the Brogan or Rudmose may allow the procedure to be made more completely automatic and still more economical.

PURPOSES AND OBJECTIVES

The CHABA Council published, as part of the report of the meeting of 1955, a summary of the purposes and objectives of audiometry in the Armed Forces. The problems are the same as for audiometry in industry. In this summary "monitoring audiometry" was first formally defined. The summary is an authoritative official expression of opinion, and we therefore quote the entire section in full:

PURPOSES AND OBJECTIVES OF AUDIOMETRY

The purposes and objectives of audiometry in the Armed Forces, including their civilian employees, fall into five major categories:

1. to select or reject men as a part of the regular initial physical examination;
2. to provide information for the otologist concerning the extent and nature, the probable cause, and the progress of individual hearing losses in relation to the disease and to the effectiveness of treatment and preventive measures;
3. to establish the amount of hearing loss for compensation purposes, including the determination of the original state of hearing before any service-connected or employment-connected hearing loss has developed;
4. to enable personnel officers to determine whether certain in-

dividuals are qualified for certain military specialties that involve special kinds of hearing ability;

5. to obtain new information as to (a) the causes and the prevention of hearing loss; (b) criteria for hazards to hearing; and (c) the effectiveness of particular tests and instruments for accomplishing the above objectives.

A clear distinction must be made between: (1) the kind of hearing test; (2) the way in which the test is administered; and (3) the particular instrument or technical means that embodies both the chosen test and the chosen method of administration. Not all types of hearing test will suit all of these purposes equally well. There is at the present time no single "best" test of hearing, and much less is there any single "best" instrument for administering hearing tests in all situations. The kind of test best suited for each purpose will depend upon the kind of information that must be obtained from the test.

For example, the most generally useful kind of hearing test is pure-tone threshold audiometry by air conduction. This was developed originally for diagnostic medical purposes and is also well suited for screening at induction centers, for monitoring hearing conservation programs, for estimating disablement and appropriate compensation, and for many types of medical research. Another kind of hearing test is speech audiometry, including tests of ability to hear speech in noise. These special tests are appropriate for determining special hearing abilities needed in particular military specialties.

It is assumed that a pure-tone test of hearing is desired. There are a number of ways in which pure-tone tests can be administered, each with its advantages and disadvantages. Furthermore, the different choices are not all mutually exclusive, but can be combined in many ways, just as an aircraft can be designed for combat, transport or reconnaissance, may be large or small, may be piloted or a robot drone, and may be powered by reciprocating, jet or turbo-prop engines.

Among methods and types of pure-tone audiometry there are major choices that must be made between: (1) screening audiometry *vs.* monitoring audiometry *vs.* diagnostic audiometry, which implies a choice between a pass-fail test, a limited audiogram, or medically-oriented audiometry including complete audiograms; (2) individual audiometry *vs.* group audiometry; and (3) manual *vs.* semiautomatic or fully automatic audiometry.

As to the means of embodying the chosen type and method in an actual instrument there are several choices at the engineering level, such as between electronic oscillators *vs.* tests recorded on discs or magnetic tape. The various choices listed above are more or less independent but, just as in the cases of aircraft, certain useful combinations are already well established. Audiometry was developed as a medical tool to assist in diagnosis and for this purpose the complete audiogram individually administered is universally employed. Further-more, nearly all audiometers for diagnostic audiometry are manually operated and contain electronic oscillators. Semiautomatic record-ing audiometers for diagnostic purposes are under development, how-ever, and may soon prove to be a useful supplementary tool in certain situations. The medical interest in diagnostic audiometry seems to lie in the development of new audiometric tests, rather than in new ways to facilitate the administration of pure-tone threshold audiometry.

For audiometry, as for aircraft, the choice of purpose is primary and the way of accomplishing the purpose depends on a balance of many factors, which include expense, personnel, and the availability of a particular instrument of established merit. The development of a means or instrument may make feasible a method that was pre-viously not possible or practical. Such development is often an essential step, but a careful review of both old methods and new developments is mandatory before commitment is made on a large scale. There have been important recent developments in pure-tone audiometry for survey, monitoring, compensation and particularly for screening purposes. Such large-scale audiometry as is obviously required by the Armed Forces should be greatly facilitated by such new methods and instruments for group and individual pure-tone audiometry, both automatic and semiautomatic.

New methods and instruments alone will not insure good audi-ometry. Three other requirements are absolutely essential for *all* forms of audiometry. They are: (1) adequate acoustic environment, which means specially sound proofed, properly located booths and/or rooms to house the instruments and subjects; (2) trained personnel to administer the tests or to service any automatic devices that may replace the trained audiometrist; and (3) provision, both instru-mentally and administratively, for periodic verification of the accuracy of audiometers in the field.

The uncertainties as to what are the best methods of audiometry for the Armed Forces appear to arise from the interplay of several factors. The most important factor is the recent laudable trend to-ward pure-tone audiometry as a required test of hearing to replace the out-moded voice and coin-click tests. The trend establishes a demand for audiometry on a large scale, but for audiometry that is quite different from the elaborate diagnostic audiometry that has for some time been employed as an adjunct to a medical specialty. Yet the concepts and the instruments for audiometry were developed for just these medical diagnostic purposes.

More recently screening audiometry, and group audiometry as a way of performing such screening, has been developed. Screen-ing audiometry arose as a part of preventive medicine with particular orientation to the conservation of hearing in school children. The ob-jective here was to identify rapidly those children who require closer examination and perhaps medical treatment. Such audiometry is roughly equivalent to the old voice tests and it has been rather taken for granted that it is the most appropriate type of audiometry for induction centers where a quick pass-or-fail test of hearing adequacy is the primary requirement. Screening audiometry, like diagnostic audiometry, is now a familiar and well-established concept.

An intermediate type of audiometry that we here term "monitoring audiometry" has more recently been developed in connection with conservation of hearing programs in industry. Its objectives are two-fold. One is to establish the state of hearing of a relatively large number of individuals and to provide reference audiograms from which subsequent changes in their hearing are measured. The reference audiograms, particularly if they are pre-employment or so-called pre-placement audiograms, may be used to determine subsequent liability for later changes in hearing in connection with workmen's compensation. Its other objective is to detect changes in the hearing of individuals, relative to their reference audiograms, before the hearing losses become a practical handicap. Monitoring audiometry thus gives warning in time for instituting effective protective measures, such as the reduction of the noise itself, the reduction of the noise exposure of the individual or the use of individual protective measures.

Monitoring audiometry is more restricted than diagnostic audi-ometry. Only air-conduction tests are required for monitoring audi-ometry and a more restricted range of frequencies and intensities [is] sufficient. It differs from screening audiometry, however, in that it must measure auditory acuity and not merely give a pass-or-fail result. Usually, within the range that it covers, it must yield an audiogram comparable in accuracy with a diagnostic audiogram. The restricted range of a monitoring audiometer favors the development of group and of automatic or semiautomatic methods of administra-tion. On the other hand, the necessity for accuracy and for an audio-gram that is complete within the chosen range imposes serious difficulties both in the design of automatic instruments (particularly automatic group instruments) and in insuring their continued ac-curacy.

It seems clear that at present it is feasible to design and develop screening audiometers and monitoring audiometers that will ex-pedite and make practical the screening and/or the monitoring of large numbers of individuals within reasonable limits of time, expense, space and trained personnel. It is not clear, however, that the same instrument should be expected to perform both functions. It is also possible that all monitoring audiometry need not be done in just the same way. In some situations an automatic individual audiometer, in other situations a manually operated group audiometer may have clear and overriding practical advantages. The general concepts of screening, monitoring, and diagnostic audiometry are well established, but there are several audiometric tests that fall in each class. There are various means or instruments for administering a given test and these differ in respect to expense, space, time and personnel required.

FREQUENCIES FOR AUDIOMETERS

In the early days of audiometry great emphasis was placed on the measurement of hearing for very low tones, such as 64 cps, and very high tones, such as 16,000 cps. The trend over the years has been to concentrate attention on the range from 500 to 6000 cps. It has gradually become clear that measurements of the extreme frequencies are unreliable and/or expensive because of various technical limitations, and, furthermore, that the hearing levels for the whole lower half of the frequency range, from 1000 cps down, can be very well predicted from the hearing level at either 500 cps or 1000 cps, while 4000 cps is the most sensitive indicator of high-tone loss. The otologist may desire measurements at 250 cps and perhaps 8000 cps, but for screening and monitoring, these frequencies are quite unnecessary. More important are the intermediate frequencies of 1500 and particularly 3000 and 6000 cps.

A recent set of recommended frequencies for various types of audiometry, based on the CHABA study of monitoring audiometry, is given in the following table.

Recommended Frequencies for Various Types of Audiometry

	250	500	1000	1500	2000	3000	4000	6000	8000
Screening audiometry:									
Single-frequency screen							4000		
Reduced screen					2000,		4000		
Full screen		500,	1000,		2000,	3000,	4000,	6000	
Monitoring audiometry:									
Retain		500,	1000,		2000,	3000,	4000,	6000	
Physical standards for general military duty:									
Retain		500,	1000,		2000,				
Retain for present							4000,	6000	
Consider for future addition						3000,			
Calculation of disability of hearing:									
Retain		500,	1000,		2000,				
Consider for addition						3000,			
Diagnostic audiometry:									
Retain	250,	500,	1000,		2000,	3000,	4000,	6000	
Consider for addition				1500,					
Consider for possible elimination									8000

Source: H. Davis, G. D. Hoople, and H. O. Parrack, "The Medical Principles of Monitoring Audiometry," *A.M.A. Archives of Industrial Health,* 17: 1–20 (1958).

REDUCED SCREENING

A convenient, although purely empirical, rule about hearing loss, particularly sensory-neural loss, is that hearing is very seldom any worse at 500, 1000, and 2000 cps than it is at 4000 cps, at least until the hearing level at 4000 cps is more than 50 db. This rule seems to be very good for men and quite good for women. It is less satisfactory for children, partly because of the greater amount of conductive as compared with sensory-neural hearing loss in children. Of course, the accuracy of the rule is limited by the variability of at least plus or minus 5 db (one step on the audiometer) that we must expect on repeated audiograms. The rule suggests, however, that we can use 4000 cps as *a single monitor* frequency to detect the beginning of noise-induced hearing loss in industry and in military situations. *Single-frequency screening* at 4000 cps may greatly simplify and expedite routine monitoring audiometry. It is very quick and it has the great advantage that it does not require an acoustic environment any quieter than that of the average office. Some audiologists prefer to employ a second frequency, usually 2000 cps, to back up the single-frequency test at 4000 cps. Of course, all soldiers or workers whose hearing levels are found to lie above the screening limit, whatever limit may be chosen, must then be tested at all the regular monitor

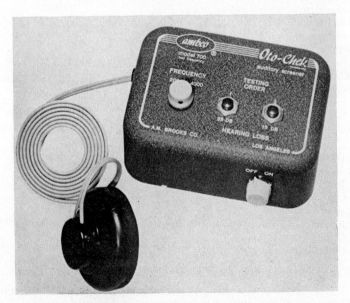

Fig. 7-14. A simple, two-tone (2000 and 4000 cps) screening audiometer can be made very compact indeed. (*Ambco, Inc.*)

frequencies, and, if the loss is confirmed, will be given a full otological examination and diagnostic audiometry.

At the present writing opinion is divided as to whether *reduced screening* at two or perhaps three frequencies is sufficiently reliable to be used to expedite conservation of hearing programs for school children as well as for adults.

Tests for Cortical Deafness

In our description of central deafness in Chapter 4 we pointed out that the impairment in this condition is not a loss of sensitivity but rather a loss of understanding. The trouble is more like a difficulty in discrimination, but it appears more clearly in an articulation test than in a test for the difference limen of pitch or of loudness. "Phonemic regression," for example, is practically defined as a very poor performance by an elderly person on a word test that is not explained by a high threshold for pure tones.

For many years, under the influence of Pavlov, we have spoken of the cerebral cortex of the brain as an "analyzer." Now we know that much if not all of the analysis, in the sense of discrimination, is carried out by the sense organs or by the lower and intermediate levels of the central nervous system. It is now more popular, and certainly more helpful, to think of the cortex as a "recognizer," a "memory file," or a "calculator" and a "synthesizer." The contrast between peripheral hearing loss on the one hand and central deafness on the other is well expressed by the familiar double demand addressed to the comedian on the stage by the man in the balcony: "Louder! Louder and funnier!"

A major job of the central nervous system is to infer a whole from some of its parts and react correctly to it. We do not need to see the *whole* of a lion or a snake to know what it is and to avoid it. Of course, we are sometimes fooled by illusions of one sort or another, but on the whole, both with vision and with hearing, we fill in gaps in familiar patterns correctly and hardly realize that the gaps were there. When we listen to someone talk there is usually a wide margin of safety for correct understanding. Not only is there usually loudness to spare but we could recognize the words if some frequencies were filtered out entirely and we could get the message even if many of the words were incomplete or missing.

It should be possible to test this recognizing action of the nervous system by using more and more garbled, fragmentary, or partially masked speech as test material. By making the task of recognition difficult, the central nervous system is made the bottleneck and its function can be assessed. The principle of such testing is clear, but specific tests of this sort have not yet been formalized and validated.

Auditory flutter has also been proposed as a test of brain injury. White noise is interrupted at varying rates and the task of the listener is to tell whether he hears the interruption or "flutter," or whether the noise sounds steady. The test has been constructed by analogy with a visual test, the critical flicker frequency, which seems to be helpful in detecting certain types of brain injury. Auditory flutter is being used experimentally in the same way but it may or may not turn out to be useful in the long run. We mention it to illustrate the possible development of auditory tests for brain injury, perhaps even of injury to parts of the brain whose function is not primarily auditory.

ADDENDUM
TO CHAPTER 7

The Zero Reference Level for Audiometers

Inasmuch as the situation concerning an International Standard for Audiometric Zero Level may remain uncertain for some time a more complete and somewhat more technical explanation of the background and the conflicting points of view is appropriate.

The first important set of normal zero values was established by the Bell Telephone Laboratories when they designed the famous Western Electric Co. 2A audiometer in the early 1920's. An otologist selected a group of eighty-one young adults working in the offices and laboratories, people whom he found to have no signs or symptoms of ear trouble. Otological examinations, medical histories, and tuning fork tests were all employed. The engineers then measured their thresholds with the laboratory model of the new instrument. The actual readings were the voltages that had to be applied to a particular earphone to produce a barely audible tone. Similar earphones were used on the production model and the instruments were adjusted or "calibrated" so that when the dial labeled "intensity" (later labeled "hearing loss") was set at zero the appropriate voltage was delivered to the earphone. (Actually the operator of this instrument had to read a different indicator on his scale, depending on the frequency he was using, but in most later models of audiometers internal adjustments of voltage are made automatically when the frequency-selector knob is turned.)

In this situation the standard for normal hearing was "stored" as we say, in the particular earphone used in the original laboratory calibration. In the early thirties several users of the 2A audiometer actually recalibrated their own particular instruments by testing their own group of "normal" listeners. They then applied corrections where necessary to the readings of the instrument. It is interesting that most of the zeros of the 2A audiometer, confirmed in general by the experience of those users who verified the values, actually lie *between* the present American Standard and the new British Standard (see Figure 2-5).

In the actual manufacture of audiometers, production control of earphones is maintained by measuring the acoustic pressure produced by each earphone in a small cavity known as a coupler or "artificial ear." The cavity is about the same size, six cubic centimeters, as the human external canal and middle ear plus the space under the diaphragm of an earphone, but the walls are metal and the shape is simple. The pressures produced in this "coupler" are not quite the same as the pressures produced in the ear by the same earphone. The coupler pressures are, however, *reproducible* and serve to show that one earphone of the same model is like another. A coupler was standardized by the National Bureau of Standards, and the present American Standard for the zero hearing level is "stored" in the form of sets of acoustic pressures produced by certain models of earphone in an "NBS-9A coupler."

A separate set of pressures must be specified for each different model of earphone. The reason is that with voltages giving the same pressure in the coupler two models of earphone may not sound equally loud to the ear. The acoustic interaction between earphone and ear is different with differences of shape and size of earphone. We cannot yet go from one model of earphone to another except by a "loudness balance." Here a jury of listeners with presumably normal ears finds what voltage applied to the new earphone produces a sound that is just as loud as the sound produced by the standard model with its standard voltage. Such a "loudness-balance transfer" is a rather laborious psychophysical procedure, but the transfer has been carried out at the National Bureau of Standards for three different models of earphone. These data, incorporated in the American Standards for Audiometers, allow manufacturers to reproduce the standard zero pressure levels in the instruments they manufacture, although if they use a different model of earphone they must carry out a loudness balance study to find how it deviates from the models for which the National Bureau of Standards has published the data.

We have now answered, in slightly simplified form, the questions of storage of the standard threshold values and of matching them in the manufacture of audiometers. There are differences between the British coupler and the American coupler, but the important international difference of opinion concerns the concept of "normal hearing."

In 1935–1936 the United States Public Health Service conducted a large health survey which included audiometry. Town, city, and country populations were proportionately represented. The measurements of hearing seem to have been very well carried out, with due precautions as to background noise in the audiometric booths, and so on. Audiometric techniques were fairly well established by that time. Questionnaires concerning age, general health, history of ear trouble and other diseases, and the like, made it possible to select from the total group the young men and women with what they themselves considered good hearing and no history of ear trouble. This group would seem to be a group of average healthy young individuals, a fair sample of "normals."

The threshold values of voltage across the earphones (WE-705A) for this group were tabulated. The value chosen for each frequency was the most common or "modal" value, i.e., the peak of the distribution curve. The seven modal values for the frequencies 125, 250, 500, 1000, 2000, 4000, and 8000 cps, stored as we have described by the National Bureau of Standards, are now the primary American Standard zero levels for audiometers. These values are a little higher than the zero values of the 2A audiometer, i.e., the Western Electric listeners had slightly more sensitive ears, but the audiologists and otologists of the United States have not complained. Our zero seems to represent normal American hearing as it walks into our hearing clinics. The values have been confirmed quite closely in a Japanese survey, in a hearing study carried out at the Wisconsin State Fair in 1954 by the Research Center of the Subcommittee on Noise (in Industry), and in similar previous but less comparable studies.

European audiologists, however, have complained for many years that the American Standard is too lenient and does not represent the best human hearing. By "best" is not meant the world's record but simply the average or mean of a selected group of young, well-motivated listeners as they listen repeatedly under the best listening conditions. The conditions of the USPHS and of the Wisconsin State Fair audiometry were good but perhaps not ideal. Above all, the attitude of the listeners was definitely rather casual.

It now seems, after several years of discussion and additional testing, that the attitude and motivation of the listeners, with perhaps a little practice effect also, make a rather large difference; as much as 10 db. A specific comparison of the "clinical" versus the "laboratory" approach was made at the Wisconsin State Fair in 1955. It showed very clearly the importance of attitude and motivation. The threshold curve for well-motivated laboratory listening has now been reproduced over and over again in various laboratories on both sides of the Atlantic, including those in the Soviet Union.

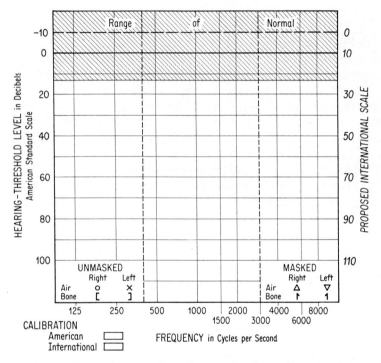

Fig. 7-15. This audiogram chart shows the relation between the present American Standard scale for audiometers and the proposed International Standard. The range of normal thresholds extends to about the 12 db hearing level on the American scale. This is the 22 db hearing level on the British and on the proposed international scale. Audiogram blanks like this could be used both for audiometers calibrated according to the present American Standard, according to the present British Standard, or according to the proposed International Standard. The calibration of the instrument would simply be checked in the lower left corner.

The symbols shown on this chart are included for illustrative purposes only. They are not part of the proposed International Standard for Audiometric Zero. The dashed vertical lines at 400 and 3000 cps are the customary reminders of the range of frequencies most important for the understanding of speech.

Probably the most complete of the recent careful studies are those that were done at the British National Physical Laboratory and at the Central Medical Establishment of the Royal Air Force. The thresholds for listening in a free field as well as for earphone listening were measured for the same listeners. (The "missing 6 db" mentioned in Chapter 2 were still missing.) These thresholds for earphone listening have been adopted as the British Standard for audiometric zero and have been proposed as an International Standard. This zero hearing level corresponds more nearly to the "minus 10" line at the top of the American audiometric charts than it does to our zero, but the difference is not quite the same at all frequencies.

As this addendum is being written (1959), efforts are being made to develop an International Standard for "normal" hearing that will incorporate American as well as British data and that will bear some simple relation to the present American Standard. If, within the limits of clinical accuracy imposed by the 5-db steps of the audiometer, we can merely shift the zero line to the top of the present audiogram chart, as indicated in Figure 7-15, the transition from the present American Standard to a new International Standard should be quite easy. In other words, we can reasonably hope that the second-order differences between the two standards (other than the obvious 10-db shift) will prove to be within the present limits of tolerance for the calibration of audiometers.

Suggested Readings

American Standards Association. *Audiometers for General Diagnostic Purposes, Z24.5-1951; Specification for Pure-Tone Audiometers for Screening Purposes, Z24.12-1952; Specification for Speech Audiometers, Z24.13-1953.* American Standards Association, Inc., 70 East 45th Street, New York City, N.Y.

BUNCH, C. C. *Clinical Audiometry.* St. Louis: C. V. Mosby Company, 1943. A monograph devoted to the development and use of the pure-tone audiometer.

DAVIS, H., and J. R. USHER. "What Is Zero Hearing Loss?" *Journal of Speech and Hearing Disorders,* 22: 662–690 (1957). This is based on a symposium of the Armed Forces–National Research Council Committee on Hearing and Bio-Acoustics (CHABA). It describes the USPHS survey and also the methods of "storing" a standard.

DAVIS, H., G. D. HOOPLE, and H.O. PARRACK. "The Medical Principles of Monitoring Audiometry," *A.M.A. Archives of Industrial Health,* 17: 1–20 (1958). This paper is based on the report of a CHABA working group to the Air Force.

EGAN, J. R. "Articulation Testing Methods," *The Laryngoscope,* 58: 955–991 (1948). This is a condensation of the reports of the same title prepared at the Psycho-Acoustic Laboratory for the Office of Scientific Research and Development. (OSRD Report No. 3802). It contains a full description of the original phonetically balanced ("PB-50") word lists.

FLETCHER, H., and J. E. STEINBERG. "Articulation Testing Methods," *Bell Systems Technical Journal,* 8: 806–854 (1929).
A classic article from the Bell Telephone Laboratories. It contains the complete list of BTL sentences.

HIRSH, I. J. *The Measurement of Hearing.* New York: McGraw-Hill Book Company, 1952.
An authoritative monograph that deals with psychoacoustic methods and principles.

————, H. DAVIS, S. R. SILVERMAN, E. G. REYNOLDS, E. ELDERT, and R. W. BENSON. "Development of Materials for Speech Audiometry," *Journal of Speech and Hearing Disorders,* 17: 321–337 (1952).
This gives the background of the CID auditory tests.

NEWBY, H. A. *Audiology: Principles and Practice.* New York: Appleton-Century-Crofts, Inc., 1958.
An excellent companion volume to Chapters 7 and 8 of this book.

SILVERMAN, S. R., and I. J. HIRSH. "Problems Related to the Use of Speech in Clinical Audiometry," *Annals of Otology, Rhinology, and Laryngology,* 64: 1234–1245 (1955).
A discussion of the purposes of speech audiometry.

WATSON, L. A., and T. TOLAN. *Hearing Tests and Hearing Instruments.* Baltimore: The Williams & Wilkins Company, 1949.
This monograph gives valuable details concerning electric audiometers and their use.

8

SPECIAL
AUDITORY TESTS

Hallowell Davis, M.D.,
and Robert Goldstein, Ph.D.

Tests of hearing, such as pure-tone audiometry and speech audiometry, are employed for many different purposes. In the foregoing chapters we have described the nature of the most widely used tests and have indicated some of the purposes for which they were designed. In the present chapter, in spite of some repetition, we shall consider the major purposes systematically and the tests appropriate to each. In the next chapter we shall also touch on the difficult questions of physical standards, handicap, and financial awards.

Diagnosis, and Assessment for Hearing Aid or Surgery

A primary reason for testing hearing is to make a medical diagnosis. On the diagnosis rest the decision as to treatment and also the forecast as to the improvement or deterioration of hearing. Advice concerning use of a hearing aid, surgery for improvement of hearing, and so on, also depends in large part on a correct medical diagnosis. Furthermore, tests of hearing may be of real assistance to the neurologist and neurosurgeon in the diagnosis of disorders of the central nervous system, whether the basic trouble is auditory or not.

The major information sought by the otologist is the anatomical and physiological distinctions already described. In particular, to what extent is the hearing loss of which a patient complains conductive? A conductive loss is a purely physical affair and something can be done about it, but sensory-neural losses are more difficult to improve by medical or surgical treatment.

If there is degeneration of nerve or sense organ the only course is

218

to make the most of what remains and, by follow-up tests, to determine whether the hearing is growing progressively worse. If it is sense-organ disease, medical treatment can be instituted, and some change for better or worse can be anticipated with or without treatment.

The otologist is always interested in the cause of the condition he finds. In order to treat it intelligently he should know not only *where* it is, but also *what* it is, and, better still, *what causes* it. Of course, the anatomical and physiological distinctions establish certain classes of possible causes. Rarely, however, even for so simple a diagnosis as conductive hearing loss, does a physician base his opinion and course of action on a single symptom, a single sign, or the result of a single test. He always seeks confirmatory evidence and he bases his final diagnosis on the balance of evidence in a total picture. Only the fully trained physician is competent to do this, although it is very tempting for an audiological specialist to begin to make diagnoses on the basis of the results of his hearing tests alone. An audiologist may be correct more often than not, but the experienced physician who considers audiometric findings as only one part of the total examination is in a better position to make a correct diagnosis; above all, the physician will usually avoid the tragic mistakes that can so easily follow from oversimplification or from dependence on a single kind of information. For him the improbable but serious alternative, such as a brain tumor or a metabolic disturbance, is a very real alternative. He is better able to recognize these conditions that actually threaten life and to realize that the auditory symptoms that result from them are of only secondary importance for the welfare of the patient.

BONE-CONDUCTION TESTS FOR CONDUCTIVE LOSS

The simple tuning fork tests—the Schwabach, the Rinne, and the Weber, described in Chapter 7—all aim to distinguish between conductive and sensory-neural hearing loss. The principle is essentially the same: in conductive loss the hearing by air conduction is impaired but by bone conduction is nearly normal, while in sensory-neural loss both are equally affected. In these tests, usually conducted in a rather noisy environment, the bone conduction of the patient is compared with that of a normal listener (Schwabach) or with his own air conduction (Rinne), or the bone conductions of his two ears are compared with one another (Weber). These tests are not quantitative, partly because the ambient noise level is so variable.

The equivalent of the tuning fork tests can, of course, be performed with an electric audiometer. A bone-conduction audiogram is taken as well as an air-conduction audiogram, and the two are compared. In principle the bone-conduction audiogram tells the degree and the distribution by frequency of the sensory-neural loss. The difference between the air and the bone audiograms, the so-called air-bone gap, tells approximately the amount and distribution of the conductive loss.

Of course, if the air-conduction audiogram is normal there is no need to take one by bone conduction. Theoretically, it cannot show more loss than the air-conduction test. If it does, it means that one test or the other has been inaccurate or improperly conducted in some way, that the audiometer is not properly calibrated, or that there has been a clerical error.

Bone-conduction tests are made *only* for diagnostic purposes. Bone-conduction vibrators are required by the American Standard for Audiometers for Diagnostic Purposes but not by the corresponding standard for screening audiometers.

SPEECH TESTS

The uncertainty of calibration of bone-conduction vibrators and the difficult problems of masking, both intentional and unintentional, in bone-conduction tests have led some otologists to seek a substitute test. One such alternative is the use of difficult word lists in speech audiometry to assess the "cochlear reserve." The score is the maximum percentage of words that the patient can repeat when the words are delivered at a high enough level to override the conductive component of his hearing loss. This, of course, is exactly what a hearing aid does. Thus the "PB maximum" test is partly a diagnostic test and partly a direct practical trial of the benefits of a hearing aid. It is often less important to know just how much of a patient's hearing loss is conductive and how much sensory-neural than to know by direct test how well the patient can do with his hearing that remains. The words are delivered at a level well above the patient's threshold for speech. If the difficult words are understood it means that the patient probably can use a hearing aid to advantage, regardless of the cause of his trouble. If his score is very poor it confirms what the tester probably had already learned from trying to talk to the patient: that he will have difficulty with, or get no benefit from, a hearing aid or even a stapes mobilization or fenestration operation. He may have a sense-organ or perhaps a central type of dysacusis with or without some conductive loss. A score that is below but not far below the average normal leaves the otologist and the audiologist both in doubt, the one as to his diagnosis, the other as to his prediction concerning the probable benefit from a hearing aid. Each will seek further evidence.

On the whole, the word lists, particularly the PB word lists, are more useful for predicting the benefit from a hearing aid than for making a medical diagnosis. Only for the most difficult recordings (Rush Hughes) have any valid claims of diagnostic usefulness been made.

The threshold tests for speech, such as the spondee word lists, are not diagnostic tests by themselves. They simply confirm the pure-tone measurements of the thresholds for the frequencies 500, 1000, and 2000 cps. They do show in addition that the patient can hear and respond to simple spoken words. A serious discrepancy between the hearing level for speech and the average level for the three pure-tone frequencies—500, 1000, and 2000 cps—strongly suggests either a sensory-neural or a central nervous system difficulty. The failure to hear, understand, or respond properly to speech is an outstanding characteristic of sense-organ and central dysacusis. The difficulty can be assessed either by formal speech audiometry or informal live-voice tests or by the effort necessary for successful two-way conversation.

SENSE-ORGAN IMPAIRMENT

Some tests aim to recognize and identify a sense-organ impairment that is distinct from presbycusis, noise-induced hearing loss, and so on, on the one hand, acoustic neuroma on the other, or central dysacusis. Noise-induced hearing loss and presbycusis are here grouped together as simple deficiency disorders that are due primarily to the loss of sensory cells and/or nerve cells. They are often indistinguishable from each other in their symptoms but they contrast in general with certain other impairments that depend on *abnormal function* of the sense organ. The distinctions are important because the prognosis and the treatment are quite different, and here tests of hearing can make important contributions to medical diagnosis.

The key words related to sense-organ impairment are *recruitment, diplacusis, discrimination loss,* and *fluctuation of symptoms.* The last refers to the variability of symptoms and of test results from day to day and from week to week. Discrimination loss for speech, discussed above, has as its symptom difficulty with many words, sometimes with even the relatively easy spondees. The characteristic statement of the patient is, "I hear the words but I can't make them out. They don't come clear." Repeated formal tests, notably the "PB maximum," or discrimination score, are useful as evidence of the fluctuation of the symptom.

Diplacusis was discussed in Chapter 7. An important symptom is a change in quality from a smooth, pure musical tone to a rough, ringing or buzzing noise. Change in pitch may be found in binaural comparison with either tuning forks or the pure-tone audiometer, because one ear is usually affected more than the other. Curiously enough, very few systematic studies of diplacusis have been reported and no test of it has been formalized and validated.

Interest has centered around *recruitment*. The word is widely misused to include not only recruitment of loudness in the original sense (Fowler) but also diplacusis and discrimination loss, as though the term were the equivalent of "sense-organ disease." The only true direct indicators of recruitment are a loudness-balance test and perhaps also a narrowed range between threshold and the maximum-comfortable-loudness level. In the loudness-balance test, if one ear is normal or nearly so, a series of comparisons are made, at one or two or even at three frequencies, of the hearing levels on the audiometer that sound equally loud to the two ears. Many audiometers designed for diagnostic purposes are equipped with two separate oscillators and at-

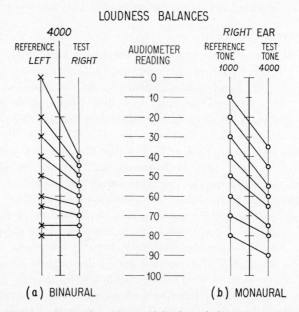

Fig. 8-1. (a) The results of binaural loudness balances at a given frequency are often plotted in this way (*Fowler*). One advantage of this form is that it can be superimposed on the regular audiogram. To do this, the values for the loudness balances are plotted about half an octave above and below the line corresponding to the frequency at which the balances are made and are joined by the straight lines. The conventional symbols for right and left are employed.

(b) The results of monaural loudness balances at two different frequencies may be plotted as shown here or in the form of Figure 8-2. The hypothetical case illustrated shows "delayed" partial recruitment at 4000 cps. The monaural balance must be used when the losses in the two ears are substantially symmetrical. The lower of the two frequencies, usually 500 to 1000 cps, should show a better hearing threshold level than the frequency to be tested.

tenuators to make loudness balancing easier. The results are usually plotted in either of the two forms illustrated in Figures 8-1 and 8-2. The key feature in Figure 8-1, showing recruitment, is the change from the sloping lines near threshold (that connect equally loud settings) to horizontal lines at high intensities. In Figure 8-2 the corresponding feature is the approach of the observed points closer and closer to the diagonal line that is the locus of equal loudness in two normal ears.

A binaural loudness balance is more difficult for the subject than a simple threshold test, but with a little practice most subjects are able to do it quite well, even though they may protest that the job is difficult and that they have little confidence in their loudness matches. A monaural balance, in which a high tone is balanced against a low tone, is more difficult but it can be done by intelligent and cooperative patients. A pitch match (binaural, of course) is quite easy for most subjects without recruitment but may be difficult when the tone sounds pure to one ear but rough, complex, or noisy to the other.

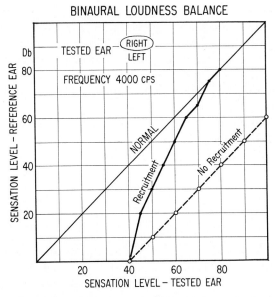

Fig. 8-2. The results of binaural loudness balances at a given frequency may also be plotted in this way (*Steinberg and Gardiner*). If, as in the ideal normal situation, the audiometer readings are equal for every intensity setting, the points fall along the diagonal line of equality labeled normal. A hypothetical case of recruitment (unilateral sensory-neural hearing loss) is also shown. A conductive hearing loss shows displacement of all points to the right, but they still fall on a diagonal line parallel to the normal line.

Monaural loudness balance depends in principle on assuming that hearing is more abnormal at one frequency than at another. The "more abnormal" is identified by its higher hearing level and usually by its more abnormal quality. A monaural loudness balance can show recruitment clearly only if there is a difference in threshold levels of 25 db or so between the two frequencies being tested.

Measurement of the *difference limen for intensity* has been suggested as a substitute for monaural loudness balance. It uses only a single tone, and the tester finds what is the smallest difference in intensity that is recognized by the subject when a stronger and a weaker tone are presented alternately. As noted in Chapter 7, it is a very plausible but apparently erroneous assumption that the difference limen should be smaller in the presence of recruitment of loudness. The method has not fulfilled the initial expectations.

The rate and amount of auditory fatigue or temporary threshold shift is probably greater in sense-organ disease than in the normal, but no test for this has been fully formalized and validated. The interesting suggestion has also been made that the dynamic range (intensity difference) between threshold and the level of harmonic distortion is abnormally small in sense-organ disease. The second harmonic, produced by the distortion within the inner ear, is recognized by listening for beats between it and a (second) exploring tone that is nearly but not exactly double the frequency of the test tone. The test as a whole seems plausible but requires validation. Some subjects have great difficulty discriminating the beats between the harmonic and the exploring tone.

The validation of all of these proposed tests proceeds slowly. No single medical center has enough independently proved cases of Ménière's syndrome, tumors that compress the auditory nerve, and central deafness to determine rapidly but with assurance the value of each new test in differential diagnosis.

Rehabilitation

The problems of auditory rehabilitation are discussed in several other chapters of this book. Assessment of hearing for purposes of rehabilitation takes several forms: first, identifying the individuals who *need* auditory rehabilitation; second, determining which individuals can *profit* by it; and, finally, assessing the degree of *success* that has been achieved. In some situations arbitrary limits of hearing level are set at which separation from active duty and the initiation of rehabilitation (if appropriate) become mandatory. An example is the Army Regulation cited in a later chapter.

The criteria for success in rehabilitation are only rarely best stated in decibels. Even the cure of a hysterical deafness or the relief of a psychogenic overlay is likely to be better described in medical or social terms. So also are the fitting of a hearing aid and the results of auditory training. It is not enough to measure the difference in speech reception threshold or in "PB maximum" discrimination scores. An assessment in terms of social adjustment and/or success in getting or holding a job is more significant. Actually, there has been a surprising lack of any validation of the methods used to select or "fit" hearing aids. (The present writers sometimes wonder whether the discrimination scores obtained with different hearing aids really measure any significant, reliable differences!) But social and economic yardsticks are difficult and cumbersome to apply, as will be seen in connection with the problem of handicap and compensation.

Malingering

In all of our discussions of tests of hearing, whether for pure-tone thresholds, speech thresholds, recruitment, or the like, we have assumed full cooperation on the part of the patient. At worst, as in the case of very young children, we assume indifference but not active hostility. Unfortunately, in cases where economic gain, "saving of face," or escape from danger is at stake, as in compensation for injury to hearing or discharge from military service, we may encounter an opposite motivation. The subject may not only make no real effort to hear; he may deliberately pretend not to hear at all or to hear much less than he really does. This behavior we call *malingering*. The detection of malingering may be a very important part of the assessment of hearing.

Many devices have been developed to catch off guard the man suspected of malingering. One consists of imparting to him in a rather low tone of voice some information that is interesting or important to him, and observing that he reacts appropriately. Typically the "test" is made outside of what appears to the subject to be the test situation. The giving of the information is made to appear unintentional. The basic principle for success of such tests is very simple: *the tester must be smarter than the malingerer, and a better actor.*

Not all audiologists are good actors, and more sophisticated tests take advantage of psychoacoustic principles which are probably unknown to the subject or which make it very difficult for him to control his behavior appropriately. One test, the *Lombard*, relies on our unconsciously increasing the volume of our voices when we are talking or reading aloud and the background noise suddenly rises, as it does, for example when an automobile passes an open window.

The presence of noise also interferes with our understanding of speech. The noise, however, must be at least as intense as the speech and usually 10 to 15 db greater for it to make speech completely unintelligible. A malinger may remember the loudness at which he pretends to begin understanding speech, but his monitor for loudness can be disrupted by the presence of noise. In the *Doerfler-Stewart tests*, both speech and noise, given to the same ear, are systematically varied in such a way that the malingerer cannot effectively retain the constant ratio of noise to speech expected from a cooperative patient and still remember at what level he is to stop "understanding."

Our monitor of loudness can also be disrupted if, while we read aloud, we are forced to listen to the sound of our own voice amplified and also delayed in time by about one syllable. In the *delayed sidetone test* the patient reads aloud into a microphone which delivers the speech to a tape recorder. The recorded speech is played back, about 0.2 second later, to earphones on the patient's ears. As long as the delayed sound is softer than the sound of the patient's speech within his own head his reading will not be disturbed. As the delayed speech is made louder the patient will stutter or stumble, drag out his words, and usually raise his voice. With this test one can usually detect rather easily the feigning of a large hearing loss, but detection of small losses and the measurement of threshold are quite difficult.

Feigned deafness in one ear can easily be detected and the amount of true hearing loss closely estimated by means of the *Stenger test*. Instead of destroying one's monitor of loudness or time, as do the other tests described, this test destroys one's monitor for whichever ear is being stimulated. The test is based on the fact that if two equally sensitive ears are stimulated simultaneously with an identical stimulus, the sound will be localized somewhere near the center of the head. If the stimulus is made more intense at one ear, then the listener will report that he hears sound only in that ear. He will not be aware of the weaker sound in the other ear. The Stenger test, originally done with tuning forks, can be performed more conveniently with an audiometer, as follows. Usually the threshold is determined on each ear for a tone of a particular frequency. The tone is then presented to the good ear alone at about 5 or 10 db above its threshold. The patient will localize the sound to that ear. The tone is also presented to the supposedly bad ear the same number of decibels above its threshold. If the bad ear is as bad as the patient claims, he will probably localize the sound somewhere near the center of his head. If threshold is better in his bad ear than what he claims for it, the tone will sound louder in that ear and will be localized there. If the patient admits that he hears the sound in his bad ear, then this is a confession that he exaggerated the loss in that ear during the threshold measurement. Rather than admit that he hears in the bad ear he may claim that he hears no sound. In this case the tester gradually lowers the intensity of the sound in the bad ear until it is less loud than the sound in the good ear, which has been constant all this time. If the patient now says that he hears the sound in his good ear, this is an admission that previously the sound in his bad ear had been strong enough to obscure the sound in the good ear. By this procedure a close estimate can be made of the actual threshold in the supposedly bad ear. The Stenger test can be modified for use with speech instead of with pure tones.

One's monitor of which ear is being stimulated can also be disrupted by the *swinging voice test* (sometimes called the shifting voice test). If speech is fed alternately (e.g., every half second) to one ear and then to the other, the speech will be very intelligible if both ears are stimulated at about the same sensation level. The listener is hardly aware that his ears are being stimulated alternately. If one ear is bad, however, the speech will lose much of its intelligibility. If a person claims a unilateral loss and still shows normal understanding of speech in this test, he can be suspected of malingering.

One modification of the swinging voice test is to present a prepared story to the listener, switching back and forth from the good ear to both ears to the poor ear. The story is presented at a level 20 to 30 db above the threshold of the good ear and is written so that if the loss is unilateral it still is perceived as a sensible story to the listener. The test is positive if the listener repeats back the part of the story presented to the poor ear. If he does this the threshold in his poor ear must be *better* than the level at which the story was presented. If he claims that he could not understand the story, even after several presentations, this should arouse the tester's suspicions. This test does not give a threshold measurement but simply an indication that the listener is not giving a true threshold.

Indirect evidence of "hearing" can be derived from electrodermal (EDA, page 231) or electroencephalic (EEA, page 235) audiometry. In cooperative patients thesholds for these electrophysiologic responses closely reproduce the thresholds determined by ordinary clinical audiometry. Consequently, when threshold by EDA or EEA is lower by 10 db or more than his behavioral threshold, the patient is suspected of malingering during the behavioral tests. Electrodermal audiometry is preferable to EEA for this purpose because of greater simplicity of equipment, of preparation of the patient, and of interpretation of the records. The Veterans Administration presently requires EDA, at least at 1000 cps, in each ear in the evaluation of social efficiency of all claimants for compensation for service-connected hearing loss.

On the whole, it is usually easy to catch the malingerer who pretends to be totally deaf. Feigned deafness in one ear is fairly easy to detect, and so is a pretended very large hearing loss. The malingering most difficult to detect is the addition of some 10 or 15 db to a genuine hearing loss of between 15 and 30 db. This, like a psychogenic overlay, can easily pass undetected and even unsuspected; yet it may make quite a difference in relation to military discharge or to the amount of workmen's compensation award.

Educational Assessment

Tests of hearing, and other tests as well, may be used to decide what method of education is appropriate for a child with seriously impaired hearing. Classically, this problem has been conceived to be to determine whether the child's deafness or dysacusis is peripheral or whether it is central. A better statement of the problem is whether the child's difficulty is a hearing impairment or deafness in the popular sense of the words or whether it is primarily a disorder of language (aphasia), or a combination of the two. The distinction is important because the methods of education appropriate for one kind of disorder may not be appropriate for the other. Furthermore, the child without auditory sense organs will be deaf for life, will never talk perfectly, but can *learn* normally. The child with what is presently called "congenital receptive aphasia" can very often be taught both to understand speech and to talk normally, but he has great difficulty in learning, particularly at first.

In addition to dysacusis, whether peripheral or central, there may be still other reasons why a child does not develop normal verbal language. Apparent deafness is more frequent among children who are severely retarded mentally or who are seriously disturbed emotionally than among children who are normally intelligent and emotionally adjusted. The audiologist must recognize mental retardation and emotional disturbance and not classify children with these disorders as deaf. They are not in the province of audiologists or of teachers of the deaf unless there is also an impairment of hearing. The distinctions are often difficult to make, however. For instance, a mentally retarded child may appear hard of hearing or even totally deaf if he cannot comprehend the auditory signals that he receives and consequently does not react to them. Of course, to the extent that he cannot comprehend auditory signals he is centrally dysacusic, but this may be a part of a general mental retardation and not a specific failure of the auditory system. Also, an emotionally disturbed child may appear to have an impairment of perception if his disturbance is manifested by "shutting out speech."

There is also the easier task of deciding whether the hearing loss of a child who is not entirely deaf is severe enough to require that he go to a special school for the deaf or whether he can probably "get by" at a regular school, perhaps with a hearing aid. For children of school age who have learned to talk, this kind of testing means simply getting the numbers by pure-tone audiometry and then combining empirical experience, good sense, assessment of the individual child, and knowledge of available educational opportunities. Sound advice can then be given on the educational problem.

Even the problem of the hard-of-hearing child is difficult, however, if we wish to test the child at a year or perhaps two years of age. Then we cannot count on the child's understanding and cooperation. Several methods have been devised to test the very young child, and particularly children suspected of some form of central dysacusis. The common feature of the tests is that they do not require any conscious, deliberate listening and signaling by the subject on the basis of verbal instructions. They have been called, rather inaptly, "objective audiometry," to indicate that no "subjective" judgment is required of the listener. We shall see, however, that plenty of subjective judgment may be required of the tester in interpreting the test that he administers.

Simple noisemakers. In Chapter 16 we mention the use of simple noisemakers. If the child is young, one simply watches for signs of startle or of attention or turning to look for the source of the noise. Unfortunately, a sound that startles or interests a child may no longer do so after two or three repetitions, and one or two doubtful responses may have to be the basis of an interpretation. For this reason it is advisable not to begin with very loud sounds. It is better to "sneak up on the child," so to speak, with louder and louder sounds until he finally startles. The first startle response may appear close to a child's threshold. Frequently the child may respond to a sound that is softer than another sound if the first sound is familiar. For example, a spoon tinkling on a dish may elicit a response while a louder sound that has no meaning to the child may be ignored. Common sources of error are vibrations or air currents from sound sources too close to the child, or a glimpse of a sudden movement that he sees from the corner of his eye. Under favorable circumstances, however, much may be learned by careful observation of these simple, primitive, unlearned reactions to sound.

Children over three years of age, of normal mentality and learning ability but limited hearing, can be taught to "play a game" with the tester. An auditory signal is used to tell the child that he may put a peg in a pegboard, turn over the leaf of a picture book, or whatever activity is likely to interest a child of his age. Loud sounds are used at first until the child understands what he is expected to do; once this is accomplished, a pure-tone audiogram can be obtained. Perhaps the number of frequencies and intensities tested must be restricted or the testing spread over two or more sessions, but if the central processes of being able to attach meaning to a sound and of being able to keep attention concentrated are normal, it is just a matter of time to map out a peripheral hearing loss. The children with auditory agnosia or "receptive aphasia" may be very erratic on this as on all auditory tests. Sometimes they seem to hear very well, sometimes not at all, sometimes rather poorly; moreover, particularly if a child has both a central and a peripheral impairment, the tests may be quite inconclusive.

"The peep show." This test is basically a formalization and standardization of the informal "play a game" type of test just discussed. Both types, incidentally, and, indeed, all forms of objective audiometry, can employ either earphones or an acoustic field. The older the child the fewer objections to earphones, and with earphones

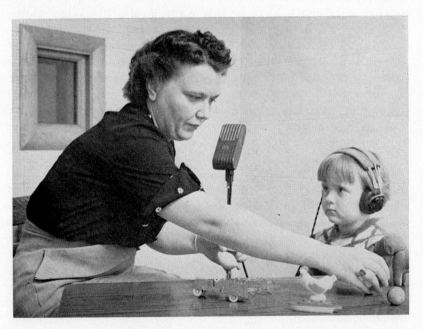

Fig. 8-3. In play audiometry the acoustic signals are controlled by an assistant in an adjoining room.

the ears can be tested separately and the sound levels known more accurately.

In one form of the "peep show" the child looks into an illuminated box at a picture. Then the light goes out. When a small signal light goes on the child can illuminate the box again and see a new picture by pushing a button, but he must wait until the signal light goes on. When he has mastered the idea, which most children over three years do quite easily, an auditory signal, usually a rather loud pure tone, is sounded along with the signal light. After several combined trials the signal light is omitted. If the child responds correctly by pushing the button when the tone is sounded alone he obviously "hears" usefully, and his hearing can be mapped out, in the same way that it is by the "play a game" method.

The numerical results and their significance are practically identical for these two methods. In each the consistency of response and the ability to understand what he is expected to do are as important for interpretation as the hearing levels in decibels.

ELECTRODERMAL AUDIOMETRY (EDA)

The "peep show" and the "play a game" forms of test are obviously modifications of experimental learning techniques and the methods of studying conditioned reflexes. In each of them the response is a conscious, directed activity in which the child participates and for which he receives a reward. The auditory signal is used to trigger a response. The close relation of all of this to learning in the usual sense of the word is perfectly obvious. Another kind of activity that can be conditioned for use in audiometry is the *electrodermal response* (EDR). By EDR is meant a change in the electrical resistance of the skin or of the electric potential between two skin areas such as the front and the back of the hand. (Many writers have called this the psychogalvanic skin response [PGSR], but electrodermal is briefer and more accurate.) The changes in electrical conductivity or electrical potential are readily recorded by a pen on a moving strip of paper; another pen indicates when electric shocks, sounds, or other stimuli are given. The electrical change reveals an unconscious reaction of the autonomic nervous system. It depends primarily on activation of the sweat glands. It occurs normally in response to any painful stimulus and it forms part of the pattern of many emotional reactions. It is one item in the battery of the famous "lie detector" tests.

The procedure with the electrodermal response may be much like that for the peep show although the so-called unconditional stimulus is unpleasant rather than pleasant. The stimulus usually begins as a mild electric shock, but it is gradually strengthened until

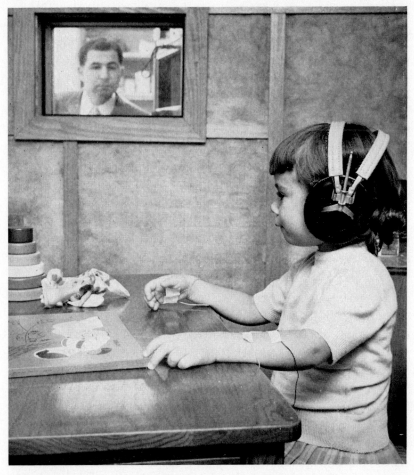

Fig. 8-4. Electrodermal audiometry may be carried out with the subject either seated or lying down. Note the electrodes taped to one palm to record the response and to the opposite forearm (or leg) to deliver the shock.

it elicits an electrodermal response. Very often it has to be annoyingly uncomfortable and even painful. Tones are sounded from time to time and shocks are given following some or all of them. With some subjects it is sufficient merely to sound the tone without using any shock. Perhaps they already fear a shock or perhaps they are sufficiently interested or startled by the sound to respond to it for its own sake. Usually, however, the acoustic signal must be combined with the shock in order to make it effective in bringing out an electrodermal response.

Some subjects respond very consistently and clearly to the test tones, and by simply observing whether or not an electrodermal response appears at the proper interval after the beginning of the stimulus, i.e., in about two seconds, we can, in principle, map out the audiogram of the subject. It helps if we reinforce the tones from time to time by giving the electric shock as well. In fact, one of the practical limitations of the test is the tendency of the response to "run down" (extinction). It gets smaller and occurs less frequently with repeated trials in spite of occasional reinforcement, and the strength of the shock usually has to be increased to keep a good conditioned response to the tones.

With sensitive subjects who respond consistently, the threshold of hearing can be mapped out with as great precision by electrodermal audiometry (EDA) as by the usual behavioral methods of clinical pure-tone audiometry, and the absolute thresholds by the two methods may be within a few decibels of each other. The theoretical advantage of this type of test is that it does not involve conscious response to the tones. The inference is that it should still be suitable for testing children (or adults) who cannot or will not respond voluntarily in conventional behavioral audiometry. No complicated process of concept formation, understanding what is wanted, or cooperating is involved. It is apparently a simple, straightforward conditioned reflex type of test in the Pavlovian tradition.

The electrodermal response has been employed in several hearing clinics with rather considerable success. In favorable cases it gives quite definite and very useful information, and positive results obtained by this method, as are those from the peep-show or informal testing, are of great value. The difficulty comes in interpreting the failures of response. It is unfortunately true, although not generally known, that many normal individuals fail completely to establish the desired association between the auditory signal and the electrodermal response. In fact, some of them give very poor electrodermal responses in the first place. Also, some individuals lose their conditioned associations very rapidly while others may be quite erratic in their responses, sometimes responding and sometimes not to the same intensity of auditory signal. In others the baseline is unsteady even without auditory stimulation, and it requires skill and experience as well as close attention to the proper latent period of response to identify the responses to the tone signals. And, most unfortunate of all, it appears that the very children who are uncertain and erratic in their responses to the peep-show or the "play the game" testing are the ones who are most likely to be erratic in their electrodermal responses.

In summary we repeat that EDA, as just described, is a very valuable method in expert hands, both as a test for children for educational assessment and as a test for possible malingering and certain forms of central dysacusis in adults, but it is neither infallible nor foolproof. Positive response means that the sound has stimulated the ear successfully and the impulses have reached at least the brain stem and have triggered off a response in the autonomic nervous system. Failure to respond, however, means little or nothing. It does not prove that there is a peripheral hearing loss.

It should also be obvious that the EDA technique described is not completely objective. The tester must constantly decide whether or not an electrodermal response was made to a particular tone. He is also influenced by the overt behavior of the patient in response to the stimulus. If a child shows an anticipatory response to a particular stimulus, such as crying or pulling at the electrodes, the tester may decide that a small movement of the pen is an EDR; if the child gives no anticipatory response, the tester may decide that the same small pen movement is not an EDR. Quite often a young child will react violently in anticipation of a shock and still give no EDR to the tone which made him react overtly. It is good clinical practice to combine one's observations of both overt and electrodermal responses in mapping out the threshold of hearing. Such a practice, however, cannot justifiably be called "objective audiometry," nor is it strictly electrodermal audiometry.

Procedures for objective electrodermal audiometry have been proposed and are practiced in several clinics. In essence these procedures require a previously prepared schedule of tones and shocks. They usually include some silent control-intervals, which are marked on the recording paper as if a stimulus had been given. In one such procedure each tone as well as each control-interval is numbered, and this number is written alongside of the mark on the paper which indicates when a tone is turned on. Only after the test has been completed are the records analyzed for possible responses to the tones. Analysis is made, therefore, without knowledge of the overt reactions of the patient at the time of the test (these are recorded, however, separately), and without knowledge of the frequency of the tone, its intensity, or which ear was stimulated or even whether there was any tone at all (control-interval). When the analysis is complete, the tester's judgment of "response" or "no response" after each number on the record is marked on the original schedule opposite the corresponding stimulus. Each stimulus is presented several times (a minimum of five or six is recommended) and the number of "responses" to each stimulus must exceed a certain proportion (according to a previously agreed criterion) before the tester considers that the patient can "hear" that stimulus. The criterion is usually based on the number of accidental responses (or false judgments of responses) which occur during the silent control-intervals. These objective procedures can readily be reproduced in any clinic that has satisfactory equipment.

This kind of objective audiometry is not always successful, but usually the threshold can be estimated with considerable certainty, even from a very few responses.

ELECTROENCEPHALIC AUDIOMETRY (EEA)

Another form of electrophysiological audiometry is *electro-encephalic audiometry (EEA)*. The brain is continually active, and in its activity it generates electric potentials like those in nerves and muscles. These potentials can be recorded by placing electrodes on a nerve or a muscle, or even in the general neighborhood of a nerve or muscle if the original signals are strong enough. The electro-cardiogram is a familiar example of the distant recording of the electrical activity of a muscle, in this case the heart. The electro-encephalogram (EEG) is to the brain what the electrocardiogram is to the heart. The electric potentials generated by the brain are strong enough to be detected by electrodes placed on the outside of the skull and even on the outside of the scalp. The potentials must be amplified, but the final patterns can be recorded by pens on a moving paper very much as the electrocardiogram or the electro-dermogram is recorded.

The brain is continually active and the pattern of electrical changes shows very well whether the subject is awake or asleep, and whether his eyes are opened or closed. Features of the pattern also depend on whether he is relaxed or very tense and anxious, whether he is a baby, a child, or an adult, and a number of other factors. The record of an adult or of an older child is usually dominated by a surprisingly rhythmic series of waves at about ten a second, known as the Berger or alpha rhythm. These waves are strongest in the part of the brain (in the back of the head) that is associated with vision and are particularly sensitive to the degree of arousal, to whether the eyes are busy looking at something or whether they are closed, and to mild startle or other emotional reactions. The stopping or "blocking" of the alpha rhythm as a result of sound stimulation is called an electroencephalic response (EER). A number of efforts have been made to use EER in audiometry, either without conditioning or with conditioning by association with flashes of light or other independently effective stimuli. These reactions (EER) have proved to be, on the whole, less satisfactory than EDR in audiometry.

It so happens that the change in the EEG pattern between

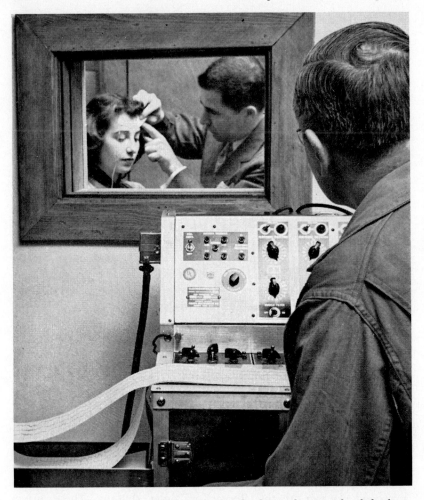

Fig. 8-5. An electroencephalograph records electrical potentials of the brain on a moving strip of paper. Electrodes are attached to the forehead of the subject in the inner shielded room. Half-silvered mirrors are usually used to provide one-way vision from the control room.

waking and sleeping is a rather striking one and, furthermore, that a person who is lightly asleep shows rather dramatic transient changes in his EEG pattern (the "K-complex" and other changes) in response to sounds. The changes are in the direction of waking up, although the subject usually does not fully awaken but sinks back to the previous level of sleep. The K-complex and other electroencephalic responses do not have to be learned. They are inborn patterns just like the electrodermal response to electric shocks.

The recognition of EER to measured auditory stimuli in sleep seemed to be a very promising tool for objective audiometry. It has now been explored rather systematically by at least two groups of investigators. Many of the original hopes have been dissipated, but electroencephalic audiometry (EEA) has proved to be of considerable value nevertheless, especially when the patient is tested asleep. Actually, one of the limitations of EEA is the same as for EDA. The greatest difficulty is that people do not give an EER to *every* sound that reaches them while they are asleep, and the more frequently a given sound is repeated, the less likely is it to produce a reaction. Conditioning of EER to an annoying stimulus such as a shock is out of the question if the patient is to remain asleep. For another thing, the fluctuations of the EEG during sleep are many and complicated, so that it may be difficult to distinguish a response to a particular signal from a spontaneous change in the EEG pattern. Some subjects react very consistently, and their audiograms can be mapped either by blocking of the alpha rhythm while they are awake or by detecting K-complexes while they are asleep. Even so, the identification of K-complexes in a rapidly moving and changing record is a really difficult task for the tester. Objective procedures such as described for EDA, however, enable a person with no previous EEG experience to make a relatively accurate analysis of responses *after the test is completed* and if he has plenty of time to study each segment of the record.

There is a distinct advantage for EEA over EDA in that electroencephalic responsiveness is not limited by age. Consistent EDR's are difficult to elicit from very young children (three years and under) but EER's seem to occur as frequently in these young children as they do in older children or adults. A child is more easily controlled in EEA than in EDA. The entire EEA, from placement of electrodes and auditory stimulation to removal of electrodes, can be completed while a child is asleep. Mild sedation to induce sleep does not significantly reduce responsiveness. In EDA the child is conscious of the wires and phones and is disturbed by the annoying shock, and the resulting agitation frequently makes testing impossible. Sedation to calm the child unfortunately reduces electrodermal responses drastically. However, EEA has not been as extensively applied and studied as EDA, and at the present time (1959) it can hardly be included in the list of generally available methods of audiometry.

EVALUATION OF EDUCATIONAL INDICATORS

A recent study of the children at Central Institute for the Deaf has evaluated many of our presently available tests for predicting the proper educational approach for children. All of the 183 children in the study had been at the Institute for at least one year, many of them for five years or longer. Their educational status and, above all, their ability to learn and make progress under one or both of two rather different methods of education had been carefully observed. In the course of their education several of the children had been transferred from one method of education to the other when careful observation of their educational progress suggested that the original placement had been inappropriate. In one section the methods of teaching are appropriate for deaf children with normal learning abilities. In the other section they are the methods we have found most successful with children whose ability to learn is impaired, particularly the ability to learn to use and understand auditory signals. (This includes the conditions called auditory agnosia and motor aphasia.) Thus the validation of the predictive tests is based on actual trial of one or both educational methods. (The methods themselves are described in Chapter 16.) One object of the study was to determine how well the group could have been divided correctly in advance on the basis of the various tests, particularly the tests made when or soon after the children entered the school.

Of course, the children studied are a carefully screened group. The only ones who had ever learned to talk normally had subsequently lost their hearing and most of their speech. About 60 per cent were judged to be deaf; the other 40 per cent were considered to have primarily a language difficulty greater than could be reasonably attributed to peripheral deafness, to mental retardation, or to psychic disturbances. None of them had any serious second handicap such as disabling paralysis or blindness. All were considered to have normal mental capabilities except for the handicaps imposed by failure to develop auditory communication and language.

Six groups of "tests" were employed. One was pure-tone audiometry, either behavioral (movements of the finger indicating "hearing," play techniques, or startle responses) or electrophysiologic tests (EDA or EEA). Another was a careful medical and developmental history from which a diagnosis of probable cause (etiology) of the handicap was made whenever possible. A third test was stimulation of the horizontal semicircular canals with cold water and observation of resultant eye movements (nystagmus). A fourth test was a full neurologic examination in which basic reflexes, coordination skills, function of the cranial nerves, and so on, were checked. A fifth test was a standard clinical electroencephalogram recorded while the child was awake. The sixth test was an X-ray photograph of the skull.

The neurological examination, the clinical electroencephalogram, and the skull X-rays proved to have little predictive value. This may be surprising until we recall that the children as a group had been screened before admission and none with major neurological symptoms or handicaps had been admitted. A major neurological defect such as cerebral palsy would obviously point to the brain rather than to the ear as the probable seat of the trouble.

The best single guide was the medical histories, and the next best was audiometry. Tests of the motor and vestibular systems were of some value, usually only confirmatory. In more detail, the authors concluded that meningitis and other severe infections in infancy and also a family history of deafness suggest that the child has a peripheral deafness. On the other hand, jaundice resulting from Rh-incompatibility, anoxia at birth, a convulsive disorder, a congenital abnormality of the brain, and a family history of disorders of speech or other neurologic disorders all rather strongly suggest a central auditory agnosia or aphasia. Maternal rubella during the first trimester of pregnancy and other complications during pregnancy may cause peripheral deafness, either alone or in combination with central dysacusis.

If good audiograms can be obtained, which is not often easy with very young children with present behavioral techniques, they are very helpful. The sharply sloping audiogram and severe hearing loss is characteristic of deaf children; normal sensitivity or a moderate hearing loss for all frequencies is characteristic of aphasic children. However, sloping audiograms with moderate to severe hearing losses occur frequently in both groups. The two methods of *electrical* audiometry—EDA and EEA—showed some merit in this study, but taken alone were not as good guides as conventional hearing tests or as the medical history and the probable etiology.

Major motor abnormalities appear more frequently in aphasic children than in deaf children. Minor motor abnormalities occur in about one fourth of both deaf and aphasic children and thus are not differentiating. Obtuseness during neurologic examination is much more frequent among the aphasic than among the deaf children.

Normal vestibular responses are more likely to occur in deaf rather than in aphasic children, with the exception that most of the children with histories of meningitis or other severe infections in infancy usually give no vestibular responses. Depressed vestibular responses in the presence of moderate or normal auditory sensitivity are more characteristic of aphasic children.

One conclusion from this study, which merely confirms a clinical impression of long standing, is that the diagnostic decision is not a simple choice between peripheral deafness *or* central dysacusis. There may be *both* peripheral and central impairment combined, and the problem is to estimate how serious each handicap is separately. The next step is to decide which method of education is appropriate for that combination of handicaps.

In the past the emphasis has usually been placed on the evaluation of peripheral hearing, particularly in terms of auditory sensitivity. Every effort has been made, including objective audiometry, to find how well the child "really hears." The choice of educational method has classically been between methods for the deaf and methods for the hard of hearing. It is clear, however, that there is another kind of handicap that we must evaluate and that can be quite as serious as peripheral deafness. This is *the inability to learn the meaning of auditory signals,* called "auditory agnosia." For this a third educational approach has been developed. For the choice of educational method the first question is not "How well does the child hear?" but *"How well can the child learn language?"* When, as often happens, there is a combination of some peripheral abnormality and some brain injury, the brain injury is likely to be the real bottleneck. Also, it is likely to make the hearing loss appear much more serious than it later turns out to be.

At present we have no direct tests to measure the ability to learn language. We badly need such a test—something to correspond to the audiogram, which is a direct measure of the function of the sense organ. It was pointed out in Chapter 7 that the audiometer is not the right tool for measuring central dysacusis. A test for the learning of language is what we need. At present we can only guess at this ability from the medical, social, and educational history, from the child's general behavior, his apparent span of attention, and the like. The only real test now is the therapeutic test. If a "deaf" child cannot learn language as fast as does the average of his classmates, perhaps he has some "central" difficulty that can be overcome by the methods that were devised originally (and quite empirically) for teaching children who could hear but who could not understand.

Suggested Readings

BARR, B. "Pure Tone Audiometry for Pre-school Children: A Clinical Study with Particular Reference to Children with Severely Impaired Hearing," *Acta Oto-Laryngologica,* 1955, Supp. 121, pp. 1–84.
This includes an excellent review of the earlier literature.

DIX, M. R., and C. S. HALLPIKE. "The Peep-Show: A New Technique for Pure-Tone Audiometry in Young Children," *British Medical Journal,* 2: 719–731 (1947).

GOLDSTEIN, R., W. M. LANDAU, and F. R. KLEFFNER. "Neurological Assessment of Some Deaf and Aphasic Children," *Annals of Otology, Rhinology, and Laryngology,* 67: 468–480 (1958).

GOLDSTEIN, R., H. LUDWIG, and R. F. NAUNTON. "Difficulty in Conditioning Galvanic Skin Responses: Its Possible Significance in Clinical Audiometry," *Acta Oto-Laryngologica,* 44: 67–77 (1954).

HIRSH, I. J., T. PALVA, and A. GOODMAN. "Difference Limen and Recruitment," *A.M.A. Archives of Otolaryngology,* 60: 525–540 (1954).
A critical study of tests of the relation of difference limens to recruitment.

NEWBY, H. A. *Audiology: Principles and Practice.* New York: Appleton-Century-Crofts, Inc., 1958.
An excellent companion volume to Chapters 7 and 8 of this book.

WATSON, L. A., and T. TOLAN. *Hearing Tests and Hearing Instruments.* Baltimore: The Williams & Wilkins Company, 1949.
This monograph gives valuable details concerning electric audiometers and their use.

WITHROW, F. B., JR., and R. GOLDSTEIN. "An Electrophysiologic Procedure for Determination of Auditory Threshold in Children," *The Laryngoscope,* 68: 1674–1699 (1958).
This paper describes and evaluates a combined method of EDA and EEA.

MILITARY STANDARDS AND MEDICOLEGAL RULES

Hallowell Davis, M.D.

Military, Economic, and Social Competence

In 1949 a very broad scale of hearing was prepared by the Committee on Hearing of the National Research Council for possible incorporation in a set of physical standards appropriate to the peacetime needs of the Army and the Navy, to partial mobilization or to total mobilization. The general principles of this broad original scale are reflected in the more recent and more detailed military standards. The scale is shown in the table.

A Scale of Military, Economic, and Social Competence of Hearing Appropriate for Incorporation in a Physical Profile Serial

Class	Name	Hearing Level for Speech in Decibels	Remarks
A	Normal	Not more than 15 in *worse* ear	Both ears within normal limits; no difficulty with faint speech
B	Near normal	More than 15 but not more than 30 in *either* ear	Has difficulty only with faint speech
C	Mild impairment	More than 30 but not more than 45 in *better* ear	Has difficulty with normal speech but not with loud speech
D	Serious impairment	More than 45 but not more than 60 in *better* ear	Has difficulty even with loud speech
E	Severe impairment	More than 60 but not more than 90 in *better* ear	Can hear only amplified speech
F	Profound impairment	More than 90 in *better* ear	Cannot understand even amplified speech
G	Total loss of hearing in both ears		Cannot hear any sounds

The following are excerpts from the explanatory comments attached to this scale:

> This scale refers solely to hearing and does not take into consideration a man's competence with hearing ads, lip reading (speech reading), etc.
>
> . . . . .
>
> The classes are defined by "decibel loss of hearing for speech." Until suitable technical facilities for direct measurement by speech audiometry are available the loss of hearing for speech shall be calculated from pure-tone air-conduction measurements by averaging the hearing losses at 500, 1000, and 2000 cps, or at 512, 1024, and 2048 cps if the available audiometers are so calibrated. A person should be classified one class lower than indicated by the average value if, with an average loss of 10 db or more, his hearing loss for any one of the three frequencies is greater by 25 db (or more) than the least of his three losses.
>
> . . . . .
>
> Special categories for special military duties (such as sonar listening) may be established, but usually the special requirements are for ability in discrimination, not in sensitivity. Such requirements should be based on job analyses and appropriate special tests. The general standard of Class A, i.e., not more than 15 db loss of hearing for speech in either ear, is sufficiently rigid for any initial screening.
>
> . . . . .
>
> The classes are defined for tests made without a hearing aid. Veterans' compensation should be awarded on this basis. For civilian and industrial purposes, however, classification should be based, if the examinee so desires, on his loss of hearing for speech (not pure tones) measured with his hearing aid in operation. No person using a hearing aid may be placed in Class A, however. The eligibility of wearers of hearing aids for limited military duties should be decided by military authorities on the basis of job analyses.

Military Physical Standards

Military service requires that a person be physically fit to perform certain required tasks and duties. Of course, there are some military duties that can be performed quite successfully by a man with a minor handicap, but a missing trigger finger, fallen arches, a leaky heart valve, a perforated ear drum, or dependence on a hearing aid quite properly disqualifies a man for unlimited service. For unlimited service a man must pass a whole series of screening tests. Failure on any one of these disqualifies him. The set of minimum requirements is known as the "physical standards." Hearing is one of the items in military physical standards.

Most of these "physical standards" could more aptly be called biological standards. They actually take their name from the doctor's "physical examination," in which he looks, feels, listens, and also measures with physical instruments such as scales, meter sticks, and blood-pressure apparatus. The audiometer is now one of these "physical" instruments.

Actually there is not just one set of physical standards but many. The military standards, however, are typical of the minimum requirements set up for their own purposes by various organizations —police and fire departments, commercial airlines, and many other groups.

There is a whole series of military physical standards. The primary set is for "unlimited" service. Then there are the more rigorous requirements for various special branches or activities such as aircraft pilot, submariner, or paratrooper. Sometimes a very specialized duty, such as sonar listening, may require the passing of special tests of hearing or other aptitude. More lenient standards are set for admission to limited duty. Still another set of standards concerns dismissal from duty entirely or from a special category. For obvious reasons a higher standard is required for admission to a particular duty status than is set for mandatory separation. Experience, the investment in special training, morale, natural deterioration to be expected from aging—all these enter the picture. The setting of initial physical standards is a difficult task of judgment, but separation involves many more conflicting interests and is even more difficult.

For many years the military physical standards for hearing were based entirely on the voice test, the whisper test, and sometimes the watch tick or the coin click (see Chapter 7). Now, however, pure-tone audiometry is also required by the Air Force, by the Navy, and, for certain purposes, by the Army.

The hearing levels adopted by the Armed Forces represent what amount to *screening levels of hearing.* As pointed out above, different screening levels are needed for different purposes and situations. It would be reasonable for the Armed Forces to be lenient, for example, when they are faced with a manpower shortage in a military emergency and are not merely selecting from among numerous volunteers or draftees during peacetime. Nevertheless, the present military and Veterans Administration physical standards for hearing are of general significance because they represent considerable experience and are among our most specific estimates of the limits of practical hearing ability.

HEARING PROFILES

The following excerpts are adapted from Army Regulation 40-115. They set the audiometric hearing standards for induction and enlistment. Three classes or "profiles" are defined. (In these excerpts "hearing level" is substituted for "hearing loss" and the specifications based on the whispered voice and spoken voice are omitted.)

H-1: Audiometer-average hearing level in each ear not more than 15 db at 500, 1000, 2000 cps and not more than 30 db at 4000 and 8000 cps.

H-2: Audiometer-average hearing level of each ear not over 20 db (no one level more than 25 db) at 500, 1000, and 2000 cps and not over 40 db (neither one over 50 db) at 4000 and 8000 cps.

H-3: Audiometer-average hearing level of each ear not over 25 db (no one level more than 30 db) at each of the frequencies 500, 1000, and 2000 cps and not over 60 db (neither one greater than 70 db) at each of the frequencies 4000 and 8000 cps. When the average level for either ear is greater than this the average level for the other ear must not be greater than prescribed for H-1.

These standards for induction and enlistment obviously stress the frequencies important for the understanding of speech and discount considerably any elevation of the hearing threshold level at 4000 and 8000 cps. The principle of averaging the levels for two or three different frequencies is recognized. If a man passes the H-1 screen, his hearing is considered fit for general unlimited duty. This screen is a reasonable definition of the "limit of normal hearing."

The following excerpts from AR 40-530-55 concern the Auditory Evaluation of Members on Active Duty:

Army members displaying evidence of hearing loss in excess of profile H-3 are referred to a medical treatment facility designated as an auditory screening center or the Army Audiology and Speech Correction Center, as indicated, for auditory evaluation, treatment, or rehabilitation.

Among the further regulations concerning possible disability is the following:

Cases of true deafness [severe persistent hearing loss] involving a hearing level in the better ear of 60 db or more in the speech range. Such patients should be considered medically unfit, processed for disability separation, and transferred to the Veterans Administration for further treatment and auditory rehabilitation.

and further (slightly paraphrased):

> Patients to be transferred to the Army Audiology and Speech
> Correction Center for evaluation, rehabilitation (if indicated) and
> final disposition will include the following:
> (1) Those cases of true deafness with hearing levels in the
> better ear of 30 db or more in the speech range which do not come
> within any of the categories of pseudo-deafness outlined above, in-
> cluding malingering, psychogenic deafness, and temporary threshold
> shift.
> (2) Patients on whom auditory screening centers are unable
> to obtain consistent findings in repeated tests.

The following Retention Standard (from AR 40-504) is an important item:

> Deafness [hearing loss] does not alter a patient's medical fitness
> for retention on active duty when the patient's hearing can be
> sufficiently improved through rehabilitation and use of a hearing aid
> to meet the medical fitness standards prescribed for retention on
> active duty. No Army member will be considered physically unfit
> for retention on active duty solely because of a hearing defect,
> provided such defect can be improved by use of a hearing aid to a
> level of 20 db or better in speech reception score.—paragraph 8,
> AR 40-504.

Disqualification of Flying Personnel

A statement by an Air Force officer at a CHABA meeting in
1955 is worth quoting almost in full:

> The physical standards for hearing in the United States Air
> Force apply to two different groups of personnel. These are com-
> missioned personnel, both flying and non-flying, and airmen or enlisted
> personnel.
> Historically, as far as hearing loss was concerned, the basic
> problem centered around the flying (or rated) personnel when it was
> realized that a certain amount of acoustic trauma occurred as a
> result of aircraft engine noise and other incident noises associated
> with aircraft. For this reason, the physical standards for personnel
> entering into flight training were set somewhat higher than the
> standards for non-flying personnel. However, when the integration
> program of 1947 began, with its consequent review of personnel
> qualifications, it was determined that the use of too stringent physical
> standards would result in a heavy attrition rate among already rated
> (flying) officers. This was obviously due to the high-frequency hear-
> ing losses that officers had apparently incurred during their hundreds
> of hours of flying experience.

As a result, it was decided that certain hearing standards would prevail *at the time of initial selection* for *all* commissioned personnel. This standard, for initial commission, flying Classes 1 and 1-A, and for pilot or observer training, permitted a maximum hearing level of 15 db for both ears at frequencies from 250 through 2000 cps, and an average of 40 db for both ears at 4000 and 8000 cps. This amounts to a permissible total sum of hearing levels of 160 db for the four high-frequency thresholds, distributed in any way between the two ears and the two frequencies, but not exceeding a total of 160 db. This obviously allowed for greater selectivity among the already rated personnel and may, in fact, be too liberal for today's needs.

It soon became apparent that, once a man had been commissioned or was actively flying, too many individuals would be disqualified or too many waivers would be granted if the standards mentioned above were maintained. As a result, rated personnel or personnel re-entering active duty may now have hearing levels that are not higher than 20 db at 250 through 2000 cps in the better ear, and no higher than 20 db at 250 and 500 cps and 40 db at 1000, and 2000 cps. No standards have been set for 4000 and 8000 cps.

Other rated personnel, not primarily in control of the aircraft and whose function will allow for some hearing loss, may have levels no higher than 20 db at 250, 500, and 1000 cps and 40 db at 2000 cps for the better ear, with no standard specified for the worse ear.

Non-rated commissioned personnel on active duty will not be summarily disqualified for active duty if they can effectively perform their duties while using a hearing aid. Trained flying personnel who have sub-standard auditory acuity are required to undergo aero-medical evaluation. This evaluation includes an estimate of ability to receive voice radio transmission over standard aircraft headsets while airborne. The examination findings are considered in determining continued qualifications for flight duty.

A general policy has been established of granting only limited waivers for marked loss of hearing acuity. Particular attention is paid to the possibility that a given hearing level may be due to a temporary threshold shift resulting from exposure to noise. The easiest method to determine this point is to remove the individual from the noise to see whether recovery occurs.

For airmen (enlisted personnel), the standards of acceptable hearing are based primarily on the whispered voice test. To be considered acceptable for an H-1 physical profile classification, an airman must have 15/15 hearing in each ear as determined by the whispered voice test. Those acceptable for H-2 profile classification must have 8/15 or better hearing in each ear, or 15/15 in one and less than 8/15 in the other, provided that the defective hearing is not due to active or progressive organic disease.

Airmen who develop an impairment of hearing greater than the H-2 limit while on active or inactive duty, who are using a hearing aid (if necessary), and who understand the spoken voice at 10 feet, may be assigned to profile classification H-3 and qualify for retention on, or recall to, active duty. Airmen, or prospective airmen, whose hearing is less than the requirements for H-2 classification are considered to be non-acceptable.

Airmen with duty assignments as control tower operators or air traffic controllers are required, by Civil Aeronautics Authority–Air Force agreement, to meet the hearing standards established for Class II flying personnel. This standard permits a maximum level of 20 db at all test frequencies through 2000 cps in the good ear, with a 20 db level at 250 and 500 cps, and 40 db at 1000 and 2000 cps in the bad ear.

SONAR LISTENING

The following excerpts from a statement by a Navy officer at the same meeting in 1955 illustrate the use of tests of hearing other than pure-tone audiometry for special duty, namely sonar listening:

. . . In the Navy the importance of measuring hearing abilities stems largely from the crucial part that hearing plays in the duties of the Sonarman. . . . Thus the anti-submarine Sonarman is responsible for detecting approximately 800 cps tonal pulses which are often weak and masked by noise and reverberations. . . . On the other hand, the sonar operator on a submarine works almost exclusively in a listening system. He normally does not employ echo ranging. He listens to a wide variety of sounds in the water over a wide range of pitch. His interpretations of objects or targets in the water are based on loudness, rhythm, and quality of sounds in a background of noise. . . . In view of these job demands . . . research workers in World War II developed two hearing measures, in addition to certain intellectual tests, as a basis for selection. One measured acuity by audiometer at octaves between 512 and 8192 cps. The second measured the ability to discriminate differences in pitch between a standard tone of about 800 cps and a variable comparison tone. . . . Today we use a standard of 20 db hearing level at frequencies 512, 1024, and 2048 cps and a 35 db level at the next two octaves. For destroyer Sonarmen, only the 20 db standard is used. For submarine Sonarmen we apply both the 20 and 35 db standard. The *pitch discrimination test* is shorter and somewhat easier than it used to be, but the cutting score is set at about half a standard deviation above the mean for an unselected recruit population. . . . Sonarmen are required to undergo an annual examination of their hearing. . . .

The Problem of Monitor Limits

The principles of monitoring audiometry have been set forth in Chapter 7. The object of monitoring audiometry is to detect, by routine periodic tests of hearing, the individuals who show signs of incurring a significant noise-induced (or other) hearing loss. It was pointed out that the specific rules and criteria for taking action or, in military language, for "medical disposition" of the cases so detected, must be evolved to fit the particular circumstances. "Monitor limits" appropriate in a military installation may be quite different from those suitable for a textile mill.

Specific monitor limits have been adopted by the Air Force in Regulation AF 160-3. The rules are quite complicated, however, and some experience is still needed to judge whether the actual hearing levels chosen are too high or too low.

Of course, monitoring audiometry overlaps with screening audiometry and the problem of physical standards. Screening is oriented toward picking out those men whose hearing is so poor that they are not suited for or can no longer perform the duties to which they are assigned and toward detecting the men whose ears require medical attention. Inspection of the audiograms made in a monitoring program can serve this medical purpose. Monitoring audiometry does more than this, however. It singles out not only those who are already in difficulty, as shown by a hearing level that is beyond some arbitrary monitor limit, but also those who are *threatened* with handicap even though their hearing levels are still below the monitor limits. This is possible if *changes for the worse* are observed, judged by comparison of the most recent monitor audiogram with a reference audiogram previously established for that individual. The practical problem is to evolve a set of rules that is effective in picking up such changes for the worse but which eliminates spurious changes due to temporary threshold shift, transient middle-ear infections, and the like. The difficulty is to keep the rules simple and yet detect the significant changes, and to do this without overburdening the diagnostic center or the consulting otologist.

Medical Rating of Physical Impairment

We shall not attempt to write a history of the important developments of the last few years in relation to the legal recognition of noise-induced hearing loss as an industrial disease that entitles a worker to compensation under workmen's compensation laws. The social wisdom of the laws and the legal justice of court decisions are irrelevant to the otologist and the audiologist in their professional capacities, but the otologist is called upon to assess or "rate" hearing for the purposes of payment of compensation. He is also asked to diagnose the type of hearing loss that a workman has so that a reasonable "causal relation" to noise-exposure can be affirmed or denied. His advice may also be asked as to the appropriate rules that should be followed by industrial commissions or even courts and legislatures in dealing with such cases. Only a very few states have so far adopted explicit rules or codes of this sort.

Questions of the evaluation of permanent impairment, of causal relation, and the like, have been considered carefully and extensively by several groups and committees, however, and a consensus now seems to be emerging on most of the controversial points. Certain confusing terms, notably "disability" and "hearing loss," have been or are being redefined with more restricted meanings. This should greatly improve communication between the medical and legal professions. The issues, and also the responsibilities, involved in the evaluation or rating of impairment and of disability have been clearly stated.

IMPAIRMENT AND DISABILITY

We have already commented on the term "hearing loss" and the clarification that is made possible by adding the term "hearing level" to our vocabulary (Chapter 4). A term that has caused particular difficulty over the entire medicolegal field is "disability." The physician has used it as almost a synonym for impairment or handicap. But *to the lawyer the term "disability" means that a person's ability to engage in gainful activity has been reduced.* In other words, disability in the legal sense is not a purely medical condition. Physicians and their affiliates, such as audiologists, should carefully respect this legal usage of the term.

A very helpful and important statement defining "impairment" and "disability" has recently been issued by the Committee on Medical Rating of Physical Impairment of the American Medical Association. It appears in the preface of the "Guides to the Evaluation of Permanent Impairment." [1] The first several paragraphs of the preface read as follows:

> Evaluation or rating of permanent disability has long been recognized as an important and complex subject. In the past much

[1] *Journal of the American Medical Association,* 168: 475 (1958).

confusion has resulted from inadequate understanding by physicians and others of (a) the scope of medical responsibility in evaluation of permanent disability; and (b) the difference between "permanent disability" and "permanent impairment."

It is vitally important for every physician to be aware of his proper role in the evaluation of permanent disability under any private or public program for the disabled. It is equally important for him to have the necessary authoritative material to assist him in competently fulfilling his particular responsibility—the evaluation of permanent impairment. It is the purpose of this and other reports by the Committee on Medical Rating of Physical Impairment to correct a past confusion of terms and to provide a series of practical guides to the evaluation of various types of permanent impairments.

The following explanations of generally used terms in programs for the disabled will suffice for all practical purposes:

1. *Permanent Disability.*—This is not a purely medical condition. A patient is "permanently disabled" or "under a permanent disability" when his actual or presumed ability to engage in gainful activity is reduced or absent because of "impairment" and no fundamental or marked change in the future can be expected.

2. *Permanent Impairment.*—This is a purely medical condition. Permanent impairment is an anatomic or functional abnormality or loss after maximal medical rehabilitation has been achieved and which abnormality or loss the physician considers stable or nonprogressive at the time evaluation is made. It is always a basic consideration in evaluation of permanent disability. It should be remembered, however, that permanent impairment is a contributing factor to, but not necessarily an indication of, the extent of a patient's permanent disability.

3. *Evaluation (Rating) of Permanent Disability.*—This is an administrative, not medical, responsibility and function. Evaluation of permanent disability is an appraisal of the patient's present and probable future ability to engage in gainful activity as it is affected by nonmedical factors, such as age, sex, education, and economic and social environment, and the medical factor—permanent impairment. Nonmedical factors have proved extremely difficult to measure. For this reason permanent impairment is, in fact, the sole or real criterion of permanent disability far more often than is readily acknowledged. A determination of permanent disability is an administrative decision as to the patient's entitlement.

4. *Evaluation (Rating) of Permanent Impairment.*—This is a function which physicians alone are competent to perform. Evaluation of permanent impairment defines the scope of medical responsibility and therefore represents the physician's role in the evaluation of permanent disability. *Evaluation of permanent impairment is an appraisal of the nature and extent of the patient's illness or injury as it affects his personal efficiency in the activities of daily living.*

These activities are *self-care, communication, normal living postures, ambulation, elevation, traveling,* and *nonspecialized hand activities.*[2] It is not and never can be the duty of physicians to evaluate the social and economic effects of permanent impairment. These effects must be evaluated by administrators in making determinations of permanent disability.

Competent evaluation of permanent impairment requires adequate and complete medical examination, accurate objective measurement of function, and avoidance of subjective impressions and nonmedical factors, such as the patient's age, sex, or employability.

The two most authoritative statements by medical authorities concerning the evaluation of permanent impairment of hearing were prepared for and approved by the Committee on Conservation of Hearing of the American Academy of Ophthalmology and Otolaryngology. The first statement has also been approved by the American Medical Association.

The following paragraphs are a paraphrase of an explanatory article about the first statement which appeared in NOISE *Control* in November, 1955.

It is not easy to construct a set of rules for translating hearing loss into dollars to be paid as industrial compensation or as veterans' benefits. Nevertheless, as the Z-24 Report of the American Standards Association (*The Relations of Hearing Loss to Noise Exposure*) pointed out, such rules are needed to take care of present cases of industrial hearing loss and also as a yardstick for any criteria that are ever to be drawn up as to what is a "dangerous" or a "permissible" noise in industrial situations.

There are four distinct steps between the hearing loss and the dollars of compensation; one is the actual measuring of hearing levels with an audiometer; another is the conversion of the hearing levels into a single figure, ultimately a percentage to apply to the value of total loss of hearing; the third is the setting of a dollar value for total permanent impairment of hearing; and the fourth is the establishment of a "causal relation" between the particular case of impairment of hearing and the noise that is presumed to have caused it.

The amount of compensation to be paid for total permanent impairment of hearing is not a medical or technical matter. It must be fixed by law, by court decisions, and by industrial commissions. It is there that the question of whether wage loss should be a necessary condition for the payment of compensation must be settled.

The method of evaluating or rating impairment of hearing and the rules for arriving at an appropriate percentage figure must be approved or accepted by proper legal authority. As yet, however, in

[2] Italics added.

spite of several attempts that have been made in the past, there is no general agreement on methods of rating hearing impairment or on the rules for calculation. In New York, for example, one set of rules is in force, in Wisconsin another set.

A statement has recently been published in the *Journal of the American Medical Association* that should go far toward clarifying the medical and technical points that are involved in writing such rules. In particular, it states a set of reasonable initial assumptions and shows how a set of logical, equitable rules can be based on these assumptions. It tries to separate the assumptions, which may be accepted or rejected by law-making bodies, from scientific facts and principles.

The most important of the basic assumptions is that the impairment of hearing which should be the basis for compensation is impairment of hearing for everyday speech. This is a middle ground between one extreme that would award compensation for any impairment of hearing, however slight or at whatever frequency, and another extreme that would make wage loss and economic disability the only yardsticks.

The statement in question is only a statement of principles, not a complete and detailed set of rules. It points out where more information is needed before final rules can be written. One large gap is a suitable tool for measuring the hearing level for speech. Such a tool we have in principle in the speech audiometer, but we do not have suitable standardized tests to use with it. Alternatively we might measure hearing levels for pure tones and translate the results into a hearing level for speech; but we need more experiments to give us a really valid set of rules for making this translation. Here, by the way, is one important point in which the present New York and Wisconsin rules differ. Experiments could show which is the better rule once we have agreed in principle on just what the rule should accomplish.

After we have measured the hearing level for speech directly or calculated it from the pure-tone levels, we must still evaluate it as an impairment in the real, everyday sense. This is a difficult step. The statement of principles recognizes that hearing levels a little above zero really lie within a medically recognized "range of normal" and that they do not cause any significant impairment of the hearing of everyday speech. But a careful, large-scale study of real men and women with real hearing losses, including many noise-induced hearing losses, must be made to find just where impairment does really begin, what hearing levels imply complete impairment of hearing (deafness) for everyday (unamplified) speech, and how much should be considered 50% impairment, and so on.

We can hope that experiments to fill these gaps will be undertaken soon. However, if the general principles are observed and the gaps are clearly recognized, it should be possible to write reasonable

rules on the basis of the best present estimates and to look forward
to a revision of the details when the necessary experiments have been
made.

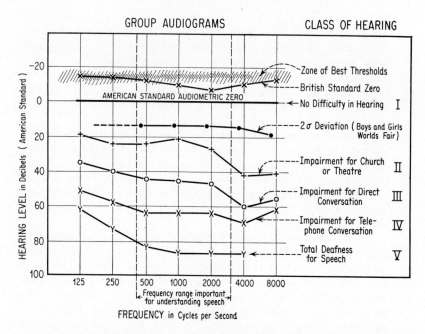

Fig. 9-1. **Self-classification of hearing impairment.** These group audiograms
show the average hearing levels of the subjects in the United States Public Health
Survey (*Beasley, 1936*), who classified their own hearing according to Captions I
to V at the right.

The means of the "normals" (after exclusion of all whose audiograms devi-
ated by 20 db or more from the mean) became the American Standard for zero
hearing level. At the top is indicated the zone of best thresholds (shaded area). The
"2 σ deviation" curve shows the dispersion of the thresholds of the boys and girls
who took the Bell Telephone Laboratories hearing tests at the World's Fair in 1939.
About 95 per cent had better hearing, 5 per cent worse hearing at each frequency.
This is a practical statistical definition of the range of normal.

The points above the zero hearing level show the British Standard zero for
audiometers. The British Standard (2497:1954) gives pressures generated in the
British Standard Coupler by a particular type of British earphone (4026A). The
points in this graph represent the corresponding pressures produced by an American earphone (WE-705A) in a National Bureau of Standards 9A coupler. (*Kind-
ness of National Bureau of Standards, based on data of J. P. Albrite, et al.*)

The Report of the Council of the American Medical Association
gives this first statement:[3]

[3] We have inserted in brackets the recommended terms "hearing level," "impairment," and so on.

PRINCIPLES FOR EVALUATING HEARING LOSS

INTRODUCTION

A method more satisfacory than those now in use is needed to evaluate hearing losses in terms of the disability [impairment] that they produce. With a pure-tone audiometer, the hearing loss itself can be measured in decibels for tones of different frequency, but this measurement does not denote the degree of disability [impairment]. Several methods have been proposed for calculating the percentage loss [impairment] of hearing from the pure-tone audiogram, but none of them has proved entirely satisfactory.

The first of these, the so-called 0.8 method,* was not intended to be a measure of economic disability or handicap. It yielded a "percentage hearing loss," useful as a descriptive medical term. In this method, and also in the method recommended in 1942 and modified in 1947 by the American Medical Association,† the basis of calculation is restricted to the "speech frequencies." In the so-called A.M.A. method,† the four test frequencies were weighted differently and greater importance was assigned to the loss [threshold shift] of a given number of decibels in the middle of the intensity range than to corresponding losses [shifts] for either very weak or very strong sounds. The weightings were adjusted in an effort to bring the results into harmony with judgments of the amount of disability [impairment] that seemed to be associated with the various hearing losses [levels]. Actually the A.M.A. method is fairly satisfactory for calculating percentage capacity to hear speech for persons who have conductive hearing losses in which the losses [hearing levels] are not very different for different frequencies. For persons with nerve deafness [neural hearing loss], however, and particularly for those in whom hearing for low and middle tones is good but the hearing for high tones is poor, the results often are in conflict with the clinical evidence.

The most valid way to measure the ability to hear speech correctly is to use words or sentences. Hearing and recognizing the spoken word is more than receiving a set of independent signals; it is a dynamic process in which time is a factor and in which there are complicated interactions. It seems logical to use speech as the material in a test of the ability to hear speech. The recent development of speech audiometers may make it practical to do so. The unaided human voice, as used in the conventional "spoken voice test" and the "whisper test," is not sufficiently accurate and is confined to too narrow a range of intensity.

* H. Fletcher, *Speech and Hearing*. Princeton, N.J.: D. Van Nostrand Company, Inc., 1929.

† Tentative Standard Procedure for Evaluating the Percentage Loss of Hearing in Medicolegal Cases: Report of the Council on Physical Medicine, J. A. M. A. 133: 396–397 (Feb. 8) 1947.

Specifications for speech audiometers have been compiled.* Lists of words and sentences for standard test material must now be selected and satisfactory recordings made of them. Methods for their use must be standardized, and rules for calculating the disability [permanent impairment] of hearing must be established. This report is intended as a first step in this task.

The next step will be to apply the proposed method to persons who have hearing losses of various types and whose hearing disability [impairment or handicap] has been estimated directly by competent and experienced observers. The disability [impairment] caused by hearing loss for these individuals will be calculated from [evaluated on the basis of] the results of speech audiometry according to tentative rules and tables, which will be adjusted until reasonable and consistent agreement is obtained. These findings will be related to tests with pure-tone audiometers and other hearing tests. The proposed method should not attempt to determine a monetary value of disability for total loss of hearing [evaluate or determine a monetary value for a permanent total disability of hearing], either for one ear alone or for both ears [binaural]. Furthermore, the determination of the percentage disability resulting from hearing loss [the evaluation or rating of a permanent impairment of hearing] is distinct from the problems of clinical diagnosis of the type of hearing loss and its probable cause.

DEFINITIONS AND PRINCIPLES

The following definitions and statements give a basis for the proposed method.

Hearing for speech. For the present purpose, hearing is defined as the ability to identify spoken words or sentences under average everyday conditions of normal living by the sense of hearing, unaided by touch or vision. The proposed method should deal with the function of hearing for speech and not with the details of injury to the ear in an anatomic sense. The functional point of view is more realistic than the anatomic and fairer to all concerned. The ability to hear very high or very low tones contributes little to the intelligibility of speech. Injury to the sense organ or the nerves that detect the highest audible tones may be real in a medical or pathological sense but usually does not cause a disability [an impairment or handicap] of economic or social importance. The tests of hearing to be recommended should give a measure, directly or indirectly, of the ability to hear correctly simple statements, commands, or questions. The ability to repeat correctly or to respond appropriately to the sentences, questions, or commands should be taken as evidence of correct hearing. In other words, the rules and schedules for calculating the percentage

* Standards of the American Standards Association, Specifications for Speech Audiometers, Standard Z24.13-1953, New York, American Standards Association, 1953.

disability [evaluating an impairment] of hearing from the results of the particular tests should be validated in terms of sentence intelligibility.

Benefits derived from hearing aids and auditory training. The probability that a particular type or degree of hearing loss may or may not be benefited by a hearing aid should not be considered in calculating the disability caused by a hearing loss [evaluating the permanent impairment of hearing]. This follows from the broad principle, which is widely accepted, that a loss [impairment] of normal function should be evaluated in the absence of any prosthetic device. The proposed schedule of percentages should not consider the possible improvement in hearing for speech that often results from the kind of prolonged training and practice known as auditory training. The percentages of disability [impairment] to be given in the schedule should therefore be the average expectations for persons of average intelligence, who originally had normal hearing, but without benefit of either a hearing aid or formal auditory training. The proposed method should not give special consideration or any unusual importance to a person's sense of hearing because of the nature of his profession or employment. In very noisy surroundings, for example, it may be difficult or impossible to communicate by speech even if the hearing of the person is normal. Furthermore, an impairment of hearing may reduce the employee's potentiality for changing his job. Everyday communication therefore should be the basis for evaluation of the disability [impairment] of hearing.

Limits of normal hearing and of total disability [impairment]. In the Minimal Requirements for Pure Tone Audiometers for Diagnostic Purposes, formerly issued by the Council on Physical Medicine and Rehabilitation, the normal threshold of hearing for pure tones is defined for audiometric purposes as "the modal value of the minimum sound pressure, at the entrance to the external auditory canal, which at that frequency produces a sensation of pitch in a large number of apparently normal hearing ears of persons in the age group from 18 to 30 years, inclusive." The average normal threshold for speech can be defined in the same way as the modal or commonest value of the threshold, once a sample of everyday speech has been chosen for reference. A full definition of normal threshold, either for pure tones or for speech, requires also a statement of the limits of normal. This concept is well established in statistical procedures as well as in medical thinking and practice. In clinical audiometry, for example, it is generally accepted that a hearing loss of 15 db for pure tones may be within the limits of normal variability. A greater loss [Levels greater] than this can be considered abnormal. Also, it is at about this level that the hearing loss usually begins to be noticed by the person. In other words, hearing losses [deviations from zero] within the limits of normal are usually unnoticed and do not cause any practical handicap. The limit of normal for the hearing of speech may reasonably be assumed for the present to be comparable to that for the hearing of pure tones in the speech-frequency range, but it should be defined more precisely in the future when more measurements and better validation become available.

At the other extreme of the hearing range, there may be a total loss of hearing or a total inability to hear speech [deafness]. As commonly used, these terms are not precise nor necessarily synonymous. It is important to define them and to determine the relation between them. This cannot be done until more experimental data are available.

The concepts of "limit of normal hearing" and of "total inability to hear speech" are fundamental. It should be possible to specify both limits in precise objective terms. When they have been established, they will constitute anchor points from which intermediate degrees of disability [impairment] can be derived.

Binaural evaluation. Measurements should be made of the hearing of each ear separately. A rule should be established for computing [evaluating] from these measurements the percentage of the total hearing disability [total permanent impairment of hearing] when both ears are used.

Detection of psychological factors and malingering. It is assumed that the individual is cooperative in the tests of his hearing and that the examiner is satisfied that the individual has understood the tests and responded honestly to them. Part of the responsibility of the examiner is to detect any failure of full cooperation or any significant psychological factors that may, in his opinion, invalidate the tests. If full and intelligent cooperation is doubted, a direct estimate of percentage of disability [a direct evaluation of his impairment of hearing] (in the functional sense) should be made on the basis of the general behavior of the individual (including his behavior during the preliminary interview) and his response to a pure-tone audiometer and to special tests designed to detect malingering. In such cases the examiner's opinion should be given weight at least equal to that of any percentage calculated from the results of routine tests.

Alternative tests for language difficulties. The standardized recorded lists of sentences and words, which may be recommended for use with a speech audiometer, should be suitable for nearly all English-speaking adults who have had the equivalent of a grammar school education. With individuals who have had less schooling or with those who are accustomed only to a strong dialect or to a language other than English, it will be the duty of the examiner to modify the tests according to his best judgment and ability but in keeping with the established principles.

Need for pure-tone audiometry. Pure-tone audiometry is essential for determination of the degree and type of hearing loss. The results of the afore-mentioned experiments may indicate that the percentage of disability [impairment of hearing] can be computed [rated] directly from such tests (the hearing levels for certain pure tones).

Problem of causal relations. A clinical diagnosis of the type of hearing loss must be made in order to determine causal relation. Pure-tone audiograms, both by air conduction and by bone conduction, should be part of the diagnostic study. The following propositions illustrate how such studies may help solve, in individual cases, the problem of causal relation.

1. Conductive hearing loss cannot be attributed to prolonged or repeated exposure to noise. Furthermore, a chronic conductive lesion tends to protect the inner ear from injury by such noise.

2. Audiometry at appropriate intervals is required to distinguish temporary from permanent hearing loss [threshold shift]. Pure-tone audiometry should be employed, as it is a delicate indicator of possible recovery or deterioration.

3. Some loss of sensitivity for high tones is to be expected with advancing age. For the frequency 2000 cps, this loss [threshold shift] on the average amounts to about 5 db in the sixth decade and 10 db in the seventh. The losses [shifts] at 4000 cps on the average are about 10 and 20 db, respectively, but there are large individual differences. These losses [shifts] may not be sufficient in themselves to reduce hearing for speech enough to cause a noticeable disability [impairment]. The type of loss that usually occurs with age is often indistinguishable by present tests from the impairment caused by exposure to noise. In the rules for determining the disability [impairment] of hearing from the results of pure-tone audiometry, an allowance for the hearing loss [threshold shift] expected with advancing age should be included.

4. The desirability of a record of the condition of the hearing of every employee made at or before the beginning of employment is obvious. Such a record is also desirable if the employee changes his type of work. In such tests a pure-tone audiogram by air conduction should be considered the minimum procedure, and, if possible, speech audiometry should also be used. If the pure-tone audiogram by air conduction indicates deviation from normal by [hearing levels of] more than 15 db for 500, 1000, or 2000 cps or 30 db for 4000 cps, a complete pure-tone audiogram by both air and bone conduction and a complete otological examination should be made and recorded. Such records would protect the interests of both employer and employee.

During the time the Council on Physical Medicine and Rehabilitation conducted an acceptance program, it compiled minimal acceptance requirements for pure-tone and speech audiometers. Substantially similar standards are still issued by the American Standards Association.* It is assumed that only instruments that conform to these standards will be employed in making the audiometric tests from which the disability of hearing is to be calculated [impairment of hearing is to be evaluated].[4]

* Audiometers for General Diagnostic Purposes, Standard Z24.5-1951.
[4] Reprinted by permission from *The Journal of the American Medical Association,* 157: 1408–1409 (1955). Copyright, 1955, by the American Medical Association.

A Guide for the Evaluation of Impairment of Hearing

More recently a specific set of simple rules that embody nearly all of the principles set forth above has been adopted (1958) and published (1959) by the Committee on Conservation of Hearing as follows:

> The following statement of principles, prepared by the Subcommittee on Noise and approved by the American Academy of Ophthalmology and Otolaryngology, is presented as a guide for the evaluation of hearing impairment * regardless of the cause or causes of such impairment. These principles are based on current medical opinion. The Subcommittee on Noise reaffirms the principles concerning the evaluation of hearing impairment already set forth jointly by it and by a cooperating subcommittee of the American Medical Association. The Subcommittee on Noise now recommends the following interim method for measurement and calculation.

> Ideally, hearing impairment should be evaluated in terms of ability to hear everyday speech under everyday conditions; the term "impairment" will be used hereinafter in this sense only. The ability to hear sentences and repeat them correctly in a quiet environment is taken as satisfactory evidence for correct hearing for everyday speech. Because of present limitations of speech audiometry, the hearing level for speech should be estimated from measurements made with a pure-tone audiometer. For this estimate, the Subcommittee recommends the simple *average* of the hearing levels at the three frequencies 500, 1000, and 2000 cps.

> In order to evaluate the hearing impairment, it must be recognized that the range of impairment is not nearly as wide as the audiometric range of human hearing. Audiometric zero, which is presumably the average normal hearing threshold level, is not the point at which impairment begins. If the average hearing level at 500, 1000, and 2000 cps is 15 db or less, usually no impairment exists in the

---

* "Impairment," is here used as defined in "Guides to the Evaluation of Permanent Impairment" approved by the Committee on Medical Rating of Physical Impairment, Journal of the American Medical Association, September 27, 1958, Volume 168, Number 4, page 475. "Impairment" as defined by the American Medical Association denotes a medical condition that affects one's personal efficiency in the activities of daily living. It is recognized that "disability" as used in various workmen's compensation laws involves nonmedical factors, since it may be related to actual or presumed reduction in ability to remain employed at full wages. Permanent impairment is, therefore, a contributing factor to, but not necessarily an indication of, the extent of a patient's permanent disability within the meaning of the workmen's compensation laws.[5]

[5] "Guide for the Evaluation of Hearing Impairment," *Transactions of the American Academy of Ophthalmology and Otolaryngology*, 63: 236–238 (1959).

ability to hear everyday speech under everyday conditions. At the other extreme, however, if the average hearing level at 500, 1000, and 2000 cps is over 82 db, the impairment for hearing everyday speech should be considered total. The Subcommittee on Noise recommends the following formula:

For every decibel that the estimated hearing level for speech exceeds 15 db, allow 1½% up to the maximum of 100%. This maximum is reached at 82 db.

At this time, the Subcommittee on Noise makes no specific recommendation regarding a correction for a shift in the hearing threshold due to age, because the relation of presbycusis to noise-induced hearing loss is not yet fully understood.*

The Subcommittee on Noise recommends that any method for the evaluation of impairment include an appropriate formula for binaural hearing which will be based on the hearing levels in each ear tested separately. Specifically, the Subcommittee on Noise recommends the following formula: The percentage of impairment in the better ear is multiplied by five (5). The resulting figure is added to the percentage of impairment in the poorer ear and the sum is divided by six (6). The final percentage represents the binaural evaluation of hearing impairment.

* For current information about the relation of hearing threshold to age, see Table XXII, 1954 Wisconsin State Fair Hearing Survey (Median Values for Office Workers). Published by the American Academy of Ophthalmology and Otolaryngology, 1957.

The statement above speaks for itself, but several points deserve emphasis or explanation. For one thing, the word "disability" in the earlier statement has now been replaced by the word "handicap." A major reason for this change was the technical legal meaning of "disability" discussed above. Actually, the recent AMA statement defines "impairment" as meaning exactly what the subcommittee intended by "handicap," and approximately what others had intended to imply in the phrases "social adequacy of hearing" and "social competence of hearing." It will be desirable for audiologists to talk only about impairment of hearing. But now a new difficulty arises: since "impairment of hearing" means "handicap" it must not be used as a synonym for "hearing loss" in the sense of an elevated threshold level or a dysacusis. In the new usage, "impairment" implies some reduction of practical everyday personal efficiency—not simply a measurable change.

The rule proposed by the Subcommittee for relating impairment to decibels of hearing level is linear between two arbitrary limits. The linear form was adopted for simplicity, and the upper and lower limits were also set with simplicity in mind. Some experts think that a sigmoid or even a more complex curve would be a little more accurate, but they cannot agree as to where or in which direction the inflections should be. There are no numerical data valid and reliable enough to be of any help here. There seems to be no doubt, however, that the lower limit of impairment in the sense of a practical handicap should be located between 15 and 20 decibels

PRACTICAL LEVELS OF HEARING

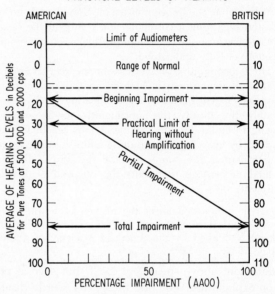

Fig. 9-2. Important practical hearing threshold levels for speech differ numerically by approximately 10 db as between the American and the British standards for audiometric zero (see Chapter 7, appendix). The hearing level for speech is estimated by taking the average of the levels for the three pure tones, 500, 1000, and 2000 cps. No standard has yet (1959) been established for an audiometric zero for speech audiometry.

The levels —10 and 0, respectively, are the lowest that are required on pure audiometers, according to the American Standard for Audiometers for Diagnostic Purposes (Z24.3-1951). Actually, a few audiometers provide fainter signals, but they are of little practical use.

The levels for beginning impairment and for total impairment and the relation, indicated by the diagonal line, between average hearing level and percentage impairment are those recommended by the Committee on Conservation of Hearing of the American Academy of Ophthalmology and Otolaryngology. The limit of the range of normal is not sharp and does not necessarily coincide either with the lowest step on the audiometer or with the beginning of impairment in the social and medicolegal sense. The practical limit of hearing at the 30 db level (American) represents a consensus of otologists and audiologists that at this level amplification is needed for successful everyday communication. The amplification may be provided by a hearing aid or by the raised voice of the talker.

hearing level for speech. This "speech" is connected discourse or simple sentences, but the level in question can be measured very well by spondee word lists.

There is one apparent discrepancy between the recent interim method and the earlier "principles." This is in regard to an allowance for presbycusis. The earlier principles advocate the inclusion of an allowance for "the hearing loss expected with advancing age." The more recent statement takes the attitude that the changes in hearing level with age and the relations of such presbycusis to noise-induced hearing loss are not yet well enough established to be made the basis of any specific rule. For the present, therefore, it remains for each commission or legislature to decide whether to omit the presbycusis correction entirely or to adopt some simple but arbitrary rule.

There are other difficulties here in addition to the uncertainty about the biological facts of presbycusis and noise-induced hearing loss. Strictly logical rules require certain assumptions about how to apportion the responsibility for an impairment of hearing. Suppose that the expected threshold shift from presbycusis is 10 db and a man's measured hearing level for speech is 25 db, and that the payment of compensation begins at 16 db. Should the 10 db be subtracted from 25 db before evaluating the impairment? If so, $25 - 10 = 15$, and there is no compensation allowed according to the rule. Or should the percentage corresponding to the 25 db hearing level be calculated first? At the rate of 1.5 per cent decibel above the 15 db hearing level, this gives 15 per cent. One might argue that because there would be no impairment from a simple presbycusic shift of 10 db, the noise should be held responsible for the entire 15 per cent. Or should the responsibility for the 15 per cent be divided between age and noise-exposure according to the fractions of the total threshold shift that each has presumably produced? A shift of 10 db is to be expected normally from presbycusis; the remainder, 15 db, is attributed to the noise-exposure. Therefore, the percentage of total compensation to be paid would be $15\% \times 15/25 = 9\%$. And, finally, if the hearing levels for a man's two ears are different, should the presbycusis correction be applied before or after his combined binaural impairment has been evaluated? These questions illustrate some of the complexities of the presbycusis problem. The answers to these questions do not lie in the area of audiology but in laws and their judicial interpretations.

Presbycusis alone does not seem to cause much impairment of hearing if we look only at the median threshold levels for various age groups. The dispersion of hearing levels is large, however, in the upper age groups, and a very significant percentage of older in-

dividuals actually does have an impairment of hearing from presbycusis in the sense of a practical handicap.

Our best present guess is that the noise-exposure somehow accelerates the process that underlies presbycusis. Certainly, the progressive development of presbycusis and that of noise-induced hearing
loss are very similar. In presbycusis the first loss is for the highest
tones, whereas for noise-induced hearing loss the elevation of threshold
usually begins at about 4000 cps, but the exact position of the noise-
induced "notch" in the audiogram depends somewhat on the frequency spectrum of the noise that induced it. In any case, the
notch deepens and then widens, and when 2000 cps and then 1000
cps are involved, the hearing level for speech may be very significantly elevated. The impairment is considerable, and so is the
percentage rating of the impairment according to the rules. The
number of individuals who have these more-than-average impairments, with or without noise-exposure, is fortunately not very large.
It may be increasing, however, and the problem of finding an equitable
rule for the presbycusis correction is very real. The total economic
stake involved is considerable from the point of view of industry as
a whole.

One can read between the lines of the "Principles for Evaluating
Hearing Loss," first drafted in 1952, the clear hope that standardized
speech audiometry was close at hand. In 1959 the trend is clearly to
rely on pure-tone audiometry and to estimate the hearing level for
speech from the hearing levels for certain frequencies. There is
considerable sentiment (1959) for including somehow the hearing
level at 3000 cps: perhaps by taking the average of 500, 1000, and
3000 cps (or 500, 1500, and 3000 cps) rather than 500, 1000, and
2000 cps, in order to recognize to a realistic extent the loss of auditory
discrimination that goes with a sharp frequency cutoff at or near
2000 cps; but more experiments are needed before such a recommendation is likely to be made by any official medical group.

Suggested Readings

There are few if any reviews, books, or monographs that deal directly with the material of this chapter. Most of the background information is in committee reports, in military regulations, or in articles
in medical journals that may not be readily available. The most significant passages and in some cases entire articles have been reproduced or paraphrased in this chapter.

"The Relations of Hearing Loss to Noise Exposure." Report of Exploratory
    Subcommittee Z24-X-2. American Standards Association, Inc., 70 East 45th
    Street, New York 17, N.Y.

10

HEARING AIDS

S. R. Silverman, Ph.D.,

S. Gordon Taylor, and

Hallowell Davis, M.D.

A hearing aid is any instrument that brings sound more effectively to the listener's ear. It may simply collect more sound energy from the air, it may prevent the scattering of sound during transmission, or it may provide additional energy, usually from the battery of an electrical amplifier.

The first objective of a hearing aid is to make speech intelligible. The "quality" or naturalness of the speech may be sacrificed if necessary. Little thought was given to quality by those who used the old ear trumpets. They were well enough satisfied if only speech could be made loud enough to be intelligible. Even with early electrical instruments, the chief difficulty was still to deliver enough energy, and any necessary compromises were acceptable as long as speech could be understood. Now, however, the arts of electronic amplification and electroacoustic engineering have made it possible to deliver as much sound as the ear can tolerate. We can therefore raise our sights and say that a hearing aid should deliver sounds loudly enough to be heard easily, but without discomfort. The listener's hearing loss should be overcome and his auditory nerve stimulated in a pattern as nearly normal as possible. Of course, the instrument should not add new "internal" noises. Distortion of the original pattern of sound should be introduced only to the extent that it assists in bringing to the listener speech that is intelligible, comfortable, and of pleasing quality.

Mechanical Hearing Aids

The simplest hearing aid, used since man became civilized enough to grow old and become hard of hearing, is the hand cupped behind the ear. The hand intercepts more of the oncoming sound wave than does the ear alone and deflects more of its energy into the external canal. The larger the scoop, the more energy can be collected. The efficiency of the scoop can be improved if it is shaped to favor the delivery of the energy into the ear canal. The broad principle of the ear trumpet is illustrated in Figure 10-1.

The ear trumpet took many forms in efforts to compromise between effectiveness, convenience, and the user's vanity. Some of the varieties of shape and style are shown in Figures 10-2, 10-4, 10-5, and 10-6, photographs of the Goldstein collection of nonelectrical hearing aids at Central Institute for the Deaf. Some instruments were small and convenient, but not very effective. Others were built into cane heads, ear ornaments, or vases. Nearly all the instruments in the collection are black, probably to be as inconspicuous as possible, and all have in common a large surface or opening to catch the sound. Some also extend toward the speaker, where his voice is louder, and carry the sound to the ear in a tube without allowing it to scatter. When we recall that the intensity of sound in open air falls off rapidly with the distance the sound travels, we can see that much more energy can be collected if the ear trumpet reaches well out toward the speaker's mouth.

Most of the old-fashioned ear trumpets were more than mere scoops to collect acoustic energy. They were also "resonators," tuned broadly to frequencies in the speech range. Sound pressures build

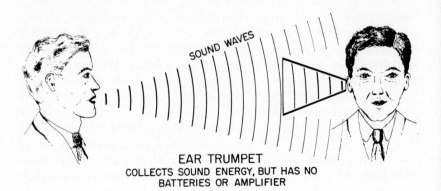

EAR TRUMPET
COLLECTS SOUND ENERGY, BUT HAS NO
BATTERIES OR AMPLIFIER

Fig. 10-1.

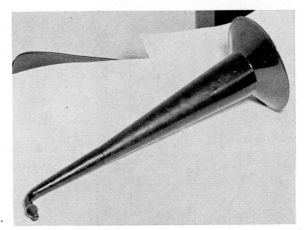

Fig. 10-2.
An old
ear trumpet.

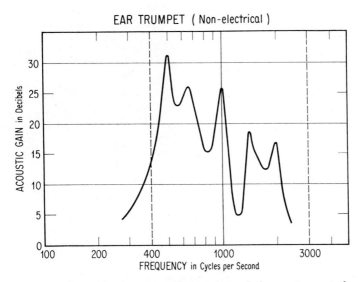

Fig. 10-3. This is the frequency characteristic of the ear trumpet shown in Fig. 10-2. The acoustic gain is the difference between the sound pressure level measured in a 2 cc coupler attached to the ear trumpet and the corresponding level measured in a 6 cc coupler mounted in a plywood baffle cut to simulate the side of the head. The baffle and microphone were placed normal to the incident sound at the position previously occupied by the mouth of the trumpet. Note the resonant peaks at 500 and 700 cps and their multiples. Sharp resonant peaks of hearing aids are exaggerated when an artificial ear (coupler) is substituted for an actual human ear. The gains for speech (spondees) of this ear trumpet, for four hard-of-hearing listeners, were 6, 11, 12, and 15 db. (*Courtesy of J. R. Cox, Jr.*)

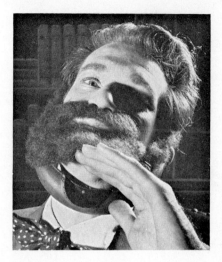

Fig. 10-4. Concealment by a beard of a large nonelectric hearing aid. (*From the Goldstein Collection, Central Institute for the Deaf. Photo, St. Louis Post-Dispatch.*)

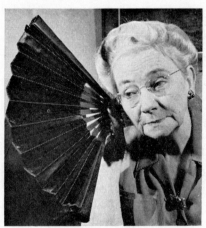

Fig. 10-5. An acoustic fan. (*From the Goldstein Collection, Central Institute for the Deaf. Photo, St. Louis Post-Dispatch.*)

up to higher levels at and near the resonant frequencies of the instrument, and at these frequencies the energy delivered to the ear may sometimes be increased in this way by as much as 10 to 20 db. The external ear canal deals with sounds at frequencies near 4000 cps in the same way. The tube of the trumpet is larger and longer than the ear canal and is thus "tuned" to a lower band of frequencies.

By empirically combining the principles of resonance and sound conduction, the ear trumpet or the speaking tube can be a fairly effective hearing aid. Those instruments are very simple and easy to use, and should not be forgotten in this electronic era. The gain for speech provided by an ear trumpet is likely to be about 10 to 15 db. Even the cupped hand behind the ear gives us 6 or 8 db. As we all know, this may make just the difference between understanding and not understanding a lecture or a sermon.

"LOUDER, PLEASE!"

The cupped hand at the ear also politely tells the speaker that the listener is having difficulty hearing him, and almost always, so universally is the sign understood, the speaker will raise his voice. An extra 10 db of voice means only a little extra effort for most speakers. We instinctively and often unconsciously raise our voices this much in noisy surroundings when we begin to have a little difficulty hearing ourselves. The intensity of the voice is increased at the source, and the hard-of-hearing listener gets the benefit.

In the Psycho-Acoustic Laboratory the wartime project dealing with hearing aids was nicknamed "Louder, Please."

EARLY BONE-CONDUCTION DEVICES

Among the mechanical hearing aids of the last century it is interesting to find one, the acoustic fan, which took advantage of bone conduction. A sheet of metal or hard rubber, shaped and decorated

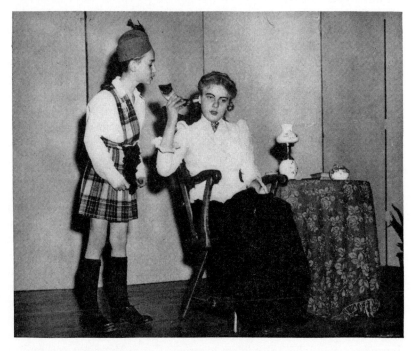

Fig. 10-6. Deaf children re-enact the story of Alexander Graham Bell. (*From the Goldstein Collection, Central Institute for the Deaf.*)

like a fan, was held with one corner against the teeth. The vibrations of the metal were transmitted through the teeth to the bones of the skull and thus to the inner ear. More recently, men have used devices resembling pipes that employ the same principle. Bone conduction can, as we have seen, by-pass a conductive deafness. The acoustic fan or pipe is unable, however, to collect enough energy from the air to be a very effective aid to hearing.

DEVICES WITHIN THE EAR

Another class of mechanical hearing aid aims to deliver more efficiently to the inner ear the sound energy that enters the external canal. Such a device may help a person whose eardrum is perforated or is missing entirely, particularly if the malleus and incus are also missing. Sometimes, but not often, a piece of flexible membrane or tissue placed over the perforation is helpful. Sometimes a wisp of cotton is placed in contact with the stapes or the round window, or a bristle with a bit of stiff membrane attached to pick up the sound waves is effective. Any such device is clearly a substitute for nature's eardrum and ossicles. Such a "prosthesis," put in place by an otologist, as described in Chapter 5, may remain in place for days, and for a time it may raise the level of hearing effectively. It is not advisable, however, for anyone except an otologist to attempt to introduce such a device into the ear. It is often difficult even for him, with all his special instruments, illumination, and knowledge of anatomy, to make contact with the "hot spot" that gives a useful improvement of hearing. Eventually the device gets out of place or must be renewed or cleaned. And only a very small minority of the hard of hearing have the particular abnormality of the middle ear that is suitable for this kind of "hearing aid." On the other hand, the reduction in the size of modern hearing aids has made the electric hearing aid within the ear a reality.

Unfortunately the occasional success of an artificial eardrum lends a glow of plausibility to the host of devices that are advertised by unscrupulous individuals in uncritical newspapers and periodicals. Complete restoration of hearing with a simple, inexpensive but miraculous gadget that fits comfortably within the ear canal is the dream of everyone who is hard of hearing. Even the most sober and rational of us dream and wish. We are not very far removed from the days when the right ear of a lion was believed to be a cure for deafness or when we bought "snake oil" from the Indian medicine man. There are still enough wishful and gullible people to keep in business a few who are willing to promise enough at not *too* high a price. A thousand-to-one chance that the wonderful gadget may be a tenth as good as it is claimed to be seems to be worth a dollar to many people. But actually there isn't such a chance. Claims of restoring hearing by "resonance" are a pseudoscientific smoke screen. Very rarely, it is true, something pushed blindly into the ear canal might open a passageway through or around a plug of wax. This might cause a real improvement; but, except for such cases, we may be quite sure that those who believed themselves benefited by mysterious, within-the-ear gadgets were either honestly self-deluded or had been suffering from the sort of psychological deafness that will be described later in Chapter 18.

One of the most rigid laws of physics (although apparently not of human society) says in effect, "You can't get something for nothing." What the hard-of-hearing man must get in order to hear is *more energy.* He may induce the speaker to provide it by saying, "Louder, please"; he may collect more and bring it more efficiently to his ear by an ear trumpet or a speaking tube; or he may provide it, as we shall see, from the battery of his electric hearing aid.

Electric Hearing Aids

An electric hearing aid is a miniature telephone. It differs fundamentally from the mechanical aids we have just described in that *its batteries, and not the human voice, supply the energy of the sound that the listener finally hears.* The voice of the speaker merely serves to control the flow of electric current in the wires to the earpiece and gives it the pattern of the voice sounds. The receiver in the listener's ear, like the telephone receiver at the end of the line, converts the electric current back into sound. The point is that the sound generated in the earpiece, like the sound from a public-address system, may be made much louder than the sound that falls upon the microphone (transmitter) because its energy comes from the battery. A telephone is designed to produce at a distance a sound nearly as loud as the original voice. The energy from the battery of the telephone is required to overcome the losses in the long wires. A hearing aid is designed to produce a louder sound in a very small receiver at the end of a very short cord. Thus the energy of the battery serves to overcome the hearing loss of the listener.

Types of Electric Hearing Aids

Electric hearing aids are of three general types: wearable, portable or desk type, and group.

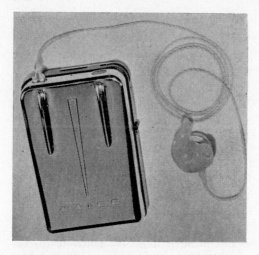

Fig. 10-7. A conventional
type of monaural hearing aid.
(*Maico Electronics, Inc.*)

Comfort, convenience, desire to conceal the instrument, and individual acoustic needs have all contributed to the development of
a variety of types of wearable hearing aids. Some types are more
popular than others, depending on what the user considers most important to him. Later in this chapter we shall comment on the
relative effectiveness of the different types in various listening situations.

Wearable instruments differ mainly in where they are worn on
the body and in whether there is a receiver in one ear or in both ears.
The following types are commercially available:

1. Conventional monaural: one instrument (microphone, amplifier, batteries) worn in the coat, shirt, or dress with receiver
   in one ear.

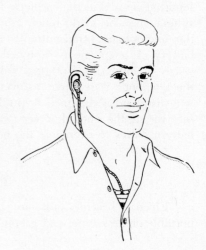

Fig. 10-8. Wearing a conventional
monaural hearing aid. Men may wear the
instrument in a pouch suspended from
the neck under the shirt or they may clip
it in a shirt, vest, or coat pocket. Women
clip the instrument to a brassière or slip
or tuck it in a pouch and pin the pouch
to a brassière strap. (*Adapted from an
illustration by Sonotone Corp.*)

2. Headtype, monaural: one instrument, housed in the temple of a pair of spectacles or in a case worn behind the ear, with receiver in one ear.

3. Pseudobinaural or Y-cord: one instrument worn in coat, shirt, or dress with a receiver in each ear.

4. Binaural with conventional "packaging": two separate conventional instruments worn on the chest, usually about eight inches apart, one for each ear.

5. Binaural spectacle: two instruments, "packaged" in the temples of spectacles, one for each ear.

6. Binaural head-mounting: two instruments on the head, usually mounted behind the ears, one for each ear.

These wearable types of hearing aids are illustrated in Figures 10-7 to 10-14.

The portable or desk type of instrument can be used by a single hard-of-hearing listener who spends much of his time in one place. It may deliver more power with better quality than wearable instruments do and it draws its power from a wall socket as a radio does.

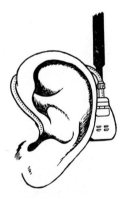

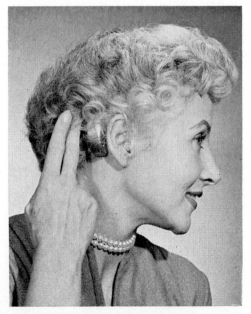

Fig. 10-9. A monaural "behind the ear" instrument. Clipped to a headband, it rests behind the ear. (*Sonotone Corp.*)

Fig. 10-10. Wearing a "behind the ear" instrument. The hearing aid is held in place by a barrette or a headband. A tube leads to the eartip in the ear. (*Sonotone Corp.*)

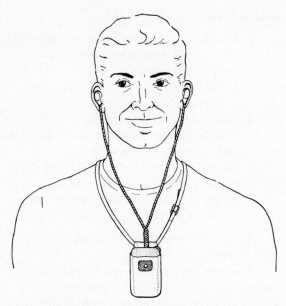

Fig. 10-11. A Y cord hearing aid. Note the single instrument, with a receiver in each ear.

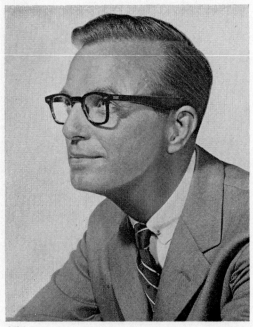

Fig. 10-12. Wearing an eyeglass type of hearing aid. (*Sonotone Corp.*)

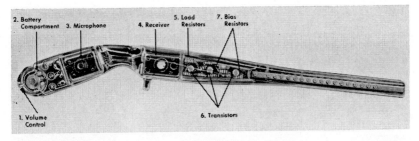

Fig. 10-13. Cutaway showing placement of components within the temple of eyeglass hearing aid. (*Maico Electronics, Inc.*)

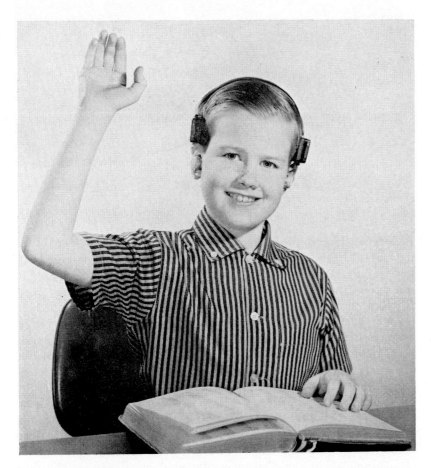

Fig. 10-14. Binaural hearing aid worn on the head. Note two transmitters and receivers. (*Beltone Hearing Aid Co.*)

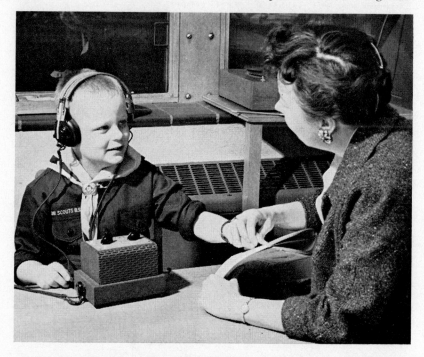

Fig. 10-15. Using a desk model hearing aid. (*Instrument by Sonotone Corp. Photo, Central Institute for the Deaf.*)

It does not require an insert receiver and frequently has two "over-the-ear" receivers. The portable hearing aid may have multiple outlets, an advantageous feature for an itinerant teacher who wants to use the instrument with two or three children.

A group hearing aid consists of one or more microphones, an amplifier, and as many as ten pairs of over-the-ear or insert receivers. Frequently a turntable is included for playing recorded speech, music, or sound effects. The effect of a group hearing aid may now be achieved with individual wearable instruments without connecting wires from the amplifier to the listeners. This is done by creating an electromagnetic field by means of an "inductance loop" around a room. Each listener wears a conventional hearing aid equipped with a magnetic "telephone" pickup. Freedom of movement around the room is not limited by connecting cords.

Group hearing aids are generally used in schools for the deaf and hard of hearing, in churches, in meeting halls, and in theaters. Binaural features are now being increasingly incorporated in these instruments.

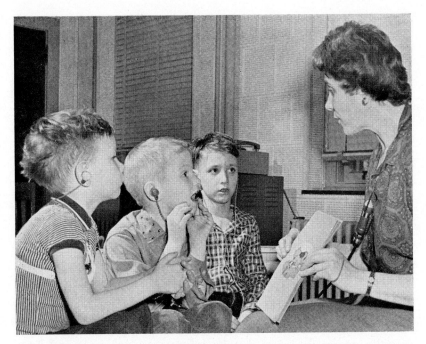

Fig. 10-16. Using a conventional group hearing aid. Note the Y cords and the "necktie" microphone on teacher. (*Central Institute for the Deaf.*)

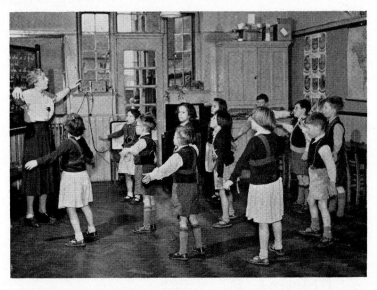

Fig. 10-17. An "inductance loop" group hearing aid. Note that the children's hearing aids are not wired to a fixed unit. The children may move about the room freely. (*Royal Residential Schools for the Deaf, Manchester, England.*)

Components of Hearing Aids

AMPLIFIERS

The "heart" of any hearing aid is its amplifier. This is the part of the hearing aid that amplifies weak electric current from the microphone to the much stronger current delivered to the receiver. We have seen a simple form of mechanical nonelectric equivalent in the ear trumpet and in the hand cupped behind the ear. Fortunately, electric amplifiers enable us to do better than this.

In the evolution of electric hearing aids, three types of amplifiers have been used: the carbon, the vacuum tube, and the transistor.

The carbon amplifier. The carbon amplifier is actually very similar to a carbon microphone, such as is generally employed in commercial telephones. It takes advantage of the change in electrical resistance between two pieces of carbon when the mechanical pressure between them varies. The more firmly they are pressed together the more easily does the electricity flow from one to the other. In the carbon amplifier this action takes place among a few grains of specially prepared carbon that lie between a fixed and a movable electrode. The moving electrode is part of, or is attached to, a diaphragm of magnetic material that moves in response to changes in the magnetic field generated by a nearby electromagnet (see Figure 10-18). A battery and a receiver are connected to the "output" leads. The changing current in the electromagnet makes the diaphragm vibrate, and as it vibrates it changes the pressure on the carbon granules. The changing electrical resistance changes the current flow in the output circuit. The changes in current in this circuit are much greater than the changes in the input current, which may come from a magnetic or carbon type of microphone and a small battery associated with it.

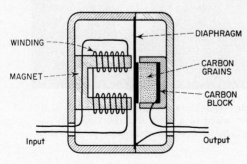

Fig. 10-18. Carbon amplifier.

Carbon amplifiers tend to be rather "noisy" because of erratic mechanical behavior and consequent changes of resistance among the carbon granules. As far as we know, carbon amplifiers are no longer used in hearing aids.

The vacuum-tube amplifier. The principle of an amplifier is the principle of a control valve. A small amount of power controls, as by a valve, the flow of a greater stream of power. The greater stream must, of course, have its own source. For the vacuum-tube amplifier this source is the B battery. The vacuum tube acts as an electrical valve, allowing more or less current to flow through it from the B battery. In fact, in Great Britain such an electronic vacuum tube is *called* a "valve." The vacuum-tube valve differs from the carbon type of amplifier in that the flow of current from the B battery is controlled directly by electric charges instead of indirectly by mechanical movements induced by the original current from the microphone. As we shall see, the transistor also controls current flow by means of electric charges.

In an ideal amplifier the flow of current from the B battery is directly proportional to the strength of the weak current or electric charge that controls it. The output of the amplifier may be thousands of times the strength of the input signal from the microphone. *There is a limit, however, to the possible output of any amplifier, no matter how strong the control signal may be.* When the input signals are very strong and "open the valve wide," the output is limited by the design of its tubes, the voltage of the B battery, and the electrical characteristics of the other elements of the circuit. For a small input signal we get a larger (amplified) output signal, and as the input signal increases, the output increases proportionally until it reaches its maximum (Figure 10-19).

A cutaway drawing of a vacuum tube and a diagram of the circuit of a simple amplifier (Figures 10-20 and 10-21) may help to clarify the valvelike action of a vacuum tube.

Inside the tube are three essential elements: filament, grid, and plate. The filament may be a single wire that runs lengthwise of the tube at its center. It is like the filament of an electric light bulb, and an electric current is passed through it to keep it red hot. Around the filament, as in Figure 10-20, is mounted a spiral of wire. This coil is the "grid." Outside the grid stands a cylinder of sheet metal, which is called the "plate" because in early tubes it was actually a flat plate. (In the early tubes the three elements were all flat and stood side by side, as they are represented in the conventional symbol used in Figure 10-21.) Some modern electronic vacuum tubes have additional elements between the filament and the plate. These ad-

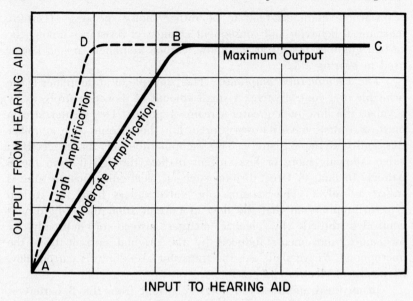

Fig. 10-19. Input-output characteristic (linear co-ordinates).

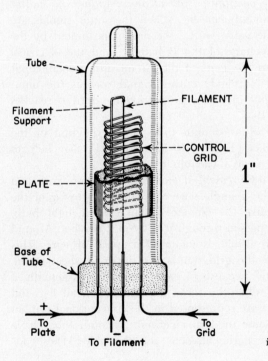

Fig. 10-20. Cutaway drawing of a vacuum tube.

ditional elements increase the stability and efficiency of the action of the tube, but we need only be concerned here with the three fundamental original elements: the filament, the grid, and the plate.

The filament must be kept hot so that it will "boil off" electrons. The A battery provides the current to heat the filament, while the B battery provides a positive charge on the plate that pulls the electrons (negative charges of electricity) across the tube from filament to plate. From the plate the electrons move along the wires and through the receiver. This movement of electrons *is* the electric current. The resistance to the movement of electrons across the space between filament and plate varies according to the electric charge on the grid. If the grid is negative (relative to the filament), many of the electrons are repelled by the grid and few pass by to the plate; but if the charge on the grid is less negative, more current will flow. Over a fairly wide range, the resistance of the tube changes in proportion to the varying charge on the grid. Therefore, if a microphone is connected, as shown in Figure 10-21, between filament and grid, the small electric charges generated by the microphone will control the current flow from the B battery across the tube and through the receiver.

To turn off the amplifier we need only turn off the A battery by means of the switch, shown in the diagram. When the filament is cold, no electrons are given off and no B current can flow. If the A current is too weak, the filament is not kept as hot as it should be; then fewer electrons are given off, and they may be given off irregularly. The irregularities may cause noise in the receiver, and

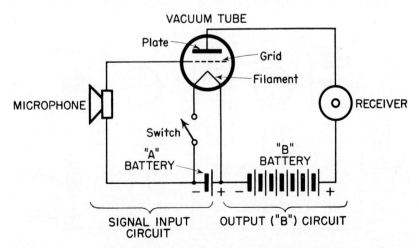

Fig. 10-21. Circuit diagram of a simple amplifier.

the smaller number of electrons available makes the B current weaker. Ultimately the B current fails altogether.

In summary, the A battery heats the filament and thus makes it possible for the vacuum tube to act as a valve. The microphone and grid control the valve action. The B battery provides the current that is controlled, and the receiver converts the varying output current into sound. A simplified diagram of a two-tube hearing aid is shown in Figure 10-22.

Although portable and group hearing aids still use vacuum-tube amplifiers, almost all wearable hearing aids now employ transistors as the "valves" of the amplifier. It is therefore useful to understand the action of a transistor.

The transistor amplifier. Many pure materials in the crystal state are very poor conductors of electricity. Some of these, however, like germanium, can be converted into *semiconductors,* capable of conducting electricity, by the addition of very small amounts of certain other elements. One part in a million of the impurity may be sufficient to make the crystal a semiconductor. When arsenic is added to the germanium crystal, the conduction takes place primarily by the flow of *negative* charges, i.e., electrons. In the pure crystal the electrons of the germanium atoms are held in a very stable pattern or "lattice." The stability of the lattice depends on the regular arrangement of the germanium atoms. When a few atoms of arsenic are added here and there, the lattice is distorted in such a way that it is easier to squeeze in a few extra electrons. The movement of electrons through the crystal takes place by the pushing out of one electron by an extra one that moves in and the migration of the displaced electrons to push

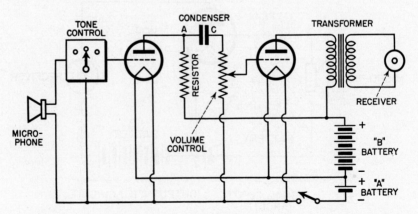

Fig. 10-22. Simplified circuit diagram of a two-tube hearing aid with tone control and volume control.

another in turn out of its place in the lattice. If, however, aluminum or indium are added as impurities instead of the arsenic, the crystal lattice is distorted in a different way. We cannot add extra electrons to it, but we may take away a few and leave vacant spaces called "holes." These "holes," being the absence of a normal negative electric charge, are the equivalent of positive charges. A "hole" can migrate through a crystal as an electron jumps from one place to fill a vacant space but leaves another vacant space behind it. A crystal which conducts primarily by the flow of *positive* charges or holes is called P type. A crystal which conducts primarily by the flow of *negative* charges or electrons is called N type.

A transistor is made from a crystal, usually germanium, that has three regions of semiconductor material arranged like a sandwich. A crystal with a very thin region of N-type conductivity sandwiched between two regions of P-type conductivity constitutes a PNP transistor. The central region is called the base. One of the outer regions, usually smaller than the other, is called the emitter, and the other outer region is called the collector. The base region is about a thousandth of an inch in diameter. The transistor is completed by providing three connections to the three regions and encasing the assembly in a hermetically sealed container.

The drawings of transistors in Figures 10-23 A, B, and C take a purely schematic form which bears little resemblance to the actual physical construction of present-day transistors. The type commonly used in hearing aids consists of a tiny slab or wafer of the base material, on each of the two flat sides of which a still tinier spot of the impurity has been fused. This fusing process results in the contaminant's combining with the immediately adjacent material of the base to form "regions" which exhibit the characteristics required for the emitter and the collector. The effect is much the same as would be obtained if a small dab of penetrating stain were placed on each side of a wood block. The block would not be physically altered but regions of discoloration having a finite depth would be present.

The base of the transistor may be of either the P type or N type of semiconductor materials. If it is N material, the emitter and collector regions will be of P material, and such a transistor will be known as the PNP type. If the base is of P material the emitter and collector will be of N material and this will be an NPN type of transistor. Functionally these two types are the same although they are not directly interchangeable in an amplifier because of their opposite polarities. Either type may be used in a hearing aid.

The operation of a transistor as an amplifier will be more readily understood by considering what happens at the junctions between the adjoining P-type and N-type regions. If we connect a battery between the P-type emitter and the N-type base with the positive end to the emitter and the negative end to the base (Figure 10-23A), the copious supply of positive charges in the P-type emitter will flow readily to the base. Very little voltage is required to move a large amount of current when the battery is thus connected in the "forward" direction. If the battery is connected with the *negative* terminal to the P-type emitter, the positive charges in the emitter cannot cross easily over the junction into the base, since once there they will be pushed back by the positive voltage of the battery. Very little current flows when the battery is thus connected "in reverse."

In normal operation, two battery voltages are connected to a transistor—a small one "forward" from emitter to base, and a large one "in reverse" from base to collector (Figure 10-23B). With these two voltages applied, an additional effect is produced. Once the positive charges have flowed across the emitter junction into the extremely thin base, instead of then flowing through the base connection to the emitter battery most of them slip across the collector junction and are removed by the high negative voltage of the collector battery. The thinner the base region, the larger the proportion of charges which slip over to the collector, and the smaller the portion going to the emitter battery. As the emitter voltage is increased (made more positive), the current in both circuits increases. It increases more in the collector than in the emitter circuit. The ratio of the collector current to base current is the current amplification or "beta" of the transistor in the common emitter configuration. The average present-day transistor has a current amplification of about 50- to 300-fold.

It is obvious from the foregoing that if provision were made, by means of another battery and a switch, for example, to increase and decrease the emitter-battery voltage at will, the resulting changes in base current would be reflected in very much greater changes in

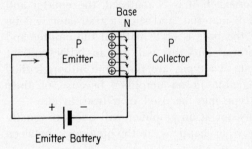

Fig. 10-23A. A transistor. Current flows (arrows) when a battery is connected to the base and the emitter only.

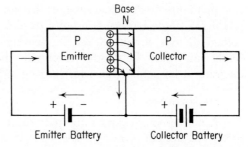

Fig. 10-23B. When the collector battery is added, the current flow from the base is decreased but a relatively heavy current flows through the transistor from the emitter to the collector.

the collector current flow. Thus the transistor could be considered as a valve capable of effecting large changes in collector current.

Figure 10-23C, a basic circuit of a transistor employed as an amplifier, shows this valve action applied in a practical manner. Instead of an added battery and switch, an input transformer is connected in series between the base and the emitter battery. An audio-frequency signal applied to the primary of this transformer will result in a voltage across the secondary terminals. If this voltage is of the same polarity as the battery it will have the effect of increasing the battery voltage. If of opposite polarity, it will serve to decrease the battery voltage. Because the signal applies a positive voltage during one half of each cycle, and a negative voltage during the other half, it will alternately aid and oppose the battery voltage. The base current will increase and decrease accordingly, and similar but very much larger changes will take place in the current in the collector circuit. Thus a minute signal applied through the input transformer activates the transistor valve, which produces a highly amplified replica at the output transformer.

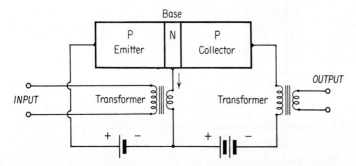

Fig. 10-23C. This basic amplifier circuit employs a PNP type of transistor. In practice a single battery is used, with its voltage divided by means of a resistance network in the circuit.

In Figure 10-23C two separate batteries are shown, but in actual practice a single battery is usually employed. By means of a resistive voltage-divider circuit within the hearing aid, the total voltage of a single battery can be divided to provide the two voltages. The circuit diagram of an actual transistor hearing aid is shown in Figure 10-34.

MICROPHONES

A microphone changes the pattern of sound waves into a similar pattern of electric current. Three types of microphone are or have been widely used in hearing aids.

The carbon microphone. The carbon microphone shown in Figure 10-24 operates on the same principle as the carbon amplifier already described. Its electrical resistance varies as the mechanical pressure on a few grains of carbon is varied. The moving electrode, instead of being driven magnetically as it is in the amplifier, is part of or is attached to a diaphragm that vibrates when sound waves fall on it. The two electrodes, one of which may be the diaphragm, are are made of electrically conducting material and a battery is connected to them. The diaphragm vibrates when sound waves fall on it and the mechanical pressure on the carbon particles therefore changes. The electrical resistance varies in turn, and accordingly more or less current flows through the microphone and its circuit.

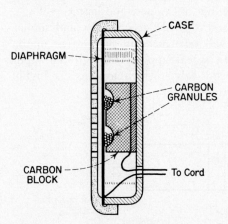

Fig. 10-24. A carbon microphone.

The crystal microphone. The crystal microphone does not vary its electrical resistance as does a carbon microphone; instead, it actually transforms some of the sound energy into electrical energy. "Crystal" does not mean that the quality of the sound that it transmits is necessarily "crystal clear" (as we might speak of a pair of glasses), although this meaning has sometimes been suggested in advertisements. It means that the essential element is an actual crystal, usually of Rochelle salt. This kind of crystal has the property of generating an electric voltage, or "potential," between opposite faces when it is mechanically twisted or bent slightly in certain directions. The voltage is proportional to the mechanical force. This *piezoelectric effect* transforms the mechanical vibrations of sound directly into corresponding electrical signals. Only a part of the energy of the sound is transformed into electricity, and the signals are weak. The signals reproduce the pattern of the mechanical movements very accurately if the latter are not too powerful; but the crystal microphone could not be used effectively in wearable hearing aids until a sufficiently small and powerful vacuum-tube amplifier could be constructed. When this was accomplished the crystal microphone came into nearly universal use for vacuum-tube hearing aids.

A common type of crystal microphone is made from a flat, rectangular slice of crystal. The slice is mounted firmly, supported by three of its corners, as shown in Figure 10-25. The sound falls upon one side of a light diaphragm, usually shaped in the form of a cone, as in the familiar radio loud-speaker. The cone is flexibly supported, so that the pressure of the sound waves can move it in and out; and it is connected by a stiff link or rod from its center to the free corner of the crystal. As the cone moves, the crystal is bent and generates a tiny charge of electricity. Tinfoil or some similar material on the large flat faces of the crystal pick up the charge, and wires carry the charges to the amplifier.

The fidelity of a crystal microphone depends not only on the crystal but also on the size, construction, and mounting of the cone. The microphone must be designed to avoid (or at least to reduce) undesired "resonance," that is, a tendency to vibrate more freely at

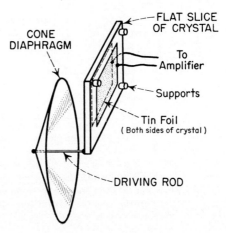

CONE DIAPHRAGM

FLAT SLICE OF CRYSTAL

To Amplifier

Supports

Tin Foil (Both sides of crystal)

DRIVING ROD

Fig. 10-25. Diagram of a crystal microphone.

some frequencies than at others. If a system is resonant, it will reproduce those frequencies more strongly than others (Figures 10-3 and 10-26) and thereby distort the original pattern of complex sounds. The result of resonant distortion is usually a "tinny," "squawky," or "boomy" quality, depending on the frequency of the peak.

The microphone is a delicate mechanical instrument. Its diaphragm (cone) and crystal must be protected from injury by hard objects; and yet its diaphragm must be freely accessible to sound. The diaphragm of a hearing aid is therefore mounted behind a protective grille, and the wearer must respect its delicacy and not injure it by ill-advised attempts to clean or adjust it. A tear or a wrinkle in the cone may change its acoustic properties considerably; and excessive heat, moisture, or dryness will spoil the crystal although these effects are minimized by suitable protection.

The magnetic microphone. With the introduction of the vacuum-tube hearing aid the crystal microphone was universally adopted. But the advent of the transistor amplifier made this type of microphone impractical. The transistor is a low-impedance device, which means it offers low resistance to alternating currents including audio-frequency currents generated in a microphone. In electrical practice the most efficient transfer of energy from one circuit to another is achieved when the impedances of two circuits are similar. The crystal

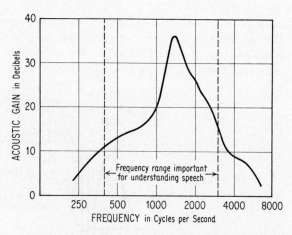

Fig. 10-26. This graph shows the relation between amplification and frequency of a hearing aid. Such a curve is called the "frequency response" or "frequency characteristic" of the instrument. The frequency response shown here is strongly "peaked" at about 1500 cps.

microphone is a high-impedance device and so is the input circuit of a vacuum tube. Thus these two made a most logical and effective team. But to connect a crystal microphone to a transistor is not unlike connecting a three-foot water main to a half-inch pipeline. Only a very small part of the water available in the main is obtainable through the small pipe.

Where the impedances of successive circuits are not too greatly different it is possible to connect them through an impedance-matching transformer. However, the impedances of the crystal microphone and a transistor are so different as to make such an arrangement impractical. A magnetic microphone, on the other hand, can be made to offer an impedance comparable to the input impedance of a transistor. Thus the magnetic microphone has been generally adopted for use in transistor hearing aids.

The magnetic microphone may be described as the equivalent of a telephone receiver in reverse. It consists essentially of a tiny coil of fine wire, a permanent magnet, and an iron diaphragm. These comprise the electromagnetic system. Attached by its apex to the center of the iron diaphragm is a larger, cone-shaped aluminum diaphragm designed to provide maximum pickup of sound energy in the limited space available in a microphone of small proportions. The vibratory motion set up in the aluminum diaphragm is mechanically transmitted to the iron diaphragm. As this moves to and fro with respect to the magnet and coil, corresponding electrical currents are set up in the coil. It is in this manner that the microphone converts sound energy into its electrical equivalent for application to the input of the first transistor.

Something of the mechanical precision employed in the manufacture of this microphone is indicated by the fact that in one type the coil, which has an outside diameter of less than one-quarter inch, and thickness of slightly over one-sixteenth inch, is made up of 3000 turns of wire so fine that it would require a bundle of five to equal the cross-sectional area of a human hair.

RECEIVERS

Receivers for hearing aids are of two general types: air conduction and bone conduction.

Air-conduction receivers. All air-conduction receivers for body-worn electric hearing aids are small enough to be worn in the ear. They are supported by an "insert" or "earpiece" of molded plastic. Even smaller than these are the type built into eyeglass hearing aids and the other tiny aids worn in or behind the ear. With the eyeglass and behind-the-ear types the sound from the self-contained receiver is carried into the ear canal through a transparent plastic tube which terminates in an individually molded ear tip. These tiny receivers represent one of the most difficult bits of electroacoustic engineering in the hearing aid. These earphones must transform electric energy efficiently into sound, and at the same time they must avoid excessive mechanical resonance, which would emphasize some one frequency too much. All this is difficult to accomplish in such a small size. An ideal hearing aid would handle all the audible frequencies with equal efficiency. Such an instrument would preserve the natural quality of sounds and also avoid the discomfort from too great amplification of any one particular frequency. The ideal is being approached more and more closely, even in instruments that employ the small insert type of receiver, but we can hardly hope that it will ever be attained completely. A rather strongly peaked over-all frequency response of an old hearing aid is shown in Figure 10-26. "Flatter" frequency responses are shown in Figures 10-31, 10-35, and 10-38. The response of a typical magnetic receiver of a hearing aid is shown in Figure 10-35. Receivers with the best acoustic characteristics, such as are used for audiometers and laboratory test instruments, are too large to be practical for wearable hearing aids. They are, however, included in many portable and group hearing aids.

The most common type of receiver is the magnetic. It operates on the principle of the ordinary telephone receiver. A thin diaphragm of magnetic material is mounted close to a permanent magnet, as shown in Figure 10-27. The electric current from the amplifier passes

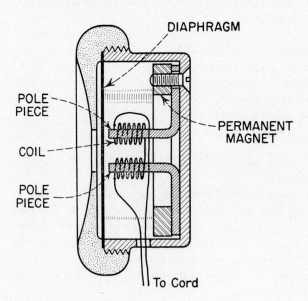

Fig. 10-27.
A magnetic
receiver.

through coils that are wound on cores of special magnetic material fastened to the permanent magnet. According to the strength and direction of the current through the coils, the magnet becomes stronger or weaker. The magnet thus pulls more or less strongly on the diaphragm. The diaphragm vibrates and sets up sound waves in the air.

The crystal type of earphone is very much like a miniature crystal microphone. The same kind of crystal is cut and mounted in the same way, and is connected mechanically to a thin metal diaphragm. The electric voltage from the output circuit of the amplifier is applied to opposite sides of the crystal, and the crystal bends in proportion to the voltage applied. The bending of the crystal moves the diaphragm and thus sets up sound waves in the air.

The moving-coil type of air-conduction receiver is known as the "dynamic" receiver. A light coil of fine wire is firmly attached to the center of a diaphragm, or cone. A strong permanent magnet is mounted so that the turns of the coil lie in its radial magnetic field. The varying electric current from the amplifier passes through the coil and causes it to move back and forth in the magnetic field in accordance with the variations in the current. The fundamental principle is used almost universally in radio and public-address loudspeakers. In the usual *magnetic* type of receiver the coil is firmly attached to the magnet and varies the strength of the field that attracts the diaphragm. In the moving-coil receiver, on the other hand, the coil moves, and the diaphragm does not need to be made of magnetic material.

The moving-coil principle, in addition to being employed in most loud-speakers, is applied in some of the large high-quality earphones used for audiometers and other special purposes. New magnetic alloys, which make possible tiny, yet permanent magnets, favor the development of this type of receiver, and a few hearing aids of the future may employ the moving-coil principle.

The most common type of *bone-conduction receiver* or *vibrator* is magnetic. It is designed to vibrate its case instead of setting up sound waves in the air (Figure 10-28). Its diaphragm is attached rigidly to a plastic case shaped to fit comfortably against the mastoid bone behind the ear. The magnetic system is supported by the edge of the diaphragm. The pull of the magnet varies with the changes in the flow of electric current through the coil, and both magnet and case move in relation to one another. The inertia of the magnet is considerable, however, and therefore the case, and with it the mastoid bone, vibrates appreciably. The case moves less than does the diaphragm of an air-conduction receiver, but it moves with con-

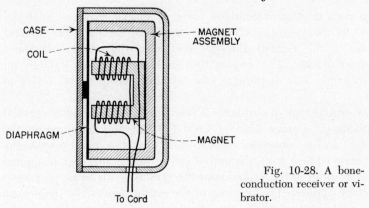

CASE
COIL
MAGNET ASSEMBLY
DIAPHRAGM
MAGNET
To Cord

Fig. 10-28. A bone-conduction receiver or vibrator.

siderable force and can therefore set up an adequate vibration in the skull. The vibrator is held in snug contact against the mastoid by means of a light spring headband, as shown in Figures 10-29 and 10-30.

Partly because of the way in which skin and bone transmit sound, it is difficult to design a bone-conduction vibrator that will deliver high frequencies to the inner ear as efficiently as it does some of the lower frequencies, but its range compares very favorably with the range of the usual air-conduction receiver.

Comparison of bone conduction and air conduction. In the chapter on the medical aspects of deafness, the principle of bone conduction was discussed. It will be recalled that bone conduction is definitely preferable to the insert type of receiver when, for any medical reason, the wearer cannot safely or comfortably use an insert earpiece. Bone conduction is most successful when the hearing loss is primarily conductive and the inner ear is still normal. We shall return to the problem of bone as compared with air in connection with the selection of a hearing aid; but it is worth noting that recent technical developments have favored air conduction somewhat more than bone conduction.

Thanks to the individually molded ear insert, a small in-the-ear air-conduction receiver can now deliver into the ear more sound of good quality than was formerly possible. A considerable fraction of the sound that reaches the inner ear from an air-conduction receiver may actually arrive by way of the bone. The faithfulness of reproduction by a good air-conduction receiver is generally better, particularly for high frequencies, than by a bone-conduction vibrator. When the bone-conduction vibrator was first introduced, it was often preferred because it was less conspicuous and perhaps more comfortable

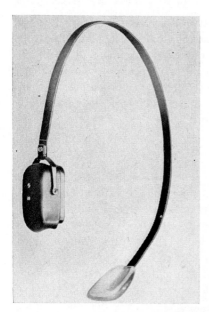

Fig. 10-29. A bone-conduction vi-brator with its spring headband. (*Sonotone Corp.*)

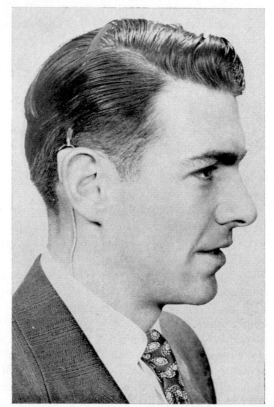

Fig. 10-30. A bone-conduction vibrator in place behind the ear. (*Sonotone Corp.*)

than large over-the-ear air-conduction receivers. Some wearers still prefer bone-conduction vibrators for the same reasons and find them perfectly adequate; but with the increased efficiency of small and less conspicuous air-conduction receivers that require no headband, the choice is based more and more often on the combination of greater convenience and simple effectiveness, and the large majority of the hard of hearing prefer air conduction.

THE VOLUME CONTROL

A volume control, or "gain control," makes it possible to adjust the over-all gain of a hearing aid to intermediate values. The volume control is usually a resistance that is provided with a sliding contact. In Figure 10-22 the upper end of the resistance is connected just beyond the condenser C and the lower end to the filament of the second tube. The full strength of the signal is impressed on the resistance, and the slider takes off more or less of the signal according to its position. When the slider is near the lower end (close to the filament), the difference in voltage between slider and filament can never be very great. If, however, the contact is at the other end, nearly the full strength of the amplified signal delivered through the condenser reaches the grid of the second tube. The strength (voltage) of the available signal falls off progressively as we move the contact from the upper to the lower end of the potentiometer.

THE TONE CONTROL

The tone control is usually a complicated arrangement of condensers and resistances. It may be placed ahead of the first stage, as shown in Figure 10-22, or between stages; and the circuits actually employed in different instruments vary considerably from one another.

The tone control changes the relative strength of the high-frequency and the low-frequency tones in the signals that pass through it (see Figure 10-31). To obtain "high-tone emphasis," a combination of condensers and resistances is chosen that transmits high frequencies efficiently and low frequencies inefficiently. The low frequencies are reduced in strength, or "attenuated," more than the high, and thus a *relative high-tone emphasis* is obtained. High-tone emphasis may really be only *low-tone suppression;* but as long as plenty of gain is available, it makes no difference. The wearer simply pushes up the volume control, thereby increasing the strength of all frequencies equally, and the net result is an increase in the high frequencies with no loss in the middle or low range.

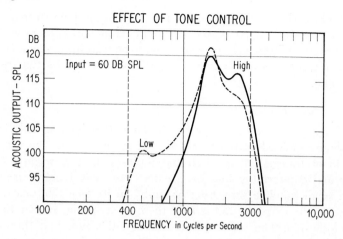

Fig. 10-31. The effect of the tone control on the frequency response of a hearing aid. (*Data from J. R. Cox, Jr.*)

Low-tone emphasis is obtained by other combinations of condensers and/or resistors chosen to suppress the high frequencies.

Some makes of instrument do not have an adjustable tone control, but instead offer several models, each with its own particular emphasis of high tones, low tones, or middle tones. The purchaser then selects the model that best suits his particular needs. Other instruments have an internal adjustment for tone, which is set by the dealer when he sells the instrument; thus he "fits" the device to the purchaser's individual requirements. Still other instruments are "fitted" by selection of the appropriate receiver.

THE OUTPUT TRANSFORMER

An output transformer provides the most efficient means for coupling a magnetic type of receiver to the amplifier circuit.

THE CORDS AND THE CASE

The cords of a hearing aid are obviously nothing more than light, flexible, insulated wires that carry the current from the amplifier to the receiver.

The problem with cords is to make them light and flexible and yet mechanically strong, durable, and electrically insulated. Furthermore, the covering must not generate static electricity or make a noise when it rubs on clothing for noise carried mechanically by cords to the amplifier case and microphone can be a source of great annoyance. In addition, the covering of a cord must keep its insulating properties when moistened by perspiration.

The case deserves mention because it, too, must be strong, light, and durable. The shape of the case and its smoothness, as well as the material of which it is made, must be carefully planned and chosen to reduce as much as possible the noise made by the friction of clothing.

THE MOLDED EARPIECE

An important accessory to all air-conduction hearing aids is the individually molded earpiece or insert (Figure 10-32). The earpiece is made of transparent or flesh-tinted plastic that is formed to fit snugly and comfortably into the wearer's ear. The receiver is made with a small tubelike projection or "nub" on its face that snaps into a recess in the earpiece and is held there by a spring, similar to that on a clothespin. The sound passes through this nub and through a hole drilled in the earpiece and is delivered well down in the external canal of the ear.

The first step in making an earpiece is to take an impression of the ear with a special elastic plastic. Dealers in hearing aids usually provide this service. They make the impressions and send them to a special laboratory, where the actual earpieces are made

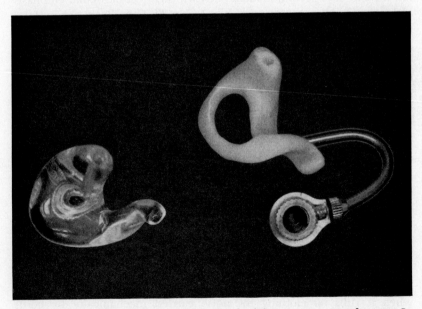

Fig. 10-32. Molded plastic eartips. On the left is a conventional eartip. In the "hideaway" type on the right the receiver may be concealed and only the eartip is visible. The size and shape of the couplers that connect receivers to eartips are standardized for all hearing aids. (*Central Institute for the Deaf.*)

according to the patterns. The manufacturers of hearing aids have standardized the nubs on receivers so that an individual earpiece fits almost any make of receiver. Rarely is an adapter needed.

The earpiece should fit the ear snugly and prevent escape of sound around it. The close fit makes the action of the receiver more efficient, as no energy is then lost through leakage. If there is a leak, the sounds reaching the eardrum will be weakened, particularly in the low frequencies.

Squeal. If a loud sound is delivered within the ear, it is important that as little as possible should escape around the earpiece. If sound escapes, it may reach the microphone of the hearing aid and be picked up and amplified. The result will be a "squeal" resulting from what is known as *acoustic feedback.* Not only is the "squeal" unpleasant; it may also drown out the sounds that the wearer wishes to hear. The development of the individually molded earpiece was an important advance. A hearing aid can deliver to the ear much louder sounds without squeal if the earpiece fits well than if it does not. Even so, even with a well-fitted earpiece, the gain of hearing aids worn at the ear is definitely limited by acoustic feedback.

The designer of a hearing aid must sacrifice some sensitivity if an instrument is to have a high acoustic output. He cannot rely on *all* the output's staying within the ear. Even if the earpiece fits well, *some* sound inevitably escapes through the back of the receiver. A very sensitive, high-gain instrument with high maximum output goes into a squeal too easily to take advantage of its high gain.

Some ways of avoiding squeal are

to improve the fit of the earpiece to the ear (and of the receiver to the earpiece);

to reduce the gain of the hearing aid;

to move the microphone farther away from the receiver; and

to adjust the tone control for the best practical compromise.

THE TELEPHONE PICKUP

A telephone pickup is a feature of many of the more elaborate conventional models of hearing aids. An inductive pickup coil is mounted within the case. A switch allows the user to substitute it for the microphone as the input to the hearing aid amplifier. Thus when the telephone pickup is in use there is no interference from the acoustic noise of the surroundings. The user simply throws the switch to the "telephone" position and holds the telephone receiver against the case of his instrument.

BATTERIES

Before the advent of the transistor, hearing-aid batteries were "dry cells" of the type that use carbon and zinc as the electrodes. The zinc electrode also serves as the case in which the electrolyte and the central carbon electrode are enclosed. Although the cell is called a "dry cell," the electrolyte is actually a moist paste. It is held in place and prevented from drying by a seal of wax, asphalt, or other suitable material. The energy is provided by a chemical reaction between the electrolyte and the zinc that takes place when current is drawn. The outer (zinc) electrode is negative (−) and the center (carbon) electrode is positive (+). The electrolyte is gradually used up by being transformed into zinc salts and other compounds. The voltage that is produced by a dry cell depends on the materials chosen for the electrodes and the freshness of the battery, not on its physical size. The combination of carbon and zinc gives about 1.5 volts when the battery is fresh and no current is being drawn.

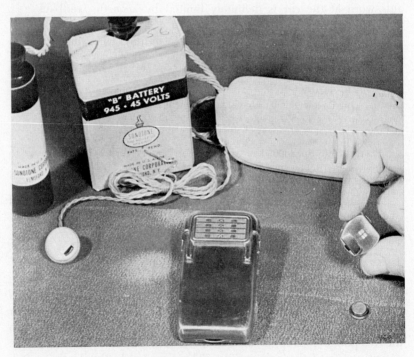

Fig. 10-33. Progress in reduction of size of hearing aids is illustrated by a 1945 model in background, a 1952 model in center foreground, and a 1957 model in fingers at right. Note change in size of batteries from upper left, 1945, to small circular battery, lower right, 1957. (*Sonotone Corp.*)

The "*mercury cell.*" The mercury type of dry cell, developed during World War II, uses compounds of mercury in its electrolyte. It works on the same principles as the zinc type of cell. Its advantage lies in the greater amount of energy that it can provide in relation to its size and in its reliability under adverse conditions of temperature, humidity, fungus growth, and the like, such as are encountered in the tropics. A fresh mercury cell operating a hearing aid has about 1.25 volts.

Practically all modern wearable hearing aids use a single mercury battery. It is difficult to specify costs of batteries for operating hearing aids because of the variety of conditions under which the instruments are used. For example, the setting of the gain control or the use of a power switch that may limit the output will influence the drain on the battery. The table shows characteristics and operating costs of some mercury batteries used under various conditions. The range is 0.07 cents per hour for a 1.25 volt battery at low level and at low

Characteristics and Operating Costs of a Particular Conventional Hearing Aid

Battery Voltage	Power Switch Setting	Full Acoustic Gain	Maximum Sound Pressure Output	Battery Life and Cost [a]					
				Low Level		Maximum Power Output		Typical Service	
		db	*db re 0.0002 Microbar*	*Hrs.*	*¢/Hr.*	*Hrs.*	*¢/Hr.*	*Hrs.*	*¢/Hr.*
	P 4	71	132	320	0.44	89	1.50	175	0.8
	P 3	71	129	320	0.44	200	0.70	270	0.52
Mercury 2.5V	P 2	71	126	320	0.44	270	0.52	300	0.46
	P 1	71	123	320	0.44	310	0.45	315	0.45
	P 4	54	126	1,910	0.07	537	0.26	1,070	0.13
	P 3	54	124	1,910	0.07	625	0.22	1,140	0.12
Mercury 1.25V	P 2	54	122	1,910	0.07	861	0.16	1,365	0.10
	P 1	54	120	1,910	0.07	1,075	0.13	1,535	0.09

[a] The current drain on the battery varies with the amount of output power the hearing aid is called upon to deliver. Thus in a quiet environment, or if the volume control is turned well down, little current is drawn, with resulting long battery life. This is the condition represented in the "Low Level" column. The "Maximum Power Output" column represents the opposite conditions, where sounds of high intensity develop full power output and consequent minimum battery life. Neither of these two extreme conditions exists continuously, of course. The figures of the "Typical Service" column represent realistic averages experienced by users.

power-limiting setting to 1.50 cents per hour for a 2.5 volt battery at high level and at high power-limiting setting. One of the most significant improvements of the transistor hearing aid over the vacuum-tube instrument has been the decrease in battery operating costs.

The Over-all Performance of Hearing Aids

The objective of hearing aid design is to amplify speech without undue distortion but at the same time to protect the user against discomfort from too loud an output. The speech sounds are "packaged" for delivery to an elevated and more or less restricted auditory area (cf. Figures 7-10 and 7-11). In addition the frequency bands above and below the important speech range are often deliberately suppressed so that noise in these bands will not annoy or distract the user.

The performance of a hearing aid is illustrated in Figures 10-34 and 10-37. Here the acoustic area of conversational speech extends from about 100 to about 8000 cps, while the range important for good understanding of speech extends from about 400 to 3000 cps. The sound pressure levels of conversational speech extend from a maximum of 66 db in the lower frequencies to 30 db or so in the high frequencies. The available auditory area of a user who has the common type of mixed hearing loss, i.e., an over-all conductive loss plus some high-tone sensory-neural loss, lies largely above this area. His threshold of discomfort is assumed to lie at 120 db, which is a likely level (Figure 10-34).

The frequency characteristic of a hearing aid is shown in Figure 10-31. This indicates how much the speech sounds will be amplified at each frequency. The "low" characteristic is repeated at the top of Figure 10-34. The flatness (or lack of flatness) of such a curve expresses the *fidelity* of the instrument. Its breadth measures the frequency range. The gain is negligible at very high and very low frequencies. The whole curve is moved up and down by changing the volume-control setting. The acoustic "gain" of a hearing aid is measured by comparing the sound pressure level developed in a 2 cc coupler with the sound pressure level (at 1000 cps) measured in a free sound field before the hearing aid is introduced into it. The gain at 1000 cps measured in this way may be 60 db or more. (It is worth noting that the "gain for speech," measured as the difference in the threshold for speech of a hard-of-hearing listener with and without the hearing aid is often considerably less than the laboratory measurement of gain.)

There is, however, a maximum acoustic output beyond which the instrument cannot go, regardless of the setting of the volume con-

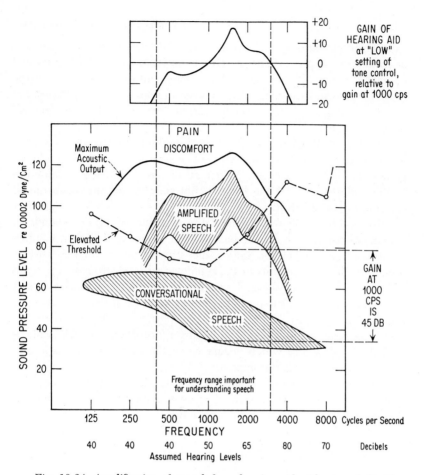

Fig. 10-34. **Amplification of speech by a hearing aid without peak limiting.**
The area of conversational speech, as measured in a free acoustic field, is shown
here with arbitrary sharp boundaries (see Fig. 2-6). The upper boundary represents the level above which the peaks of speech, at that frequency, very seldom
rise. The speech elements below the lower boundary contribute very little to intelligibility and can be disregarded. All of the measurements of output are made
in a 2 cc coupler. *The "gain" of a hearing aid* at 1000 cps is the difference between
the sound pressure level measured in the field before the hearing aid is introduced
and the sound pressure level measured in the 2 cc coupler. *The area of amplified
speech* in this figure was found by moving the speech area upward by 45 db at
1000 cps and then modifying the shape of the area according to the over-all frequency characteristic of the hearing aid, as drawn above. This is the curve shown
for the "low" setting of the tone control in Fig. 10-31. The shape of the curve of
maximum acoustic output is determined by the receiver, shown separately in
Fig. 10-35. The level of maximum acoustic output is measured at 1000 cps, and
is here assumed to be 120 db SPL, measured in a 2 cc coupler. This is close to
the usual threshold of discomfort. Only occasional peaks of pressure at frequencies
near 1500 cps reach this level. The limited auditory area for a hypothetical case of
mixed hearing loss is shown. The amplified speech is delivered efficiently and with
a minimum of distortion to this reduced "target area."

trol or the strength of the input signal. The frequency characteristic
at maximum output (Figure 10-34) is flatter than it is in the normal
operating range, but it has one or more maxima, because of the
resonant peaks of the magnetic receiver (Figure 10-35). The position
of this limiting maximum acoustic output curve describes the "power"
of the instrument.

In Figure 10-34 we see how the "area" of conversational speech
is elevated and modified in shape by a hearing aid set to moderate
gain and "low" tone control. Nearly all of the speech sounds now fall
in the auditory area of the listener, but they do not encroach on his
threshold of discomfort.

In Figure 10-37 we see how the distribution of the sounds of
conversational speech would be modified by using a higher volume-
control setting and at the same time altering the frequency characteristic to "high" by means of the tone control. The stronger low tones
of speech are now deliberately amplified less that the weaker higher
tones. The fidelity of the output is not as good as in the first example,
but the speech may be easier for this particular listener to understand because another kind of acoustic distortion (which will be
described below and which occurs when the maximum acoustic output is approached) is minimized.

In terms of these measures of performance—fidelity and frequency range, gain, and maximum power output—we can judge the
performance of present-day hearing aids.

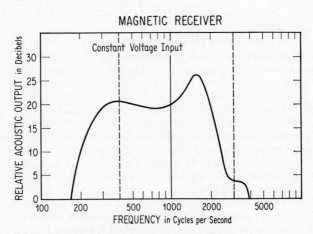

Fig. 10-35. Frequency characteristic of a magnetic receiver. The voltage of the electrical input is held constant;
the acoustic output is measured in a 2 cc coupler. (*Courtesy
of J. R. Cox, Jr.*)

FREQUENCY RANGE

The frequency range of the hearing aid is determined mostly by the characteristics of the microphone and the earphone. The microphone becomes inefficient at the lower frequencies and the earphone will not reproduce the higher frequencies. Both the microphone and the earphone have one or more resonant "humps" or "peaks." These are usually so located as to supplement one another and to give a relatively smooth and fairly flat frequency characteristic with quite acceptable fidelity over the middle range that is most important for speech. Modern hearing aids give ample practical coverage of the speech frequencies.

GAIN

An acoustic gain of at least 60 db for the frequencies near the peak of the frequency characteristic is easily provided by a magnetic microphone, a transistor amplifier, and a magnetic receiver. The maximum *usable* gain is less likely to be limited by the electroacoustic apparatus than by an inadequate seal achieved at the ear. The individually fitted earmold has contributed greatly toward increasing the maximum usable gain of hearing aids. The volume control provides a variable gain in most aids so that a range of gain of 30 to as much as 60 db or more is available in many instruments. Sufficient gain is no longer a problem.

POWER

The maximum output of a hearing aid is controlled by the inherent limitations set by the power available in its battery and the power-handling capacities of its component parts. The acoustic distortion produced as maximum output is reached will be considered in more detail in the next section. Here compromises must be made, and both the designer of the hearing aid on the one hand and the user on the other are faced with a series of practical problems that involve the size and the expense as well as the performance of the instrument. Fortunately, for most users of hearing aids with moderate hearing losses, these problems are not often serious, as they rarely need to push their instruments to the limit of maximum acoustic output. On the whole, modern hearing aids are very well-designed and effective instruments, within the limits set by their objectives and by the engineering difficulties imposed by the desirability of making the instruments themselves as small and as comfortable to wear as possible.

Hearing Aids and Auditory Training for Deaf Children

Electronic hearing aids for use with deaf children may be one of many varieties of three basic types: group, desk, or wearable. The advantages of a group hearing aid are its greater power output and a more desirable frequency response than the wearable aid and the possibility of minimizing acoustic feedback by keeping the microphone at a reasonable distance from the earphones. The improvements in wearable hearing aids, however, are increasingly reducing the differences.

Dr. E. Wedenberg of Sweden has suggested the principle of inserting appropriate filters "to compensate the lack of balance between the high and low portions of the speech frequency spectrum which accompanies auditory impairment. Thus the formant areas of higher frequencies valuable . . . to perceptibility may be 'raised' to a level at which they are audible along with the lower speech spectrum areas." This principle may be useful for children whom we can expect to achieve refined auditory discrimination. Whether this type of frequency response or the simple rising frequency characteristic suggested by the Harvard Report (see page 327) is best for hearing aids for deaf children remains to be investigated.

The major advantage of a wearable hearing aid for the child is that he can have it with him at all times and benefit continuously from auditory stimulation. Frequently, children are first taught to appreciate sound over group instruments and then use their own wearable instrument outside the classroom.

There are a number of problems concerning features of group hearing aids for deaf children about which there is little experimental information. The desirability of compression amplification (described below) is generally recognized, but how restricted the dynamic intensity range of the compressed signal should be is another matter. For the deaf child who cannot make fine discriminations, the information contained in intensity changes in speech is important.

We also need more information about the value of binaural hearing aids for deaf children. The reference here is not to pseudobinaural hearing aids that use one microphone, one amplifier, and two earphones, which are little better than a monaural system, especially for localization of sound. A true binaural hearing aid is possible if each ear is aided by a system that is fed from a microphone mounted at that ear. Its advantage for a deaf child, in addition to his not too primary need for localization of sound sources, is yet to be determined.

Other features of group hearing aids that are proving useful in practice are the insert type of earphones to increase comfort and to reduce acoustic feedback, ceiling-mounted microphones or inductance loops to increase freedom of action for the teacher and the pupils, acoustically treated rooms to reduce reverberation and distortion, visual aids to indicate intensity or pitch changes, and outlet boxes at blackboards.

Hearing Aids Cannot Do Everything

No hearing aid can ever compensate completely for a hearing loss. Everyone who is thinking of getting a hearing aid should realize at the outset that there are limits to what *any* hearing aid can possibly do. Some limits are imposed by the ear and others by the nature of the sounds that we wish to hear. There are practical limits also, set by size, weight, and expense, to what can be built into a wearable hearing aid at the present time.

For example, an ear with sensory-neural deafness may be unable to hear high tones no matter how much they are amplified. If *all* the nerve fibers that are normally stimulated by tones above 3000 cps have degenerated, then no conceivable hearing aid can ever make sounds above 3000 cps audible again, except by transforming them to some lower frequency. This is the fundamental reason why hearing aids are often of little or no assistance in the "abrupt" type of high-tone sensory-neural deafness.

Until about 1940 a practical limit of performance was set by the inability to provide enough amplification without undue distortion. Now, however, a powerful instrument can deliver a sound as loud as most wearers are willing to tolerate even after they have become accustomed to loud sounds. The limit of useful power is now set by the ear. A good hearing aid must, of course, bring sound above the threshold of audibility, but its output must never exceed the listener's threshold of discomfort.

In the hard-of-hearing ear the thresholds of discomfort and pain usually stay near the normal levels, so that *the range (in decibels) between the faintest audible tone and the loudest tolerable tone is diminished.* Now if we amplify all sounds equally, the strong sounds may become intolerable before the weak sounds are powerful enough to be heard. *Some suppression of the strong sounds may therefore be necessary if the weak ones are to be made audible.*

Speech is a mixture of sounds of different intensity, and the weakest sounds may be as much as 30 db below the strongest (see Figure 10-34). If the range between audibility and discomfort is less (as it may be with a severe hearing loss) it may be possible to make speech audible and intelligible as well as tolerable, but only at the sacrifice of some "naturalness" or "quality." Fortunately, however, this compromise is necessary only when the hearing loss is very severe.

"LIMITING" OF OUTPUT

The necessary protection against discomfort can be provided automatically. We have pointed out that an amplifier can deliver only just so much current through its last stage even when the "valve" is open wide. *One of the fundamental principles of selecting a hearing aid is to pick an instrument that has enough amplification but also has a maximum output that will be tolerable.*

When a hearing aid is used near its maximum output, as may be necessary if the hearing loss is severe, the strongest peaks of the electric waves will reach the maximum output of the instrument. We may think of the maximum output as a ceiling. The peaks of speech cannot surpass this limit, and the waves are therefore squared off, or "clipped," as shown in Figure 10-36. These clipped waves are tolerable, but obviously they are distorted in shape. That is why the quality of the sound suffers.

EFFECTS OF PEAK CLIPPING

Fortunately a considerable amount of simple peak clipping does not greatly reduce the intelligibility of speech even though it may make the voice sound harsh, rough, and unnatural. Ordinarily the low frequencies of vowel sounds, which are the most powerful of the speech sounds, as indicated in Figures 10-34 and 10-37, reach the limiting maximum acoustic output first and consequently suffer from peak clipping. The change of quality in the speech is most noticeable in these vowel sounds. It is actually rather surprising, however, to see on an oscilloscope how severely the speech waves may be squared off and distorted by simple peak clipping before the speech becomes really difficult to understand.

In order to reduce or avoid the distortion and loss of quality introduced by peak clipping it is desirable to amplify the higher fre-

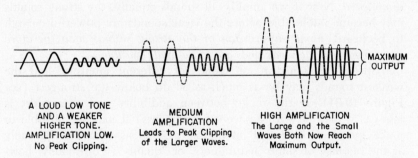

A LOUD LOW TONE AND A WEAKER HIGHER TONE. AMPLIFICATION LOW. No Peak Clipping.

MEDIUM AMPLIFICATION Leads to Peak Clipping of the Larger Waves.

HIGH AMPLIFICATION The Large and the Small Waves Both Now Reach Maximum Output.

MAXIMUM OUTPUT

Fig. 10-36. Diagram showing various degrees of "peak clipping" of speech waves.

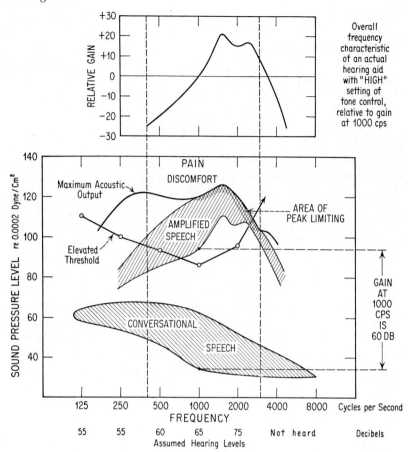

Fig. 10-37. **Amplified speech with peak limiting.** The hearing aid is now set for maximum volume, assumed to be 60 db gain at 1000 cps, and for HIGH tone control (see Fig. 10-31). The hypothetical hearing levels, shown below, leave only a small target area below the threshold of discomfort. The maximum acoustic output is 120 db, at 1000 cps, as in Fig. 10-34. The amplified speech (shaded area) is delivered efficiently to the target area. Peak limiting occurs at frequencies above 1000 cps, but not below. This holds distortion to a minimum. This result is achieved by the sharply rising frequency characteristic of the microphone-amplifier combination. The input is assumed to be ordinary conversational speech. Of course, with loud speech there would be more peak limiting.

quencies of speech more than the lower frequencies, so that both the high frequencies and the low frequencies reach the limit of maximum acoustic output together. Such "high-tone emphasis" is introduced by reducing the amplification of low tones, as shown in Figure 10-31. This moderate high-tone emphasis allows for the use of the greatest gain before the clipping level is reached. It uses most efficiently the restricted auditory area of most hard-of-hearing listeners, as illustrated in Figure 10-37.

One reason that the intelligibility of speech suffers so much more from peak clipping of the low tones than from corresponding clipping of the high tones is that some of the harmonics that are introduced by the peak clipping of low frequencies are clearly audible, while for high frequencies most of the harmonics lie above the range of speech frequencies and are very inefficiently transmitted by the receiver of the hearing aid. If the listener has a high-tone hearing loss, these high-frequency distortion products are doubly excluded and of no consequence.

With the proper combination of high-tone pre-emphasis and appropriate limiting of the output by peak clipping, plenty of amplification can be used in a hearing aid to make faint sounds audible while at the same time the ear is protected against discomfort. Intelligibility is well, although not completely, preserved. There is some deterioration of quality when the peak clipping becomes severe. We must pay for the protection, so to speak, but the price in quality need not be very high. The high-tone emphasis must be introduced *before* the peaks are clipped, as was pointed out in the Harvard Report. That is why we speak of high-tone *pre*-emphasis. No additional high-tone or low-tone emphasis should be put in by the receiver *after* the clipping.

In order to get the best combination of protection and intelligibility, a receiver with good acoustic characteristics must be used. Some hearing aid receivers are too "resonant," meaning that they respond too well to one particular band of frequencies. After the amplifier has clipped the peaks of the waves electrically, the receiver should deliver all parts of the speech spectrum to the ear at about the same maximum level, a little below the threshold of tolerance.

A receiver that has a resonant peak will amplify not only that frequency of the input but also the second, the third, or even the fourth harmonics that are introduced by the peak clipping of lower frequencies. Not only may the resulting high peak pressures reach the threshold of discomfort; they also cause a further deterioration of the intelligibility of certain vowel sounds, to say nothing of the unpleasant ringing quality that it introduces. For example, a receiver with a resonant peak at 1500 cps, shown in Figure 10-35, gave a strong response at this frequency to inputs in the neighborhood of 750, of 500, and of 375 cps when these were strong enough to reach the clipping level. The output wave forms are shown in Figure 10-38.

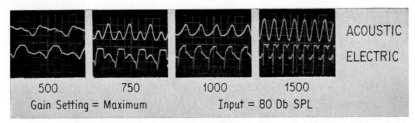

Fig. 10-38. For this figure the electrical waves were recorded at the output of a transistor hearing aid across the terminals of the receiver. The peak clipping in this instrument is unsymmetrical, and a sharp transient peak is introduced by the output transformer. The receiver, the frequency characteristic of which is shown in Fig. 10-35, has a resonant peak at 1500 cps. It smooths out the sharp irregularities of the electrical waves, but it accentuates the first two or three harmonics of frequencies that are an octave or more below its resonant peak. For these oscillograms the input was 80 db SPL, gain setting was maximum, and the tone control at "low." The over-all frequency response of this instrument is shown in Fig. 10-31. (*Courtesy of J. R. Cox, Jr.*)

COMPRESSION AMPLIFICATION

Another way of limiting the output of a hearing aid is by *compression amplification*. Compression amplification is equivalent to a rapidly acting automatic volume control. The strong sound waves themselves reduce the gain of the amplifier. The output of the instrument is limited to a definite maximum, and the method has the advantage that the wave form is less distorted than it is by simple peak clipping. Automatic gain control is now incorporated in some conventional hearing aids.

Over-all Circuit of a Four-Transistor Hearing Aid

The separate components of hearing aids and the principles of their action have been described in foregoing sections. Here we shall see how they are assembled and operate in a particular four-transistor instrument.

Figure 10-41 shows the complete schematic circuit diagram of the hearing aid. The three panels indicate the three major functional divisions, namely (left to right) the input and first transistor gain stage, the second transistor gain stage, and the push-pull transistor output stage.

INPUT

At the extreme left is the magnetic microphone of the type

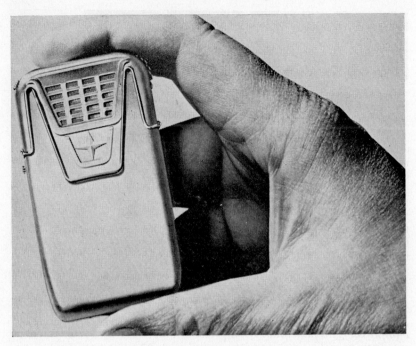

Fig. 10-39. The "Model 200" hearing aid, which is here discussed and analyzed. (*Sonotone Corp.*)

described above. It converts sound energy into its electrical equivalent for application to the input of the first transistor.

Immediately adjacent and to the right of the microphone is the telephone pickup coil. A switch permits application of the output of either the microphone or the pickup to the first transistor. Thus, during a telephone conversation, the microphone is cut out and all air-borne interfering sounds are eliminated—a blessing indeed when one is telephoning in a noisy location.

When the telephone receiver is held near the telephone pickup coil, the voice currents flowing in the coil of its magnetic system induce corresponding currents in the pickup coil. These are amplified in the transistor circuits, and reach the ear of the user at approximately the same levels as would normal speech entering through the microphone. They can be regulated by the VOLUME control as well as by the position of the telephone with respect to the pickup.

The pickup coil consists of a magnetic core around which are wound 8500 turns of the same wire used in the microphone coil. The over-all dimensions of this entire assembly are only five sixteenths of an inch high by a quarter inch outside diameter.

FIRST TRANSISTOR GAIN STAGE

The MIC-TEL switch is shown connecting the microphone to the first transistor in the circuit of Figure 10-41. The very small currents generated in the microphone and applied to the transistor are there amplified approximately one hundred times. The output currents flow through the primary of the transformer, T1, shown just to the right of the transistor. This transformer, because of the unequal turns-ratio of its two windings, has the effect of stepping up the current twofold. The result is that the current flow in the input circuit of the second transistor is twice that in the output circuit of the first transistor.

SECOND TRANSISTOR GAIN STAGE

Intervening between the transformer T1 and the second gain transistor are the VOLUME control, the external LO-CUT, and the internal LO-CUT and HI-CUT circuits.

Volume control. The VOLUME control (technically the "manual gain control") is located here, rather than later in the circuit, because loud sounds impinging on the microphone might otherwise be amplified to such magnitude in the first gain stage as to overload the second transistor, with resulting distortion. This control circuit consists of the variable resistor labeled VOLUME CONTROL and the fixed resistor R1 connected across the secondary of the first transformer. As the slider (arrow) is moved toward the top end of the variable resistor the signal current to the second transistor input is decreased.

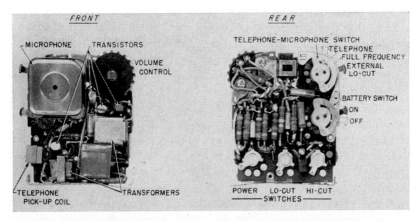

Fig. 10-40. Front and rear views of the chassis ("Model 200") with the major parts identified. The chassis occupies approximately two thirds of the space provided by the hearing aid case, the battery the other third. (*Sonotone Corp.*)

Tone control. From the VOLUME CONTROL, the signal path is completed through the two capacitors, C1 and C2, to the emitter of the second transistor, provided the TONE CONTROL switch is not in its center position. When the TONE CONTROL switch is placed in the center, or FULL TONE, position as shown in Figure 10-41, it short-circuits the first of these capacitors, C1, leaving only the second one in the signal path. This second capacitor, C2, is not important to the present consideration of the circuits. The first capacitor, however, plays a part in the function of the TONE CONTROL. Audio-frequency currents can pass through a capacitor but the efficiency with which they do so depends on the size (in microfarads) of the capacitor and the frequency of the signal. High frequencies are passed more readily than low. The selection of a capacitor of sufficiently low value for C1 partially blocks the passage of low frequencies, but the higher frequencies pass freely. Thus we have an effective low-cut arrangement. When the TONE CONTROL is in its FULL TONE position the signal currents are by-passed around C1 and its blocking effect on the lower frequencies is thus eliminated. The following capacitor, C2, has no significant effect on the frequency response of the hearing aid because of its relatively large capacity.

Notice that the MIC-TEL switch and the TONE CONTROL switch are mechanically connected to one another so that the wearer has only a single three-position control to operate. The choices open to him are (1) microphone + low cut, (2) microphone + full tone, or (3) telephone + full tone.

Internal LO-CUT circuit. One of the design problems met by this particular circuit is the provision of two low-frequency cutting circuits: one internal, for use as a permanent adjustment to suit the hearing of the individual user; the other external, to be used when needed to aid in understanding speech in the presence of interfering noise. The problem was to make these two functions independent of one another so that either or both could be used, in the latter case their effects being additive. This could not be accomplished by simply inserting another capacitor in the signal path because sufficient independence could not thus be achieved. The solution was found in the circuit comprised of the LO-CUT switch, the resistor R2, the capacitor C3, and the center-tapped resistor below and to the right of C3.

The signal current is applied to the second transistor between its base and the emitter. The amplified output signal path includes the collector, the battery, the primary of the transformer T2, and the emitter. However, a second path for a portion of the output signal

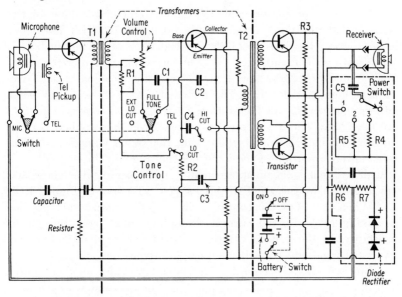

Fig. 10-41. The schematic circuit diagram of the "Model 200" hearing aid. (*Sonotone Corp.*)

is from the collector, through the center-tapped resistor and capacitor C3 to the emitter. If the LO-CUT switch is closed upward, instead of to the left as in the diagram, part of the current from this second path is fed back into the input circuit of the transistor. It is, however, 180 degrees out of phase with the input signal and thus opposes the latter. This is the principle known as "inverse feedback." Now, if a means were found to feed back only the low-frequency portion of the output signal and thus cancel out some of the low-frequency energy of the input signal, the desired low-cut effect would be achieved. This is precisely the principle employed in this LO-CUT circuit.

It was explained earlier that capacitors will pass the higher frequencies of a signal current more readily than the low. This is another way of saying that a capacitor offers greater impedance (resistance to the flow of alternating current) for the low frequencies than for the high. It is basic that when current flows through a resistance there is a voltage drop across the resistance. This voltage drop is proportional to the values of the resistance and the current. It follows then that when a signal current passes through a capacitor the resulting voltage drop will be greater for low frequencies and also that the voltage drop across a small capacitor will be greater than that across a large one.

We can now consider the LO-CUT circuit in the light of this. Assume that the switch is closed upward in the LO-CUT position so as to connect the resistor (R2) and capacitor (C3) to the base of the transistor. The capacitor C3 is of low value and therefore offers high impedance (resistance) to low-frequency signals, with consequent high voltage drop. The impedance to high-frequency signal currents, however, and therefore the voltage drop they will produce are negligible. The low-frequency voltage drop thus applied between emitter and base is out of phase with the signal voltage and therefore cancels a portion of the low-frequency signal. The over-all result is a decrease in gain of approximately 6 db per octave below 2000 cps as shown by the INTERNAL LOW CUT curve of Figure 10-42.

When the LO-CUT control is in its "off" (horizontal) position, as in Figure 10-41, the current through it must pass through the resistances of the volume control. It is thus reduced in amount and has little or no effect on the frequency response.

Internal HI-CUT circuit. This circuit provides another internal adjustment of the frequency response of this instrument to the user's requirements. Like the internal LO-CUT circuit just described, the HI-CUT circuit also employs inverse feedback. A portion of the output signal is passed back into the input circuit through the HI-CUT switch and the capacitor C4 of Figure 10-41. Because the capacity of C4 is small, only frequencies above about 800 cps are passed with

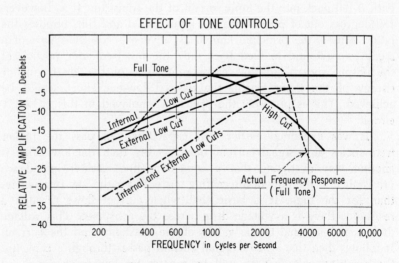

Fig. 10-42. The effects of internal and external tone adjustments on the frequency response. These effects are independent of those provided by the different receivers represented in Fig. 10-45. (*Sonotone Corp.*)

sufficient magnitude to affect the frequency response. The higher the frequencies the more easily they pass. Thus the higher the frequencies in the input signal the more opposition they meet from the feedback circuit. The over-all effect is illustrated in the curve labeled HIGH-CUT of Figure 10-42.

At first glance it might appear from Figure 10-41 that the LO-CUT and the HI-CUT circuits are simply alternative pathways from the emitter to the base, each with a condenser in series in the circuit. It might seem, therefore, that they should have the same, not opposite, effects. There are, however, important differences in the positions of the condensers relative to the resistances and the transformer (T2) which cause one feedback loop to have a rising and the other a falling frequency response, as described above.

Note on transistor connections. There is one more point of interest in the second transistor stage. Referring to the circuit of Figure 10-41, the primary of the following transformer is in the emitter leg, whereas in the first transistor stage the transformer primary is in the collector leg. Actually in each of these cases the primaries are connected between emitter and collector and the circuits are therefore basically alike. This can be checked by tracing the circuits. In the first transistor stage the output signal current path includes the collector, primary winding, battery, and emitter. In the second transistor circuit the circuit elements remain the same although they are in different order. This difference is purposeful but the reasons are beyond the scope of this book. The important fact is that the circuits are functionally identical.

OUTPUT STAGE

There are a number of features incorporated in this portion of the circuit which are of special interest because they contribute to battery economy, higher amplification and power output, and reduced distortion.

Push-pull circuit. Two transistors are employed in what is known as a "push-pull" circuit arrangement, which operates as follows. In each cycle of a sound wave there is a period of compression of the air, followed by a period of rarefaction. When the sound wave is converted into an electrical counterpart the resulting electrical wave constitutes an alternating current which flows in one direction during one half of the cycle, then reverses and flows in the opposite direction for the other half cycle. These are designated as the positive and negative halves of the cycle.

Now if, in Figure 10-41, we consider the primary of the second transformer (T2) in this way, it is apparent that, as a result of the alternating current flowing through it, one end of the winding is positive and the other negative during a portion of each cycle. A half cycle later in time, the polarity is reversed. Similarly, the current induced in each half of the secondary of this transformer also reverses its direction twice in each cycle.

During the half cycle when the top of the transformer (T2) secondary is negative, the upper transistor will pass current. The input signal path consists of the transistor base, the upper half of the transformer secondary, a series resistor (R3), and the emitter of the upper transistor. The amplified output signal current flow is from the collector through the upper half of the battery and back through the receiver to the emitter. The current drives the receiver diaphragm through half a cycle.

During the next half cycle the upper transistor passes very little current, but the lower transistor can pass current readily. The output signal path is then from its collector through the receiver and the lower half of the battery back to the emitter. Again the receiver diaphragm is driven through half a cycle, but this time the direction of current flow through the receiver is reversed and its diaphragm is therefore driven in the opposite direction. If it was pushed during the first half cycle, it is pulled during the second. This suggests the term "push-pull."

The total amplitude of movement of the diaphragm during the full cycle is a mechanical replica of the electrical input to T2. Instead of only one transistor in the output, one benefit of the push-pull arrangement of two transistors is its ability to handle at least twice as much input signal without overloading the transistors. Overloading would cause distortion of the output signal. This higher power-handling ability is principally due to the use of two transistors instead of one. Two transistors connected in parallel rather than in push-pull would achieve approximately this same purpose. But the push-pull arrangement offers other advantages. One of the most important is that when the signal level is such as to drive the output stage to its limit, equal clipping of the positive and the negative peaks takes place. This symmetrical peak clipping substantially improves speech intelligibility as compared with a single-transistor output stage or one with two transistors in parallel. If the peak clipping is symmetrical (as in Figure 10-36), only odd-numbered harmonics are present as distortion products in the output signal. If it is unsymmetrical (as in Figure 10-38), the even-numbered harmonics are present also. The second harmonic is the greatest offender with respect to the intelligibility of speech. A push-pull circuit does overload and cause peak clipping if the input signal is high enough, but because the clipping is symmetrical the troublesome second harmonic is eliminated, together with all other even ones.

Battery-saving Class AB operation. Another important advantage of the push-pull arrangement is what is known as "Class AB operation." This class of operation automatically regulates the flow of battery current according to the intensity of the input sound. In quiet surroundings the current drawn from the battery is at a low level, known as the "idling current level." When sounds cause alternating current to flow in transformer T2, first one transistor, then the other, draws more current from the battery. The total current with loud sounds is considerably higher than the idling current level. In practice, of course, the average drain is somewhere between the idling current level and the level reached with really loud sounds. The practical effect of the Class AB operation on battery life and operating cost is shown in the table on page 299.

The usual single transistor or vacuum-tube class of operation is Class A. Battery voltages, grid bias voltages, emitter currents, and so on, are adjusted so that considerable current flows at all times through the tube or transistor. This current is modulated, i.e., made stronger or weaker, by the control signal. The operation of the push-pull stage as described above would be "Class B" operation if each transistor closed off completely and drew no current at all when no alternating current at all is delivered to it from the transformer and each one drew current *only* during one half of each cycle. In practice the transistors are allowed to draw a small idling current when there is no input sound, and this compromise is called "Class AB operation." The compromise is made because as a practical matter the amount of distortion can be made less with Class AB than with complete Class B operation.

Automatic gain control (AGC) circuit. The AGC circuit is shown as a separate section within the output stage area of Figure 10-41. A small amount of the output of the final push-pull stage is delivered to this circuit through the capacitor C5 and the POWER switch when the latter is in Positions 1, 2, or 3. When in Position 4, it will be noted, the connection between the output and the AGC circuit is broken and the AGC circuit does not operate. At low output levels the current flow in the AGC circuit is very small but at high levels there is sufficient current flow through it to the base of the first transistor to alter the operation of this transistor and decrease the amount of amplification that it provides.

In Figure 10-41 it will be seen that the biasing voltage normally applied to the base of the first transistor, by way of the hollow line from R6 and R7 to the microphone, is taken from a voltage divider

(R6 and R7), which is connected across one half the battery. The values of these two resistors are selected to apply just the right proportion of the battery voltage to the transistor to provide the maximum practical gain ever desired from this stage. The portion of the alternating current output of the final stage that flows through R6 and R7 adds to the bias current in question. The diode rectifiers allow the output current to flow in this part of the circuit in one direction only, as a series of half waves. The condenser across the terminals of R6 and R7 smooths the flow. This smoothed flow adds with the flow from the battery and increases the base bias to change in such direction as to lower the first stage current and thus reduce the gain of this stage. The additional bias voltage decreases the amount of amplification provided by the first transistor.

The amount of automatic regulation provided in this manner depends upon the position of the POWER switch. Maximum AGC is obtained with this switch in Position 1, which places no resistance in the path of the current. In Position 2 the current flow encounters a moderate amount of resistance (R4) and in Position 3 still more resistance (R5). The amount of AGC action decreases accordingly. This is illustrated in Figure 10-43.

One advantage offered to the user by AGC is that the maximum output of the hearing aid can be adjusted to his tolerance threshold without sacrificing the gain that is needed to make weak sounds

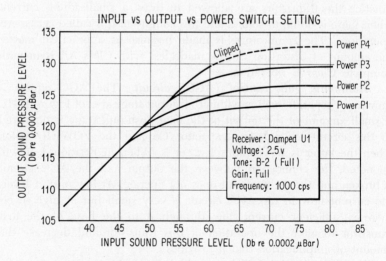

Fig. 10-43. The effects of the automatic gain control circuit. "Tender ears" are protected by the limits of maximum power output imposed by the different positions of the POWER switch. (*Sonotone Corp.*)

audible. Some users of conventional hearing aids are constantly fiddling with their volume controls. Usually they do so because with the gain too low they fail to hear weak speech but when it is turned higher loud speech and other sounds cause distortion and/or discomfort. Automatic gain control is a boon to such users because it allows maximum gain as long as only soft to moderate sounds are impressed on the microphone. When a loud sound does occur, however, the gain is decreased automatically, thus avoiding overloading and also possible discomfort. The improved hearing and freedom from discomfort create greater ease and confidence in the user, especially if he is a new user or is inclined to be a nervous one.

The effect of AGC in providing better intelligibility of speech in the presence of noise is illustrated in Figure 10-44. When noise is present at a level higher than that of normal speech, a talker will

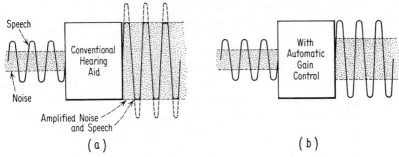

Fig. 10-44. Automatic gain control (b) reduces the gain for loud sounds so that the sound waves do not suffer the distortion of peak clipping, as they do (a) in a conventional hearing aid. The background noise is also reduced as long as stronger speech sounds are also present.

automatically raise his voice in order to be understood by normal-hearing people. But a problem is introduced for the user of a conventional hearing aid because if the noise (and speech) levels are high it is quite possible that they will drive his hearing aid to its overload point. This tends to drop the speech he wishes to hear down into the noise. In Figure 10-44 such a condition is shown at (a). Here the amplified noise has reached the full output capacity of the hearing aid. The speech, although initially of higher level than the noise, cannot exceed the same output capacity and therefore becomes submerged in the noise.

This condition could be improved, provided the noise background were reasonably constant, by turning down the gain control of the hearing aid so that the noise would not be amplified to capacity and some leeway would remain for the speech to exceed the noise level in the output. But in a variable noise background, with the talker's voice rising and falling accordingly, it is difficult to keep pace with the changes by manually manipulating the gain control. But the AGC circuit can and does respond automatically to changes of input level within a small fraction of a second. The result is as shown in (b) of Figure 10-44.

Receivers. The receiver employed in the hearing aid illustrated in Figures 10-39, 10-40, and 10-41 is one of the magnetic type described earlier in this chapter. It therefore calls for no further description here. However, the selection of the most suitable receiver is an important step in choosing a hearing aid for an individual. The principle involved here is illustrated in the curves of Figure 10-45.

The solid curve labeled "U1 DAMPED" shows the over-all response of the hearing aid here described when this, the receiver most commonly employed, is in the circuit. The U1 receiver has a small plastic liner inserted in the hole in its nub through which the sound issues into the user's ear. With this damping removed, the frequencies in the range between about 1200 and 3000 cps are emphasized. If a user needs such extra emphasis it can be provided in this way in addition to the flexibility and variety offered by the tone adjustments provided in the hearing aid itself.

Even greater accentuation of the high frequencies is provided by the U2 receiver, as shown by the lowest curve. This is particularly appropriate for individuals whose hearing for low frequencies may approach normal but whose impairment for high frequencies is severe. The 8080 receiver provides still another variation, suitable for some types of impairment.

The receivers represented in Figure 10-45 vary considerably in their sensitivity, but this does not mean that the less sensitive ones cannot be used by individuals with severe hearing impairments. The measurements on which the curves of Figure 10-45 are based were all made with the same input sound level to the hearing aid. In normal use of the hearing aid the user of a U2 receiver, for example, would simply set his VOLUME CONTROL at a somewhat higher level to compensate for the lesser sensitivity of this type of receiver.

Basic Principles for the Selection of Hearing Aids

Of course, a hearing aid should be as small, light, durable, and inexpensive as possible, and it should amplify sound without unnecessary impairment of quality. But when we use the terms "as possible" and "unnecessary," we admit that we are prepared to

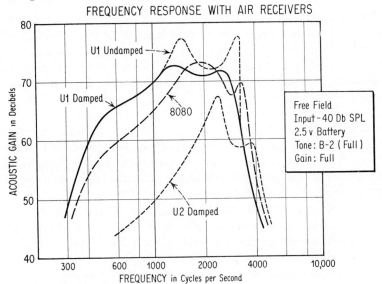

Fig. 10-45. The effects of different receivers on the over-all response of the hearing aid. (*Sonotone Corp.*)

compromise. If he cannot have both the user will sacrifice quality in order to obtain intelligibility. We have pointed out some of the features that make a hearing aid "good" in general, but exactly the same instrument may not be the best for everyone. People differ too much in their hearing losses and in the loudness of the sounds that they will tolerate, not to mention in the size of their pocketbooks! Different features will be more important for one man than for another. Let us illustrate with a few examples.

Miss Brown has a moderate, uniform hearing loss of about 45 db. Remember that the maximum intensity of average speech is about 65 db. Her hearing loss reduces this 65 db to 20 db. A glance at Figure 10-34 shows that this is too low for her to understand more than a rare word or two. But a hearing aid that provides 30 db of amplification raises the 65-db speech to 95 db. Her hearing loss makes it sound to her like 50 db, but this is loud enough for her to understand nearly everything. She will do well in ordinary social situations. This 30 db of assistance is Miss Brown's first requirement.

Miss Brown's second requirement is that the amplified sound must not reach her threshold of discomfort. Most persons, whether their hearing is normal or subnormal, feel discomfort only when speech reaches 115 db or even higher. If 115 db are Miss Brown's threshold of discomfort, she should select a hearing aid that has a maximum output just under 115 db. There is no conflict between her two requirements. The 30 db of amplification raises average speech from 65 db to only 95 db. There is still a margin of 20 db before the hearing aid's maximum output of 115 db is reached. This margin will allow Miss Brown to hear loud speech naturally and without noticeable peak clipping. The distortion of peak clipping will seldom occur, and Miss Brown is therefore not much concerned about how the instrument sounds when it is "overloaded." The limiting feature is for her merely an emergency protection that guards her against great discomfort from sudden unexpected noises. She should easily find an instrument that gives her practically perfect intelligibility whether the speaker talks loudly or softly.

Miss Brown will probably find, if she shops around, that several different makes of instrument are about equally effective, clear-toned, and attractive. Certain models may not sound as pleasant as others, but two models or combinations of the same brand may very well differ more in "how they sound" than two similar models made by different companies.

Suppose that Miss Brown goes to a laboratory and is tested with different hearing aids by elaborate and time-consuming articulation tests. She would probably make a nearly perfect score with each of several instruments. Then even the expert who tested her would be unable to say with certainty that *one* instrument is better for her than any other. Miss Brown is easy to "fit."

But consider Mr. Jones, who has a really severe hearing loss. He has not been able to find an instrument that can "get through" to him without hurting his ears. His audiogram shows about 80 db loss for low and middle frequencies, and he cannot hear 4000 cps at all. He obviously needs a great deal of amplification. The critical point for him is to find an instrument which will provide this high gain, and yet not be uncomfortably loud even when it is driven to its maximum output. The 65 db or so of amplification that Mr. Jones requires, added to the original 65 db of average speech, makes a total of 130 db. This total is at least 10 db more than the normal threshold of discomfort. The fact that Mr. Jones is hard of hearing does not mean that his ear is any "tougher" than normal. We will assume that his threshold of discomfort is 120 db. For comfort, therefore, Mr. Jones must be satisfied with less than the full amplification that he apparently needs. He must find a hearing aid with just the right maximum output. The instrument must "package" speech accurately by clipping its peaks or by compression, and must deliver it into the very restricted range between Mr. Jones's threshold of hearing and his threshold of discomfort. Success or failure may depend on whether the receiver is "flat" instead of "resonant" and on whether the tone control suppresses the low frequencies enough to keep speech intelligible when it is distorted by peak clipping. Mr. Jones is difficult to "fit."

If Mr. Jones has not used a powerful hearing aid before, he is likely to profit considerably by auditory training. Listening systematically to sound that is loud but not quite uncomfortable may increase his tolerance so that he can use an instrument with greater maximum output. Such an instrument will have more "elbow room" and will not clip the peaks of speech so heavily. Speech will then sound more natural and probably be more intelligible; but Mr. Jones's high-tone loss is severe, and he must not expect any instrument to give him a perfect articulation score.

Mrs. Smith is quite hard of hearing, but she is not so badly off as Mr. Jones. She has a loss of 60 db at 1000 cps, increasing to 80 db at 4000 cps. A fairly powerful hearing aid should make speech loud enough for her. She can probably find several instruments that

1) are tolerable, even for loud speech when the gain control is well up,

2) make faint or distant conversation intelligible,

3) make nearly all words intelligible under good listening conditions, and

4) have a "quality" that is acceptable to her.

In making comparisons of instruments, Mrs. Smith should listen at both low and high levels. Two hearing aids may sound very much alike at low levels; and yet one may be obviously superior to the other when loud sounds drive them to the limit of their output and force them to clip and distort some of the sound waves. On the whole, Mrs. Smith will probably do best with an instrument that has a definite high-tone emphasis, but she may prefer the quality of an instrument without the high-tone emphasis. This compromise is probably best settled by Mrs. Smith herself, but her decision is easier if she can choose an instrument that has an adjustable tone control. Then she can increase or decrease its high-tone emphasis according to the situation.

We will not discuss the special problems of old Grandpa Tompkins or little Mary Johnson, but the same general principles of compromise apply to all of them. Additional practical hints regarding the selection and use of hearing aids are given in the next chapter.

SELECTIVE AMPLIFICATION AND INDIVIDUAL FITTING

We have deliberately spoken of "selecting" rather than "fitting" a hearing aid. "Fitting" suggests too strongly the fitting of a pair of eyeglasses or a suit of clothes. The differences among hearing aids are not as large and as obvious as they are among eyeglass lenses and suits of clothes. Therefore it is difficult to judge with sufficient precision the success of the "fitting" of a hearing aid.

Selecting a suitable hearing aid is, first, a series of tests of adequacy in fundamentals, and then a series of judgments of intangibles or a series of compromises. There is usually no one best fit that is demonstrably best under all circumstances.

The idea of precise individual fitting is a survival from the days of feeble amplifiers and sharply resonant receivers and microphones. Perhaps we should explain in more detail that a mechanical vibrating system like the diaphragm of a telephone receiver operates most efficiently near its "natural period," but may be much less efficient for frequencies that are an octave or two higher or lower. Resonance may be made less sharp by "damping" the diaphragm, but the maximum efficiency is reduced at the same time. When amplifiers were weak, the necessary efficiency was obtained by deliberately making the receiver and the microphone quite sharply resonant without much damping. The same compromise was made in the early telephones. The quality was poor, as all of us who remember the telephones of fifty years ago can testify, but the sound was loud enough to be heard and most words could be understood. A reasonable compromise was achieved by making the microphone and the receiver resonant for different frequencies so that a wider band of frequencies was transmitted with fair but adequate efficiency. For the early electrical hearing aids an assortment of receivers and microphones, resonant at different frequencies, was provided, and the wearer determined by trial which combination gave *him* the best quality and intelligibility with adequate loudness. There was actually considerable variation among receivers of the same model, more variation than there is in modern instruments; and "fitting" was a three-way trial-and-error effort to get the best combination of microphone, amplifier, and receiver for the particular listener. The intelligibility was sometimes so poor that small differences in instruments might be quite important. Speech might be usefully intelligible with one combination and nearly unintelligible with another.

The idea of "fitting" a hearing aid was supported by the very plausible argument that a hearing aid should compensate for each person's particular hearing loss by amplifying some frequencies more than others. The audiogram was taken as the guide to show which frequencies needed "selective amplification." This principle seems obvious, but for several reasons it does not work out in practice.

In the first place, if we should compensate fully for the abnormality of the audiogram, we would usually compensate too much.

It was pointed out in Chapter 4 that *the hearing for loud tones is usually more normal than the hearing at threshold,* particularly with sensory-neural hearing loss. If we correct strictly according to the audiogram, we are therefore likely to get a caricature of the proper correction.

Really accurate compensation for the audiogram has never been tried. Most audiograms are irregular and the frequency characteristics of a hearing aid are nearly always irregular also. Only by chance can an exact compensation at all frequencies ever be achieved.

Finally, the principle of selective amplification overlooks the effects on the intelligibility of speech when the hearing aid is operated at high gain and peak clipping occurs.

In a series of wartime studies at the Psycho-Acoustic Laboratory, at Harvard University, it was found that an instrument with good over-all characteristics and true square-top peak clipping that amplified a wide range of frequencies about evenly or with moderate emphasis of the high tones gave the best results. Hard-of-hearing listeners made as good (or better) articulation scores with it and had more "elbow room" than they had with any other combination that was tried. This was true for all of the common types of hearing loss. Other "compensations" that were tried (but with no better results) included several that more nearly followed the principle of selective amplification. The details of these experiments are now available in book form for the technical reader (see Suggested Readings at the end of this chapter).

In general, similar results were obtained by British investigators (1947) and were made the basis of the design of the Medresco (Medical Research Council) hearing aid that is manufactured for and distributed by the British government.

THE AUDIOGRAM AS AN AID TO SELECTION

What remains of the principle of selective amplification and of fitting according to the audiogram boils down to something like this: It doesn't work out well to give a real low-tone boost. The choice for the best understanding of speech lies between undistorted reproduction and a moderate low-tone suppression (or high-tone emphasis). Hard-of-hearing listeners are likely to prefer natural reproduction as the best for quality, but with a high-tone hearing loss, speech is often better understood if moderate high-tone emphasis is given. If the hearing loss is severe, regardless of whether it is "flat" or "high-tone," a high-tone emphasis (introduced by the microphone or the amplifier) is very desirable because it preserves the intelligibility of speech when the hearing aid is pushed to its maximum output. In the selection of a hearing aid the audiogram is most useful as a guide to *how powerful* an instrument will probably be needed —not as a guide to the best frequency characteristics. The audiogram also reveals the cases of abrupt high-tone nerve deafness that cannot be helped much by any hearing aid because their ability to hear high tones has been lost completely.

Other tests were developed during the 1940's that employed measurements of the threshold and discrimination for speech described in Chapter 7. We shall mention one fallacy that is common to several tests, so that the hard of hearing and their advisers alike may be warned.

It was suggested, for example, that if, with instrument A, a listener can *understand fainter speech* than with instrument B, then instrument A is the better instrument for him. *The weakness of this type of test lies in the setting of the gain control of the hearing aids.* The listener is usually instructed to set it himself so that average speech comes to him at "the most comfortable loudness." Unfortunately, many subjects on repeated trials do not duplicate their own settings for most comfortable loudness. "Most comfortable" seems to cover a range of a good many decibels. Of course, if instrument A happens to have its gain control set higher than B, it has just this much advantage when the final test is made. It will be able to pick up fainter speech than can instrument B. Tests of this sort are likely to be tests of how the listener happens to set the gain control, not of how well the instrument "fits" or how "efficient" it is. All that we can usefully find out with faint speech is whether an instrument has *some* gain setting that will allow the wearer to pick up speech that is as faint as he is likely to encounter in everyday life. Most present-day hearing aids can do this. Of course there will always be the unusual case with unusual requirements. Our comments apply, however, to the large majority of people with impaired hearing.

Another frequent misunderstanding concerns the "noisiness" of a hearing aid. Of course, any crackling or hissing generated in the instrument is undesirable, but sometimes instruments with high amplification are wrongly rejected as "noisy." The trouble may be that the wearer has happened to set the gain control higher than he needs to, and all the background noises therefore sound unpleasantly loud. Perhaps a different setting of the tone control may make the noise less annoying. It is not the fault of the instrument that it amplifies all the sounds that reach it and that it cannot pick out the voice and

11

THE CHOICE AND USE
OF HEARING AIDS

S. R. Silverman, Ph.D.,
and S. Gordon Taylor

A hearing aid may be ridiculed as a "tin ear." It may be thought to detract from a person's appearance or suggest premature old age. But the man or woman whose hearing is failing should want so earnestly to hear that he will not worry about such real or imaginary trifles. His friends will welcome his use of a hearing aid because it spares them the painful necessity of having to shout and repeat for him. In fact, *it shows lack of consideration for his family and friends when the hard-of-hearing person does not wear a hearing aid if he can possibly do so and benefit by it.* Moreover, his hearing aid opens to him a broad vista of enriched social experiences which every person, hard of hearing or otherwise, needs for a happy adjustment to our complex world. Let it not be said of the hard of hearing, "Vanity, vanity, all is vanity."

To Wear or Not to Wear a Hearing Aid

According to a publication of the hearing aid industry, there were to be an estimated 1,950,000 hearing aid wearers in the United States in 1959. Probably from two to three times this many are potential users. Of course, we are aware that many individuals who own hearing aids are not constant wearers.

It is interesting to estimate the proportion of users as related to age. In Figure 11-1 we present our rough guess of this relationship. As our criterion of those who can be "helped" by a hearing aid, we have chosen a loss of 30 db or more at one end of the scale and the ability to receive communication satisfactorily (socially) at the

329

other end. We note that the greatest percentage of people who need help fall between the ages of twenty and sixty. In the top portion of the figure we have attempted to indicate when certain conditions related to hearing impairment manifest themselves. This information essentially leads us to the rationale of the graph.

We do not mean to imply that all individuals with such conditions as noise-induced hearing loss and presbycusis can be helped substantially by hearing aids, but we feel it is important to keep in mind the prevalence of these circumstances in arriving at estimates of the distribution of potential users.

Whoever has difficulty with his hearing in everyday conversations should think seriously of getting a hearing aid. The difficulty may vary with different situations, depending on the distance from the source of sound; the surrounding noises; the clarity of the speech or music; the lighting, which may help or interfere with speechreading; and many other factors. For example, someone with a moderate hear-

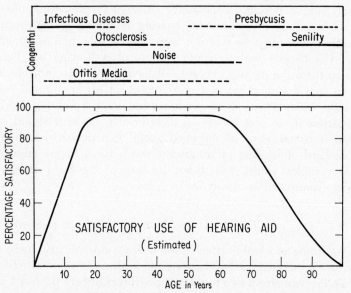

Fig. 11-1. The graph shows as a function of age the estimated percentage of individuals with hearing levels for speech of 30 db or worse who can receive social communication satisfactorily through a hearing aid.

The chart above indicates the incidence of hearing loss by age and major cause. The solid lines indicate the age periods during which the hearing loss is usually first noticed. This chart includes cases with hearing levels for speech better than 30 db but who have levels of 30 db or worse at frequencies above the range most important for speech, as in presbycusis and noise-induced hearing loss.

ing loss may not need amplification for ordinary conversation but may need it for lectures, sound movies, and church, and in social gatherings where there is likely to be a background of many voices. Also, obviously, the accurate understanding of speech is more important for some than for others. The businessman who must know exactly what goes on in conferences needs it more than the elderly person who merely wishes to hear the radio, the television, or casual conversation more easily. In the long run, each man and woman must decide for himself whether his hearing loss makes him socially (or economically) inadequate.

If a man is in doubt as to his need for a hearing aid, the audiogram is a very helpful guide. Generally, *if the hearing level for speech in the better ear is worse than 30 db, a hearing aid is needed.* But the prospective user must realize that, in spite of optimistic advertisements, a hearing aid is not a perfect instrument. It does not provide complete compensation for hearing impairment. It will benefit the wearer only in proportion to his willingness to accept it short of unattainable perfection and to his patience and effort in learning to make the most of it.

Some types of hearing loss are less favorable than others for benefit from a hearing aid. For example, a man's audiogram may show a slight loss (10 to 20 db) in the low frequencies and a precipitate drop beginning at 1000 cps. He will probably complain, "I hear, but I can't make out what you are saying." This is understandable, since the frequencies above 1000 cps convey sounds which are very important for the intelligibility of speech. For example, "fin" may sound the same as "thin" or "sin." Ordinarily, a hearing aid alone is of little value in overcoming this difficulty. However, even in such a case a proper hearing aid, *supplemented by a program of intensive auditory training* in discrimination of the sounds which make up speech, can be of great assistance. This is true even if the auditory training and instruction in speech turn out to be more helpful than the hearing aid!

HEARING AIDS FOR THE AGED

The use of hearing aids by elderly people is likely to present another special problem. Their deafness is usually of the sensory-neural type, technically known as *presbycusis*. Their ability to hear high frequencies decreases with advancing age. As we have just pointed out, such a pattern of hearing loss often results in imperfect discrimination. In younger people, intensive auditory training and constant use of an instrument help the listener learn to make use of all auditory clues.

When the other problems of advancing age are added to deafness, the situation becomes still more difficult. We must frequently reckon with poor health and gradual failure of other faculties, particularly of vision, which is so helpful as a supplement to hearing. Not only do old people often become very dependent on others; they may also find themselves unable to "keep up with the times." In addition, many of them live alone or with children who "have their own lives to lead." All these factors may lead to tensions, fears, and general nervousness, which are hardly conducive to the concentration essential for effective and comfortable use of a hearing aid. Nevertheless, we should be encouraged by the favorable reports of the Veterans Administration of its experience with elderly users of hearing aids (see Chapter 19).

Each elderly person should be evaluated in terms of his particular temperament and way of living. Where there appears to be any possibility of benefit, we strongly suggest a trial period with a hearing aid during which the person is encouraged but not forced to use the instrument. If he himself then expresses a desire to have the hearing aid, it should be purchased.

HEARING AIDS FOR CHILDREN

There is a great difference of opinion, again without much supporting evidence, as to when a child is ready to wear a hearing aid. One point of view holds that the early years are the years in which the child learns the meaning of sounds, particularly speech, and hence he should wear a hearing aid at all times from the moment it is discovered that he is deaf. On the other hand, some workers believe that the child must be trained to some degree of awareness and discrimination of sound, since failure to benefit from the instrument will discourage its use. Furthermore, some young children may fear the loud sound of an instrument and may become conditioned against it. Some suggest the possibility of damage to an ear exposed to the high sound pressure levels generated by a hearing aid. This is certainly a remote possibility. As we have seen in previous chapters, the cause of lack of response to sound may be elsewhere than in the periphery and it would be unfortunate to damage an intact end organ.

WILL A HEARING AID ENDANGER HEARING?

The prospective user of a hearing aid often asks, "Will the use of a hearing aid destroy the remainder of my hearing by overloading it?" We want to emphasize that *a hearing aid neither injures nor cures an abnormal ear*. Nor does it alter the status of impaired hearing (see also Chapter 4). It merely enables the user to make better use of the hearing that he possesses and keeps his hearing in practice. He remains attentive to sound. If, however, the new hearing aid makes the wearer "nervous," he should break it in by using it for short periods daily, gradually increasing the length of each period of use. We have to repeat that we must be cautious when we are not sure of our assessment of hearing in a very young child.

HEARING AIDS AND SPEECHREADING

There is no truth in the rather prevalent notion that the use of a hearing aid will diminish one's skill in speechreading. On the contrary, the hearing of speech is likely to reinforce speechreading because auditory clues assist in the discrimination of words that look alike on the lips. For example, in the sentence, "The package is heavy," the word "baggage" might be substituted for "package." The context, which the speechreader ordinarily uses to distinguish words that look alike on the lips, is no help here, since both words fit the context. But a hearing aid might enable the speechreader to discriminate between the initial "p" and "b" and between the "ck" and "g" in the two words. Of course we have chosen an extreme example, but long-time users of hearing aids generally report that *the continuous association of hearing and seeing speech is mutually advantageous.* Even in cases of extreme hearing loss, where complete understanding of speech is not attainable, a hearing aid may furnish enough auditory clues, such as stress patterns, to supplement speechreading quite effectively.

AIR CONDUCTION AND BONE CONDUCTION COMPARED

Air- and bone-conduction hearing aids differ in the construction of their receivers and in the pathways over which the amplified sound is delivered to the inner ear. The buttonlike air-conduction receiver, coupled to the external auditory canal by a fitted plastic earmold, delivers sound through the normal pathway. The rectangular bone-conduction vibrator, on the other hand, makes contact with the mastoid bone behind the ear, and its vibrations are transmitted by the bone directly to the inner ear. (See also Chapter 10.)

We might suppose that a bone-conduction instrument is indicated whenever the deafness is of the conductive middle-ear type. The obstruction that interferes with the passage of sound presumably can be by-passed by bone conduction, and the intact nerve endings can pick up the sound waves as they come, relatively unimpeded, directly through the bones of the skull. However, physical difficulties limit the performance of bone-conduction units. Bones and the skin that covers them vary in density and elasticity and, therefore, in their ability to transmit sound. It is more difficult to get efficient delivery of speech sounds by bone conduction than by air conduction. Disinterested and experienced clinicians generally report that from 5 to 10 per cent of their cases can use bone conduction more satisfactorily than air conduction. This rather small percentage suggests that if the prospective user of a hearing aid is still in doubt after listening by both air and bone conduction, unless he has competent advice to the contrary, he should choose air conduction.

Bone conduction is definitely preferable, however, when the user suffers from chronically discharging ears. Also, a few users who can hear over the telephone without a hearing aid, but who cannot quite follow face-to-face or group conversation, find it a great convenience to have the ear free for direct contact with the telephone receiver. However, a telephone pickup, described in Chapter 10, makes an air-conduction instrument also very convenient for telephone conversations.

THE INDIVIDUALLY MOLDED EARPIECE

Anyone who expects to use an air-conduction hearing aid should have an earmold that has been fitted to the contours of his own external ear; an earpiece that is not properly fitted may irritate the ear canal and may also interfere with the efficient transmission of sound. As was pointed out in the preceding chapter, a well-fitting individual earmold not only is more comfortable and more secure; it allows the hearing aid to deliver sounds as it is designed to deliver them, that is, with the greatest efficiency and fidelity. Even for the person who has not yet made his final selection of a hearing aid, a molded earpiece is a good investment because it will fit almost any make of air-conduction receiver to which it is attached. For adults the fit is permanent, but growing children obviously require a periodic change of earmolds.

MONAURAL OR BINAURAL?

Of great interest to hearing aid users is the advent of the binaural hearing aid. We need to remind ourselves of the illustrations in Chapter 10 which distinguish between the Y cord and binaural instruments. The Y-cord hearing aid consists of one microphone and amplifier with a receiver going to each ear. A binaural aid is made up of two complete instruments, one for each ear. Since the microphone is the new ear for the user, the binaural aid attempts to duplicate nature by providing two "ears." The conventional means of "packaging" the binaural aid is to house an instrument in each temple of a pair of spectacles as shown in Figures 10-12 and 10-13.

Of course, individual aids of the type shown in Figures 10-9 and 10-10 can be worn behind the ears. As will be pointed out in Chapter 13, binaural hearing aids may make localization of sound and discrimination in noise easier for some listeners. It is important to remember, however, that the single hearing aid worn at the ear permits the listener to take advantage of head movement in seeking out the source of sound. Therefore, in making comparisons between monaural and binaural hearing aids, it is wise to be sure that the difference is due to whether one or two hearing aids are worn and not to *where* the instrument is worn. The monaural hearing aid worn on the chest is likely to give different results from one worn behind the ear. Theoretically, binaural hearing aids should make it much easier to discriminate the voice of a particular talker from background noises from other sources. It is still too early to judge how well and for which hard-of-hearing individuals these possibilities are fulfilled.

RIGHT EAR OR LEFT?

The audiogram is a useful guide to the choice of the ear on which to wear the hearing aid. If both ears show hearing levels for speech between 30 and 65 db, the hearing aid should be worn on the *worse* ear. The better ear is left free, and it is still good enough to be of some use without a hearing aid. If, however, one ear or both ears have a hearing level worse (numerically greater) than 65 db, the *better* ear should be fitted. If the level is worse than 65 db, it is difficult enough to get good hearing with the better ear. There is usually a good deal of sensory-neural hearing loss in such a case, and intelligibility may be poor even with a powerful instrument. Furthermore, the margin between the threshold of hearing and the threshold of discomfort begins to get rather narrow when the hearing level is worse than 65 db. Of course, there are exceptions to these rules, but experience has shown this rule to be a good guide in a large majority of cases. If an audiogram is not available, the user should wear the aid on the worse ear if his hearing loss is only mild, but on the better ear if he is severely handicapped without any aid at all.

How to Choose a Hearing Aid

The medical aspects of deafness have been discussed in Chapter 5. In summarizing these rules for the choice of hearing aids we assume that the prospective user has consulted his family physician or, better, an otologist, and that the medical profession has done all that it can do. The otologist will presumably take an audiogram for his records and to assist him in his diagnosis, and he will give reliable advice as to whether a hearing aid is indicated.

We believe that a qualified audiologist should be consulted in all decisions about hearing aids for children. As mentioned in Chapter 10, there are now many clinics that offer unbiased advice on the selection of hearing aids, whether for children or for adults. These problems are complicated, and it is difficult even for an expert audiologist to pick out objectively and scientifically the hearing aids which best "fit" each individual. Furthermore, many persons are forced to rely on themselves, their friends, and the distributors of hearing aids in making their selection. Otologists will continue to give assistance.

The hearing aid dealer is obviously not a disinterested party except for assisting in the selection of the most suitable model from among his own particular offerings. Most purchasers must rely very largely on their own judgment and be prepared to discount some of the claims for special methods of "fitting" put forward by competing manufacturers. For this reason auditory tests and the basic principles of selection were described at length in the preceding chapters. Now let us consider how a person who wants to buy a hearing aid may, without the benefit of expert advice or special apparatus, make a reasonably satisfactory selection from among the makes and models of instrument that may be available in his community. Fortunately, the selection among the better instruments is no longer as critical as it once was or as is suggested by some advertisements. *Any one of several choices is likely to be a good one,* thanks to the great advances in recent years by the hearing aid industry and its distributors.

AVAILABLE DEALERS

It is generally not wise to buy a hearing aid by mail if there is any practical alternative. Direct personal contact with the dealer is most desirable. The prospective user should find out first, therefore, which hearing aid companies have local representatives in his district. His choice is practically restricted to the makes of instrument which are available to him for inspection and trial. Nearness to a dealer is also a great advantage for subsequent repair and replacement service.

SERVICE, BATTERIES, AND EARMOLDS

Specific inquiry should be made about the availability, quality, and cost of service, including the replacement of batteries. Hearing aids, like automobiles, must sometimes be repaired. If repair service is not immediately available, the user may be deprived of his instrument for long periods of time. Some dealers replace the entire hearing aid, others lend an instrument while an aid is at the factory for service, and others may be able to replace immediately such major parts as transistors, microphone, receiver, or even the entire amplifier assembly. Unnecessary repairs at exorbitant prices are to be avoided, and the user is cautioned against being "high-pressured" into buying a new model of an instrument to substitute for an older model that happens to get out of order. It is wise to look into the company's policy regarding trade-in value of old instruments in the event that new models appear on the market.

Some spare parts, particularly cords, should be purchased, particularly if the dealer is not easily reached. As a matter of fact, *we suggest a complete spare hearing aid if the cost is not prohibitive.*

Dealers in hearing aids arrange for the manufacture of the individually molded earpiece. The contract of purchase should clearly indicate whether the cost of the earpiece is included in the final price of the instrument.

SIZE, COST, AND CONVENIENCE

Even when expert advice is available, the decision as to size, weight, cost, style, color, and convenience of the instrument is the user's own. Only he can strike the balance of his preferences. He must, however, weigh these items against the performance of the various instruments in overcoming his own particular hearing loss. There are three major items of expense in a hearing aid: the initial cost, repairs and replacements, and battery operation. Low cost of one of these items does not necessarily mean low costs of the others.

SIMPLE TESTS OF THE PERFORMANCE OF A HEARING AID

In general the prospective user may rely on the dealer to recommend the particular combinations of amplifier, earphone, and tone-control setting that are most likely to be suitable for him. An audiogram will usually help the dealer arrive at his conclusions, and some dealers make their own audiometric tests. Each company that relies on the audiogram or other tests usually has a system or formula to show which of its several instruments or combinations is most likely to give satisfaction. The systems have been worked out with care, partly on theory and partly from the experience of actual users, and the choices based on them are usually rather good. It is advisable to try the first two or three combinations suggested by a dealer, but it is rarely necessary to try more.

No simple set of rules for self-selection will do for everyone, because some people are much more seriously handicapped than others. The following method should work well, however, for someone who is just becoming really hard of hearing but can still "get by" if people will only speak up loudly enough. The principles have been explained in the previous chapter; if the rules obviously do not fit your case, you can probably judge readily enough what feature of a hearing aid is most important for you and how to test for it. The general principle is this: Test for the essentials; follow your preferences thereafter.

The features of performance that should be tested when a hearing aid is chosen are

Tolerability
Intelligibility of ordinary speech
Intelligibility of faint speech
Intelligibility of difficult words
Freedom from internal noise
Aesthetic "quality"
Intelligibility under difficult conditions

It is not possible to test these items *accurately* without elaborate apparatus; but with the help of a friend, it is not difficult to come to a useful opinion on most of them. The assistance of a friend is essential, however, because *the tests should all be made under similar conditions and with the same voice and the same set of words and sentences.*

The ideal arrangement is a loan or trial period with each of several instruments, so that they may all be tested at leisure at home under the same conditions and in the same place, and the more promising ones tried in actual everyday situations. Trial periods are not generally encouraged by dealers because some unscrupulous "prospects" have no intention of purchasing the instrument and because others will not take responsibility for damage. A compromise can be worked out in most instances. Perhaps it may be possible to rent an instrument or to make a deposit for the trial period that will be applied to payment for the hearing aid if it is purchased, but will be sacrificed otherwise.

If arrangements cannot be made for home testing, the prospective user should ask a friend to go with him to the various agencies and try to carry out the same trials and tests in each case under as nearly the same conditions as possible. The friend must have a good, normal voice and be willing to practice the trick of speaking test words and reading some selected passage from a book or magazine over and over in just the same tone and *with the same loudness.* If he can standardize three different voices—average, faint, and loud—so much the better. During the trials he must keep his distance with care. A distance of five feet, which is an average conversation distance, is good, but three feet is better if the room is small or if there is some unavoidable noise. For most of the tests a quiet room is very important.

The desirability of obtaining an individually molded earpiece has been mentioned. For the very first trials one of the "universal" earmolds provided by the various companies will have to do. With them, however, it may not be able to test the instruments at full gain, because, as has been explained, a hearing aid is more likely to "squeal" if the earpiece does not fit snugly.

Each of the instruments should be worn as they are meant to be worn. They should not merely be held in the hand. The body reflects, absorbs, and distorts sound waves and is part of the acoustic system of the hearing aid when the instrument is actually in use. During the actual tests the friend should be faced, but the eyes should be closed to avoid unconscious speechreading.

TOLERABILITY

Tolerability is very important but is very difficult to test unless you are already an experienced user of a hearing aid. Sounds that are uncomfortably loud at first become tolerable with a little practice. The unfamiliar experience of hearing a really loud noise may be terrifying to someone who has been hard of hearing for a long time. Therefore, feel your way with a little care. Unless your hearing loss is quite severe, an instrument of only medium or low power may be better at first. However, with your friend, you should cautiously *try the maximum output of the instrument before the final choice is made.* But remember: *An otherwise satisfactory instrument should not be rejected simply because it is very loud, but only if it is really intolerable.* Unless your hearing loss is severe and you must use nearly full gain, you will rarely hear the loudest output except by accident, as when a door slams, and then only for a very short time.

INTELLIGIBILITY

Intelligibility of speech can be tested in three ways. First, your friend reads a selected passage from a book or newspaper, over and over again if necessary, in an ordinary but even voice. Experiment with the volume control and the tone control to *be sure that you can find a combination that makes it easy to understand what he is reading.*

If more than one instrument makes ordinary speech easily intelligible to you, the test can be made more difficult. Let your friend read in a *very quiet voice*. This is, of course, equivalent to "hearing at a distance." A higher setting of the volume control may be necessary, but be sure that you can find *some* setting that will do the job. Some instruments may fail on this test. Eliminate them from the competition, and center your attention on those that pass.

Now comes the test with difficult words. You should have prepared in advance a set of word lists with each word written on a separate card. These can be prepared from the lists in the Appendix. Shuffle the cards each time they have been read. Prepare a number of such little packs with the words in each pack alike except for one sound. A series of words to test the vowels is *bat, bite, boot, beat, boat, bout, bit, bait, but, bet, bought*. For consonants, the following words can be used: *vie, by, high, thy, shy, why, thigh, die, lie, tie, rye, pie, fie, my, sigh, guy, nigh*. If you know that you have difficulty with certain kinds of sounds, it is easy enough to make up a list that is heavily loaded with just the words that you find most confusing.

Your friend should read the words in an ordinary voice and all at the same volume. It may help him to say "now" before each word to get his voice going smoothly. You should set the volume control so that the words come to you quite loudly, but not uncomfortably so. This is not a test of sensitivity of the instrument but a test of how well it enables you to discriminate among and recognize correctly the sounds that ordinarily are difficult for you. Loud sounds are easier to discriminate than faint ones, so the instrument is "given a break" by being set so that words will not be missed simply because they are too faint.

It is a good plan to put some words two or three times over on the same list. The important points to keep in mind are these:

Use the same list, reshuffled each time, for all instruments.
Your friend must keep his voice, his distance, and all other conditions as nearly the same as possible.
Avoid speechreading.
Keep score systematically.

This test is about as elaborate and rigorous as is practical without special apparatus. The remaining "tests" depend much more on your opinions and preferences, but your friend can be very helpful by making sure that all points are considered systematically, and by noting your comments. Let him be scorekeeper. Without some sort of score card, it is very difficult to compare the performance of one instrument heard in one shop with another heard somewhere else and perhaps on another day. Remember, however, as we have said in Chapter 10, hearing aids cannot do everything.

INTERNAL NOISE

By the time you have finished the tests of intelligibility, you have probably formed some opinion of the "quality" of the instrument, that is, whether or not you "like its sound." If the instrument has any great internal noise, either electrical or from friction against your clothing, you will certainly have noticed it by this time and will have scored a black mark against that instrument.

QUALITY

As to "quality," it is well known that men and women who have heard high tones poorly for some time, as well as many with normal hearing, prefer the quality of a hearing aid (or radio) that does not emphasize—and may even suppress—high tones. They describe its sound as "smoother, more mellow, more comfortable, more pleasing." When the high tones are emphasized, or even merely restored to their normal strength, such listeners say the voice or music is harsh and unpleasant, even though words may be crisper and easier to understand. Remember, therefore, that if your hearing has been subnormal for some time, you are likely to prefer the instrument with the "full, smooth tone," even though the word test may show that you understand difficult words better with an instrument that emphasizes the high tones a bit. Your friend will probably remind you of the importance of understanding correctly. He represents your "talking public." Other people, too, are interested in having you understand them readily, and to them *your ability to understand is more important than how mellow their voices sound.* If the word tests do not show any great difference, then pick the instrument that "sounds best" by all means, but remember that *the quality preferences of those who have heard poorly for some time are notoriously misleading.* You may have forgotten how speech *should* sound.

As a final word of advice, when you are scoring an instrument on quality, lean toward the crisp rather than the mellow. You are likely to get the best results with it in the long run, even though some practice will probably be necessary before you realize the full benefits.

DIFFICULT CONDITIONS

But it is not enough to judge the quality of an instrument under good conditions only. An instrument may work very well when its volume control is set low or when your friend talks in an ordinary voice; but it may lose its clarity when the control is set high or when your friend suddenly raises his voice. The reasons for this were explained in the preceding chapter. The point to remember is this: Compare instruments for *loud* as well as for average voices *without moving the volume control from the position that makes the average voice easy to understand.* This test gives some idea of the leeway the instrument has before it either loses quality from "overloading" or else becomes intolerably loud. Plenty of leeway, technically called a "good operating range," is important for those whose auditory area has been much restricted by a severe hearing loss. But, in this test, your friend should raise his voice by degrees. Don't invite someone with a distorted sense of humor to help on this one!

One of the most frequent complaints of a new hearing aid user is that his instrument does not help him in noisy places like restaurants or social gatherings where many people are talking at once, as at a typical cocktail party. In such noisy surroundings a binaural hearing aid of the spectacle or head-mount type may help you to pick out and pay attention to one particular voice. You will be aware like a normal-hearing listener, that the voices or noises come from different directions and this makes it easier to keep them separate and listen to just one of them. This is the "stereophonic effect."

There is no very good way to find out without actual trial periods how different hearing aids sound in noisy places. Your friend may have a fairly standard voice, but he cannot carry a kit of sound effects with him. We have mentioned the desirability of a trial period if the dealer will consent. It is not necessary to make such trial of *every* available instrument. The tests that you and a friend can do on the spot should be enough to narrow the field down to two or three leading instruments.

It is an open question whether anyone who has not already had experience in wearing a hearing aid is really qualified to judge the performance of an instrument in noise. The novice is likely at first to suppress the high frequencies with the tone control, then turn down the gain control, and end by "throwing out the baby with the bath." If there is much noise around you, you must listen to noise if you are to hear voices also. Normal listeners must put up with the noise and often must struggle to understand. The tone control of a hearing aid make take some of the sting out of the noise, but no instrument can magically sort out speech from noise or one voice from another when both sounds occupy the same part of the frequency spectrum. Therefore, do not lean much on judgment of performance in noise in an on-the-spot test.

A trial period gives a better idea of the strong and the weak points of an instrument; but *play fair with the first instrument you try. Give it another trial after you have tried other instruments.* You are likely to do better in everyday situations with the second or third instrument and also to like them better because you are learning how to wear and use them. After you have gained this experience, a second trial of the first instrument may show that it is better than you thought.

The Use of a Hearing Aid

MECHANICAL PROTECTION

The hearing aid as a whole is a complicated and necessarily delicate electrical and mechanical instrument and should be guarded accordingly against unnecessary rough treatment. Actually, it is surprising how much mechanical abuse an instrument will often tolerate, thanks to modern engineering and careful design, but do not tempt fate too far. The dealer will suggest convenient ways of wearing the hearing aid without imparing its efficiency too greatly.

The receiver cord is the most vulnerable part of the hearing aid from the standpoint of wear. The cord should be worn with sufficient slack to prevent strain and to lessen noise caused by rubbing against clothing. It is particularly desirable to allow some slack near the terminals of the cord, which is where the greatest possibility of breakage exists. In disconnecting the cord from the hearing aid or the receiver be extremely careful not to tug at the cord itself. In such an operation the cord should be withdrawn by firmly grasping its terminal plug.

Exposure to excessive perspiration sometimes renders a hearing aid temporarily inoperative as a result of moisture working its way into the instrument. In extreme cases this may happen even though the hearing aid is slung in a bag, unless the bag is a waterproof one. Trouble can be avoided by inserting a sheet of waterproofing material between the hearing aid and its bag or between the bag and the body.

Also to be avoided is violent jarring which causes a hearing aid suspended around the neck to strike violently against the body. When strenuous activities are contemplated it is advisable to add a strap or belt to hold the hearing aid snugly against the body.

USE AND CARE OF THE EARPIECE

Users of bone-conduction units do not need individual earpieces. They soon learn the most desirable pressure and location for the vibrator on the mastoid prominence of the temporal bone just behind the ear.

To insert the earpiece of an air-conduction receiver, put the long piece of the earpiece gently into the external canal, at the same time pulling the top of the external ear gently upward and back. Insert the earpiece slowly so that no extra pressure is created within the canal. The earpiece is then seated by twisting it slightly backward and finally forward again to engage the contours of the external ear.

If a poorly fitting earpiece causes irritation of the external ear, try a little petrolatum on the earpiece. If this is not effective return the earpiece to the dealer, who can buff it down to smooth off irritating projections. This is what a dentist does with a dental plate which may not fit perfectly on the first trial.

Since wax may plug the sound channel, the earpiece should be cleaned regularly with soap and warm water and a nail brush with long bristles that reach down into the holes. Dry the earpiece thoroughly and blow the last drop of water out of the hole, where a tiny drop of water will block the passage of sound. A pipe cleaner is another very handy and effective tool for cleaning out the sound channel. Do not boil the earpiece or let it stand for long in hot water, as heat may soften or damage the plastic material. If you want to disinfect the earpiece, rinse it thoroughly in 70 per cent alcohol in water. A clean and sanitary earpiece is a good safeguard against infections of the external canal.

The coupling holes on all earpieces and the nubs on all air-conduction receivers are standardized so that any combination should fit well. Occasionally the fit of the coupling is not quite snug, and leakage of sound, particularly sound of low frequency, occurs. Some loudness is lost and "squeal" is more likely to occur. An excellent remedy is to insert rubber, plastic, or cloth reinforcers (of the type used in loose-leaf note books) like washers between the receiver and the earpiece to ensure a snug fit and a good acoustic seal.

TONE AND VOLUME CONTROL

The tone control modifies the quality of sound and may help to reduce the annoyance of background noises. The volume control regulates the loudness of sound, and it should be turned "up" when increased volume is desired. Usually, however, it should not be turned up much higher than necessary or "peak clipping," explained in the last chapter, may begin too soon and reduce the quality of sounds. In general, the user, through trial and error, learns the best combinations of tone and volume-control settings for various situations.

It is likely, for example, that one combination may be satisfactory for ordinary conversation in a quiet room, and another combination may be desirable at a dinner party or on a streetcar.

Even though a hard-of-hearing person cannot hear the high-pitched sounds of the doorbell, the alarm clock, or the telephone, he may still be able to hear a low-pitched *buzzer*. The substitution of such buzzers may be a great convenience to him and may make it possible for him to hear the signals even when he is not wearing his hearing aid.

It is also helpful to have *signal lights* in strategic parts of offices and homes connected to the doorbell and telephone. Alarm clocks that throw a strong light into the eyes of a sleeper at a set time are available for people who cannot be roused by any form of auditory signal.

Families and associates of hearing aid users *should not shout* into the microphones. It is better to speak naturally but distinctly and to face the listener so that he can take full advantage of speech-reading. Slamming of doors and pounding, which are nerve-racking to most wearers of hearing aids, should be avoided.

If a hearing-aid user has difficulty hearing the radio or television clearly enough for his enjoyment, he should consider having his set equipped with a socket into which he can plug an earphone. High-grade telephone receivers are now available, and they may reproduce music and voice even more faithfully than can a hearing aid. It may be very helpful to avoid the unnecessary transformations, first into sound by the radio and then back into electrical signals by the hearing aid. All noises in the room are thus excluded. The arrangement should offer no difficulty for a good radio or television service-man.

Some persons with a long-standing hearing loss may not like a hearing aid simply because it sounds "strange." They have often forgotten what it means to hear well, and therefore their judgment as to how things should sound is not very reliable. They must be as patient with a hearing aid as they are with a new pair of shoes, and their families must be equally patient with them.

If you are just starting to wear a hearing aid, you probably do not know some of the tricks of troubleshooting that are well known to many veteran users of the instruments. To save you time in mastering them we have collected a few here in condensed form as a practical guide.

There are several "symptoms" of trouble in a hearing aid:

It may squeal.
It may sound noisy or "scratchy."
It may sound weaker than usual.
It may have an unusual tone quality.
It may go on and off intermittently.
Or it may fail to operate at all.

Broadly these boil down to either "sounds different" or "no sound." This difference is the first important guide in your search for the trouble. If there is no sound at all or if the sound goes on and off, you should think of a break somewhere in the electric circuit. If the sound is weak or is unusual, the instrument is operating, but its batteries may be weak, the microphone or receiver may be damaged, or something, such as wax clogging the earpiece, may prevent the sound from reaching your ear as effectively as usual.

With this general suggestion as to where to begin, try to find what part of the instrument is not working properly. The most likely trouble spots are weak batteries, dirty contacts, or a broken cord.

The sure method of locating the source of trouble is to replace one accessory part of the instrument after another with spare parts that you keep in reserve. Of course, this suggestion does not apply to all types of hearing aids. For example, in the tiny hearing aids which fit directly into the ear and in which the microphone, amplifier, receiver, and battery compartment are built-in parts, there are no accessories to cause trouble that is correctable by the user.

You should certainly have on hand at least a spare cord and spare batteries. It is a very good plan to have a spare receiver and, better still, a complete instrument if you can afford it. The complete reserve instrument also insures you against being left without a hearing aid if something goes wrong in your regular amplifier and you have to return it to the maker for repair or replacement. Again, spare cords are a "must." Cords fail sooner or later. Even servicemen do not try to repair them. Repair is difficult and the expense of replacement is relatively small.

Substitute the spare parts one at a time: fresh batteries, a new cord, then the spare receiver. And do not forget to look for a plug of wax or a drop of water in the earpiece. Your battery tester, if you use one, will confirm or disprove your suspicion that a battery has run down.

If your hearing aid works properly after you have substituted a spare cord or battery, try the old part again. Often the trouble is merely a loose or dirty contact; or simply taking the cord off or replacing a battery may remedy the trouble.

We suggest a word of caution concerning spare batteries of the mercury type. When carried in a pocket or a purse, or wherever it is likely to come in contact with any metal object, including another battery, each battery should be enclosed in some form of nonmetallic container or individually wrapped in insulating material, such as paper, cloth, or plastic. Otherwise, any metal, such as a coin or key, that comes in contact with the battery may cause a short circuit and drain away the battery's life. Two or more similar batteries loose in a container may in this way short-circuit one another. Frequently, a hearing aid user suspects that his batteries do not give uniform service or are of poor quality when actually the fault lies in his own carelessness. Incidentally, an ordinary pencil eraser is useful for cleaning corrosion from the surfaces of a battery or from the battery contacts in the hearing aid.

Here is the troubleshooting chart, with the suggestions grouped roughly by symptoms. Under each symptom are listed possible causes of the trouble, tests to determine which of the possible causes applies, and the remedy to employ when the cause has been found. Brief though it is, this chart should enable you to diagnose and remedy any trouble that does not necessitate the attention of a skilled repairman. Some of the suggestions are worth memorizing, as they may enable you to locate and correct trouble even when away from home with no replacement parts available.

TROUBLESHOOTING CHART

Symptoms	*See Paragraphs*
Hearing aid dead:	1, 2, 3, 4, 5, 7, 10, 14, 15
Working, but weak:	1, 2, 3, 4, 5, 6, 7, 8, 9, 10, 13
Works intermittently or fades:	1, 3, 4, 5, 10, 15, 16
Whistles, continuously or occasionally:	6, 9, 11, 12, 13, 15, 17, 18
Sounds noisy, raspy, shrill:	1, 3, 4, 5, 8, 9, 10, 11, 12, 17
Sounds hollow, mushy, muffled:	1, 2, 7, 15, 16
Other kinds of bad quality:	1, 7, 10, 15, 17
Noise when the wearer moves:	19, 20, 21

Causes, Tests, and Remedies

1. *Cause*—Dead, run down, or wrong type of battery. *Test*—Substitute new battery. *Remedy*—Replace battery.

2. *Cause*—Battery reversed in holder so that (+) terminal is where (−) terminal should be. *Test*—Examine. *Remedy*—Insert battery correctly.

3. *Cause*—Poor contacts at receiver-cord plugs due to dirty pins or springs. *Test*—With hearing aid turned on, wiggle plugs in receptacles and withdraw and reinsert each plug. *Remedy*—Rub accessible contacts briskly with lead-pencil eraser, then wipe with clean cloth slightly moistened with Energine or similar cleaning fluid. Inaccessible contacts usually can be cleaned with broom straw moistened with cleaning fluid.

4. *Cause*—Break or near break inside receiver cord. *Test*—While listening, flex all parts of cord by running fingers along entire length and wiggling cord at terminals. Intermittent or raspy sounds indicate broken wires. *Remedy*—Replace cord with new one. Worn ones cannot be repaired satisfactorily.

5. *Cause*—Plugs not fully or firmly inserted in receptacles. *Test*—While listening, withdraw and firmly reinsert each plug in turn. *Remedy*—Obvious.

6. *Cause*—Eartip too small or not properly seated in ear. *Test*—With the fingers press the receiver firmly into the ear and twist back and forth slightly to make sure that the eartip is properly positioned. *Remedy*—Obvious.

7. *Cause*—Eartip plugged with wax, or with drop of water from cleaning. *Test*—Remove eartip, examine visually, and blow through it to determine whether passage is open. *Remedy*—If wax obstructed, wash eartip in lukewarm water and soap, using pipe cleaner or long-bristle brush to reach down into the canal. Rinse with clear water and dry. A dry pipe cleaner may be used to dry out the canal, or blowing through the canal will remove surplus water.

8. *Cause*—Loose receiver cap. *Test*—Examine. Shake. *Remedy*—If cap is of the screw type, turn tight with fingers. If cap is cemented on or crimped, and has become loose, it can be repaired only by the manufacturer.

9. *Cause*—Insufficient pressure of bone vibrator on mastoid. *Test*—While listening press the bone receiver more tightly against the head with the fingers. *Remedy*—Bend the bone-vibrator headband to provide greater pressure. This is preferably done by the dealer, who is more skilled in maintaining conformation with the head.

10. *Cause*—Battery leakage (resulting in poor battery connections) or corroded battery contacts. *Test*—Examine battery and battery holder for evidence of leakage in the form of a powder or corrosion. *Remedy*—Discard the battery and wipe the holder ter-

minals carefully with cloth dampened (not wet) in warm water
to remove loose powder. Then clean with pencil eraser.

11. *Cause*—Receiver close to wall or other sound-reflecting surfaces.
Test—Examine. *Remedy*—Avoid sitting with the fitted side of the
head near a wall or other surface. Such surfaces close by tend to
reflect the sound from the receiver so that it is more readily picked
up by the microphone, thus causing whistling.

12. *Cause*—Microphone worn too close to receiver. *Test*—Try moving
instrument to provide wider separation between it and the receiver. *Remedy*—Avoid wearing microphone and receiver on same
side of body, or close together.

13. *Cause*—Microphone facing the body. *Test* and *Remedy*—obvious.

14. *Cause*—Telephone-mike switch in wrong position. *Test* and *Remedy*—Place switch in desired position.

15. *Cause*—Faulty receiver. *Test*—Examine receiver for possible
breaks, cracks, etc. *Remedy*—Replace with a new receiver.

16. *Cause*—Collapse of tubing. *Test*—Check to see if tube bends
(either when head is in a satisfactory position or is moved.)
Remedy—Shorten or replace tube.

17. *Cause*—Volume control turned too high. *Test*—Reduce volume
until speech sounds clearer. *Remedy*—Obvious.

18. *Cause*—Air leak between earmold and receiver. *Test*—Check
ring, retainer of earmold, receiver nozzle, and plastic seal washer.
Remedy—Replace defective part.

19. *Cause*—Clothing noise from loose clothing clip. *Test*—Check.
Remedy—Tighten or replace clip.

20. *Cause*—Clothing noise from improper placement of aid. *Test*—
Experiment by placing aid in different positions on the body.
Remedy—Obvious.

21. *Cause*—Clothing noise because garment bag is not used. *Remedy*
—Obvious.

**If the above tests do not disclose the source of trouble, the difficulty
is probably internal in the receiver, microphone, or amplifier and the
instrument should be serviced by your dealer.**

A Word to the Wise

No one but an expert should ever open the case of a hearing-aid amplifier.
Even opening and closing it may cause trouble, and to poke around inside
may cause severe damage that will be expensive to repair. If you must
satisfy your curiosity and see the inside, your dealer will be glad to show it
to you. Remember, if you do damage through opening up the case (and
don't think your dealer will fail to detect it), it is liable to void your service
guarantee!

Suggested Readings

CARHART, R. "Hearing Aid Selection by University Clinics," *Journal of Speech and Hearing Disorders,* 15: 106–113 (1950).

An exposition of the role of an audiology clinic in a university, with particular reference to the selection of hearing aids.

HIRSH, I. J. "Binaural Hearing Aids: A Review of Some Experiments," *Journal of Speech and Hearing Disorders,* 15: 114–123 (1950).

NEWBY, H. A. *Audiology.* New York: Appleton-Century-Crofts, Inc., 1958.

Chapter 9 contains a description of procedures used by the audiologist in selecting a hearing aid.

PATTEE, H. L., and M. P. DOWNS. "A Survey of Hearing Centers in the United States," *Archives of Otolaryngology,* 59: 413–430 (1954).

SHORE, I., R. C. BILGER, and I. J. HIRSH. "Hearing Aid Evaluation: Reliability of Repeated Measurements," *Journal of Speech and Hearing Disorders.* In press.

See also Suggested Readings for Chapter 10.

PART 4

REHABILITATION
FOR HEARING LOSS

12

SPEECHREADING

Miriam D. Pauls, Ph.D.

By nature man is a gregarious animal whose entire well-being is closely related to his ability to communicate freely with his fellows. Out of this need evolved one of the most remarkable achievements of all times, the development of language to facilitate the interchange of ideas, feelings, desires, and the like. Obviously, communication requires not only the verbalization of language by the speaker, but its intelligent reception by the listener. The actions and reactions of each participant in a conversation are colored by the ease with which he can exchange ideas, and any interference with any part of the process has far-reaching effects.

For example, we are all only too well aware today of the difficulties that arise in international conferences because of the lack of a common language. Let us visualize an important conference with an American, a Russian, and an Arab who are separated not only by national and ideational differences, but by a language barrier. To settle any problem they are forced to exchange views, argue points, and attempt to come to an agreement, not in their native language, but in still a fourth language, diplomatic French. Each speaker must attempt to express his thoughts and emotions in the less familiar French. Each listener must go through a similar process to decode the message from French into his native language, in which he thinks most readily. An interpreter only adds complications, since his facility or his errors in translating from one language to another color every sentence. There is no quick or sure flow of ideas; so it is small wonder that misunderstandings, confusion, irritation, and even hostility are the result.

A comparable situation exists when a physical defect, such as deafness, blindness, or a speech disorder, hinders the expression or reception of language. Each of these handicaps interferes with com-

353

municative exchange and so tends to isolate the individual from his fellow men.

In most conversation we employ both sight and hearing. Hearing is so predominant for most of us, however, that we seldom appreciate the importance of sight. The information that we get by watching not only the movements of the speaker's lips, but also his gestures and the expression of his face, is realized only when we hear with difficulty and are unable to see the speaker to our satisfaction.

Contrary to popular opinion, the man who is deaf or blind does not miraculously acquire a "supersense" to compensate for his particular handicap. Instead, he must learn to utilize to the utmost what he has left to work with. It is a shift of attention that enables him to work seeming miracles. For example, a blinded man must learn to rely principally on the cues that can be supplied by his ears and his sense of touch. Similarly, the deafened man must compensate for his loss of hearing by giving greater attention to the use of his eyes and to his interpretation of the situation of the moment. Keen observation and intelligent synthesis are the basis of speechreading.

Prior to 1940, when help for the hard of hearing was limited to a course of speechreading lessons ("lip reading" is the older, less inclusive term), several systems had been developed. The originator of each system made an analysis of the formation of the sounds in the English language in terms of visibility, and outlined a course of lessons designed to present the material in logical sequence. Several of the systems went a step further and correlated what was *heard* and *felt* with what was *seen*. This approach is being more generally applied as we better apprehend what is involved in the communicative process; communicative rehabilitation as a total concept is being clarified.

Speechreading is the skill that enables a person, regardless of whether he possesses normal or impaired hearing, to understand language by attentively observing the speaker. So much for the simple definition. Let us analyze it to appreciate all that is implied by "attentively observing."

The basic assumption underlying this analysis is that the individual has language facility (the mind's reflexive use of verbal symbols) as well as an adequate vocabularly. If one's language is limited, one cannot hope to speech-read no matter how attentively he observes!

Spoken language is a rapid succession of utterances that are composed of some forty-odd meaningful sounds, or phonemes, of varying degrees of visibility. These sounds have been divided by phoneticians into two major categories: vowels and consonants. The speechreader must be able to recognize instantly all the visible movements and fill in those that are invisible. Fortunately, the sounds like *f, s, th, ch,* which are difficult to hear, are easy to see on the lips. Likewise, the sounds that are difficult to see, like the short vowels, are easier to hear because they have more energy in the lower- and mid-frequency range, where the majority of hard-of-hearing people have useful residual hearing. These forty-odd sounds are produced by changing the shape of the mouth and the relative position of the tongue, teeth, lips, and jaw. It is these visible movements that the speechreader must observe and interpret. To help him fill in the gaps and make the most of what he hears and sees (for only about a third of speech sounds are clearly visible) the speechreader can learn to use the sensations that he feels in his own speech muscles as he watches the speaker. Notice what even an expert speechreader does when puzzled. He silently imitates the movements he sees. This repetition helps him translate a visual image into a motor-speech image and usually gives him the needed clue. This use of the muscle-feeling sense is a valuable training and checking device and is used in teaching.

It may seem impossible to read speech when only one third of the sounds are visible, but we are all accustomed to the same sort of confusion, albeit to a lesser degree. Two or more words like "ice" and "eyes," or "up," "cup," "come," and "gum" may *look* alike or nearly so, and the speechreader must recognize by the context, and other clues, which one is intended. This is no different from what all of us must do with words that *sound* alike, such as "their" and "there," or "so," "sow," and "sew," or the many meanings of some single words that not only look alike and sound alike but are even spelled alike. The speechreader simply has many more choices to make than the rest of us, as well as blanks to fill in, and he must learn to anticipate and integrate all cues.

In conversation there is no pause between words as there is on the printed page. For example, the phrase "plenty of potatoes" has the same number of movements as the jawbreaking word "plenipotentiary," but both are tripped off the tongue with equal speed and lack of division between syllables. The division into words is an interpretive process that takes place in the mind. It is never seen on the lips.

In addition, the speechreader must observe the rhythm of the sentences: each language has a characteristic flow that is determined by its syntactical patterns as well as by the pronunciation of words. An appreciation of this cadence helps him to fill subconsciously the many gaps in what he actually sees and hears.

Stress and accent also affect what the speechreader sees. By watching the timing of syllables and the pauses between them, he gets additional meaning. The same sentence said with different stress and inflection has its meaning changed entirely. Read aloud the following sentences, stressing the italicized word, and note the result. Then watch to see the differences in timing as someone else says them, and you will have a better appreciation of this point:

> *Good!* By God we're going to Kansas.
> Good-by, *God,* we're going to Kansas.
> Good-by, God. We're going to *Kansas.*

In addition to these factors, the cues provided by the general situation are very helpful. Facial expression, gestures, and reactions are frequently more expressive than the words that are uttered. Often an object handled or pointed to gives a valuable clue, while the place and the particular speaker shed light on the topic under discussion. For example, we can easily anticipate what the clerk behind the counter at the grocery store will say, or the remarks of the conductor coming down the aisle punching tickets, or the comments of the motorcycle cop who has signaled us over to the side of the road for running through a red light.

The deaf and the hard of hearing must learn to recognize and employ these details of every speech situation. The more limited his hearing, the greater the strain on the speechreader, for his attention is concentrated on this rapid succession of ever-changing movements that vary with every speaker. This rapid flow of speech must be grasped in a fleeting instant, for there is no opportunity for review. Interpretation must be instantaneous. Attentive observation of all these factors demands such alertness that tension and fatigue are produced in a relatively short time. Then, too, poor lighting, distance, noise, confusion, and distracting movements can defeat even the most experienced speechreader. Many a deafened person, dependent on speechreading alone, has been so fatigued by the demands of his daily job that a social evening is an impossible ordeal for him.

For the majority of hard-of-hearing persons, these difficulties can best be helped by use of an appropriate hearing aid. For the individual with a moderate to severe conductive and/or sensory-neural loss, amplification appropriate to the nature and degree of his loss can bring him within the range of good auditory function.

Unfortunately, there are some individuals who by the very nature of their problems cannot use amplification, or can profit from it only to a minimal degree. Its value may be limited to auditory support without additional clarity, or it may merely help to alert the speechreader to the source of voice. One of the major benefits may be to help him monitor his own voice. There are individuals with central dysacusis whose ability to discriminate speech is seriously affected. Still others may have mild sensory-neural losses and cannot tolerate increased loudness in the noise and confusion of daily living.

On the other hand, the use of a hearing aid does not eliminate the need to learn speechreading. We communicate best with a combination of looking and listening, and the two are complementary. All this emphasizes the need for a careful diagnostic study before training is started.

SPEECHREADING AND AURAL REHABILITATION

Advances in the medicine and surgery of the ear, and the emergence of clinical audiology as a professional field, have done much to improve our understanding and management of auditory disorders. Speechreading is no longer recommended as a panacea, but is used as an integral part of a total program.

We should be able to take it for granted that a careful diagnostic evaluation by an otologist and an audiologist is the basic first step in any aural rehabilitation program. In complicated cases, a complete physical examination, with various specialists contributing to the total picture, is indicated. Any medical or surgical treatment should be carried out. The audiologic evaluation should not only measure the nature and degree of the impairment but, what is even more important, assess the total communicative function of the individual.

If a hearing aid is indicated in terms of the otologic and audiologic findings, its selection should be guided by the audiologist, and he should help the individual learn to use it. With this information and preparation, it is possible to plan a training program that will help the particular person meet his specific problems. Two problems are rarely identical; we deal with people, not with "ears."

The experience gained in the military rehabilitation programs during World War II laid the groundwork for current concepts of aural rehabilitation, but certain modifications were inevitable. In a military organization control over the patient and his time is complete. Thus it was possible to have concentrated daily instruction for a four- to eight-week period. Such a program is not practical for the average adult engaged in earning a living or managing a busy household. Thus any program must be arranged in terms of feasibility as well as need.

A concentrated course of instruction might profitably be considered for hard-of-hearing children in the public schools for whom no special help is available in the local community. With a concentrated short-term course of instruction, located in a state school for the deaf or in other residential facilities, many children who are floundering could stay in a regular educational course.

The major role of the speech and hearing therapist in the public schools is not just to teach the child speechreading or auditory training or to correct an off-pressure "s," but to be sure that the child's vocabulary and language are expanding. Most youngsters can understand language that is familiar. The greatest need is supportive help and, possibly, academic tutoring so that the youngster can keep up with his group. Speechreading lessons, once or twice a week for years on end, can scarcely meet his needs.

If one is to achieve a satisfactory adjustment through training, two basic approaches are required. First, the individual must understand the nature of his hearing impairment and face objectively the problems it poses, and he must be led to assume responsibility in meeting them. It is also profitable to instruct the members of his family so that they will better understand the problem and how they can help. With school children, this information needs to be given to the classroom teacher as well as to the parents. Secondly, the three aspects of the communicative process—speechreading, auditory training, and speech correction—must be developed in a close-knit fashion with emphasis on whichever aspect is most pertinent for that individual. A predetermined, set curriculum is usually fruitless.

Just as important as the initial otologic and audiologic evaluation is regular reassessment over the years, by both the otologist and the audiologist, with further guidance and recommendations. The physical status may change, the hearing loss may shift, and hearing aids wear out.

THE TEACHER OF SPEECHREADING

Experience has shown that in order to carry through such a program successfully the teacher must meet reasonably high educational and professional qualifications. It is important that the teacher be a stable, emotionally mature individual, possessed of sound clinical judgment and the ability to guide objectively the complete readjustment of the student. Fundamental requirements are a good voice, natural, intelligible speech, and no peculiar mannerisms. Wide cultural interests, a pleasing personality, and a sense of humor are essential. The teacher should be trained in both hearing and speech so that she has the fundamental philosophy and the wide knowledge of communication that is required. This last presupposes that satisfactory grounding has been acquired in the theory and methods of speechreading, phonetics, speech correction, auditory training, audiometry and hearing aids, anatomy, physiology, and pathology of the ear and vocal mechanisms, as well as the related areas of psychology and education. The teacher with such training and experience will avoid putting undue emphasis on speechreading to the detriment of the other skills of communication.

It is not likely, nor is it essential, that the teacher be a proficient speechreader, unless perchance she herself has impaired hearing. *The basic factor is her ability to teach,* which implies knowledge of her subject and the capacity to present it in such a way that it will meet the needs of each pupil.

Competent teachers are all too few, but they may be found. To begin with, many colleges and universities have established hearing and speech clinics whose facilities are open to the public. More and more large hospitals, particularly those connected with medical schools, have audiologists and speech pathologists on their staffs. The Veterans Administration has its own audiologic centers (see Chapter 19), and, in areas that are not covered, it purchases services for veterans from some thirty authorized clinics. The Armed Forces have maintained their aural rehabilitation units for service personnel. Public schools frequently employ hearing and speech therapists for the children, and on request these instructors might offer night classes for adults. A similar arrangement might be made with a school for the deaf. There are also some teachers of speechreading in private practice. Many of them also teach at the local chapters of the American Hearing Society.

Methods of Teaching Speechreading

Speechreading is not a mysterious skill. Extensive screening tests, given before a student has had any instruction whatsoever, have shown that most persons possess some potential ability. Everyone unconsciously practices some small degree of speechreading. Consider the difficulty experienced in understanding a lecturer when his face is obstructed. We naturally rely on visual cues for easy understanding. This is really speechreading. While facility is usually developed to a high degree only by formal instruction, necessity can produce a spectacular skill.

This was vividly illustrated by a young marine who was a patient at a naval hospital. He had been captured on Bataan and confined for three and a half years in a Japanese prison camp. Shortly after capture, he was profoundly deafened by shell explosion at close range and, on regaining consciousness in a Japanese hospital, he found that he was cut off from his fellows except through the medium of writing.

Put back to hard labor, he strove unsuccessfully to participate in the camp life and became more and more frustrated and baffled. Then, two months later, he saw an officer in conversation with another prisoner and thought he understood the word "China." Excitedly, he made inquiry and found he was right.

This was his first hint that he might understand conversation if he watched closely. He realized that if he set the conversational stage he could anticipate and understand the reply. He began saying, "Good morning," and his fellow prisoners replied in kind. His buddies joined in the game, and since common camp topics were usually limited to home, food, and escape, he had ample opportunity for practice. The grim struggle for survival, "Either you do, or you don't," furnished the most powerful motivation.

After release, he was sent to the Philadelphia Naval Hospital for treatment. There he was fitted with a hearing aid, but his loss was so profound that the aid served merely to give him awareness of sound and to help him control his own voice. With systematic instruction, his skill in speechreading became phenomenal. Because he could converse so readily, once his attention was secured, one almost forgot that he couldn't hear. Even though few people can, or need to, achieve this marine's unusual skill, his example may well offer inspiration and incentive to any hard-of-hearing person.

This experience suggests the pattern that is followed by the teacher of speechreading, the progress from the known to the unknown, dealing first with generalities and then advancing to specific details as the student makes progress. Everyday topics of conversation are used so that the pupil feels that he is making progress and that he can use his new skill outside the classroom. He also realizes that all normal conversations provide him with much-needed practice. The teacher should see to it that all basic material used in the lessons is phrased in everyday idiom and in a simple conversational style. There is no place for stilted, bookish phraseology.

GROUP TEACHING

Group teaching is effective if the group is homogeneous. A class of four to eight has been found to be a good working unit for both teacher and pupil. The effectiveness of group instruction was clearly demonstrated in the Army and Navy Hearing Rehabilitation Programs, where it was necessary, because of the pressure of circumstances, to plan with a limited staff the most efficient and effective program

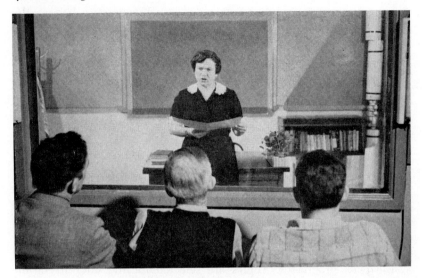

Fig. 12-1. Group instruction in speechreading through a glass partition. The partition prevents the pupils from getting auditory clues and enables the instructor to talk naturally. (*Veterans Administration.*)

for a large turnover of patients. It meant adapting old techniques and creating new ones. However, the advantages of well-planned group instruction were retained on their own merits. Results can be obtained with a group that are difficult to achieve with individual instruction. This is particularly true in the development of the right attitudes.

The association with others who are similarly handicapped continually reminds the pupil that his case is not unique. He becomes less inclined to self-pity, and he profits by the successes, the observations, the comments, and even the errors of his classmates.

The group method fosters more varied and interesting lessons because greater leeway is allowed both the teacher and the student. The element of competition enters, and the interplay of personalities, as well as the spontaneous comments of the group, produces the easy, natural atmosphere favorable for learning. These same comments develop the student's ability to anticipate, as well as the mental flexibility to deal with, abrupt changes of subject. There is rich experience with the conversation of the varied personalities within the group.

As long as the group is kept small, the teacher can evaluate and meet the needs of each student. Individual work may be indicated for the very slow, or the very superior student.

Before any formal instruction in speechreading is begun, the essentials of communication are explained to the group in much the same terms as are used in this discussion. The objectives, the training to be undertaken, and the method of instruction are described. This groundwork has two desirable purposes: it gives the student understanding of the task confronting him and confidence in its ultimate goal; and for the teacher, it secures the intelligent cooperation of the group.

Each lesson is devoted to a single topic. Thus, one lesson may center on a discussion of dining out, another on shopping. Such subjects as banking, travel, movies, and sports are other possibilities. Interest is sustained by the unity of the topic, and valuable experience is gained in anticipating the turn of conversation, since there is a central theme to guide the students' thoughts. Obviously, the needs of the group determine the degree of complexity of the material, and more complicated sentences and ideas are introduced as the class progresses. Topics are selected for the interests of the group and should contain a wealth of informative and amusing material.

Speechreading is demonstrated in the classroom in two ways. The first is with normal or subdued voice. Whispering is avoided for it fails to demonstrate a normal speech pattern. In fact, it exaggerates and distorts the pattern. Then, practice with no sound is given by the use of a large glass partition between speaker and observer. The speaker converses behind the glass in normal tones, with no distortion resulting from attempted muffling, and the speechreader discovers that he has followed the conversation, despite the complete absence of auditory cues. It is a dramatic demonstration and has the psychological effect of accentuating the situation by the effective concentration of group attention.

Amplified sound is freely employed in order to give instructions and explanations. With these clearly and easily understood, teacher and students can relax.

The speechreader is given practice in following speech at distances varying from three to approximately thirty feet. At the same time, the various speakers may be either seated, standing, or moving about.

There are a variety of ways to supplement the regular classroom procedures. Original skits are written that involve two or more characters in an amusing situation. These skits hold the attention of the audience and serve to develop the students' ability to follow rapid dialogue as well as to utilize the entire situation to clarify meaning. The skits also provide splendid practice in reading the

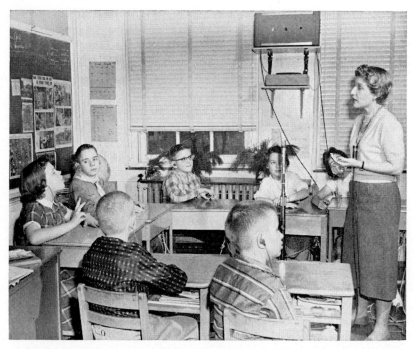

Fig. 12-2. Group instruction that combines speechreading and auditory training. (*Central Institute for the Deaf.*)

speech from every angle—full front, profile, and all the degrees in between—of a variety of people in action.

Likewise, motion pictures are excellent for instruction and practice in speechreading. At present this is a relatively undeveloped field, for only a few specially produced speechreading films are available. This author has used carefully selected and edited commercial shorts, cuttings from feature pictures, and also certain Navy training films. These films are well acted and well photographed. They have the advantage of a sound track, making it possible to run them interchangeably as sound or as silent films, thus giving needed practice in combining sight and hearing. Such films hold great possibilities, not only as a means of providing supplementary practice, but also as an excellent way to illustrate forcefully many of the problems of the speechreader. They can also be used as standardized tests of a student's progress.

A study of simplified English phonetics is one of the best ways to make the student aware of the details of speech and to show him the close interrelationships among the many avenues that are employed in communication. A rapid analysis of English sounds and the grouping of these sounds into broad categories help the student acquire a definite feeling for the auditory, visual, and kinesthetic forms of speech. The consonants, for instance, are grouped into three categories, referred to as *ports,* according to where he *feels* the sounds as he and the teacher say them together.

In Port I are placed the sounds that are felt on the lips, such as *p*ie, *m*ama, *f*ive, *v*ase, *wh*ite, *w*indow.

In Port II are grouped the sounds that are felt in the front of the mouth because they are made by the tip of the tongue, the teeth, and the palate, such as *t*ie, *n*o, *s*ix, *d*o, *sh*oe, *ch*ew, *th*ree, *l*emon, *r*abbit.

In Port III are grouped the sounds that are felt in the back of the mouth because they are made by the back of the tongue against the palate, such as *k*ind, *c*ut, *g*o, *k*ing.

By repeating simultaneously with the teacher groups of words containing the same initial sound, such as *box, baby, boy, but, book,* the visual, auditory, and kinesthetic (muscle sense) images of that sound are imprinted on the student's mind. He learns that Port I sounds are very visible, that Port II sounds are less visible, and that Port III sounds are, for all practical purposes, invisible. Such systematic groupings emphasize the sounds that look alike on the lips and give an effective method of attacking the problem of speechreading.

The so-called imitation exercises, or "talking together" exercises, offer another valuable way of developing this awareness of the various forms of speech. The students talk in unison with the speaker so that they simultaneously *see, hear,* and *feel* the speech pattern. This is immediately followed by silent review of the same material while the student watches and endeavors to recall all the sensations he had while talking aloud with the speaker. In short, motor memories related to speech are built up in response to visual and auditory cues.

This type of training is done with simple sequences of words or phrases that enable the student to anticipate a probable sequence, such as counting, months, the days of the week, cities, states, and the like. The drills are presented in such a way as to make him aware of, and responsive to, the rhythm and flow of language. These exercises are particularly valuable for slow groups.

PRACTICAL CONSIDERATIONS FOR THE SPEECHREADER

Speechreading is never easy, because so many vital factors are beyond control. A poorly lighted room that throws deep shadows on the speaker's face, a seating arrangement that forces the speechreader to look into a bright light—these are unsatisfactory. The friend who attempts to help by buttonholing the speechreader merely presents an additional problem. At close range the speechreader cannot readily follow the speech, nor can he observe any situational cues. A distance of approximately six feet has been found to be the most comfortable one. Furthermore, it is well worth the speechreader's efforts to seek a position from which he can most comfortably observe all members of the group without facing the light. Confusing and disturbing movements and noises only serve to divert his attention and increase his fatigue.

The very character of speech itself presents a major problem. Ideas must be grasped in a fleeting instant, for speech is never static. Much of it is invisible and every new combination of syllables produces minor changes in the individual sounds. No two mouths are alike; no two individuals' speech patterns are identical. Poor speakers impose a burden, for their articulation is careless and indistinct and therefore hard to see. *The greatest help is quiet, good speech.* The well-intentioned person who shouts or who uses exaggerated speech only increases the difficulties. One who covers his mouth, turns away while talking, or has annoying mannerisms presents similar problems. Likewise, it is well-nigh impossible to follow the speech of a man who has his teeth clamped on a pipe or has a cigarette dangling from his lips. An impassive, expressionless face is more difficult than a mobile one. The considerate speaker, however, can materially reduce all these problems.

The sociable person, keenly interested in people and events, usually makes rapid progress in speechreading, while the shy, reserved individual and the unimaginative, phlegmatic type are at a disadvantage. The secret of successful speechreading lies in the ability to grasp an idea intuitively and develop its meaning without attempting to follow every word. A too literal person, or one who clings tenaciously to a preconceived idea about where the conversation is headed, always has serious difficulties. An illuminating answer was given this author by a relatively uneducated pupil. Pressed for an explanation of his unusual skill in speechreading, he replied, "Well, Missy, I figures out where you're going and I beats you there!"

Essential as it is to be on the alert to catch significant trends and changes in a conversation, it is also true that undue tension and fatigue may cause a mental "block." Therefore the speechreader must strive to maintain a happy balance.

From the outset, a speechreader needs a sense of humor to help him surmount many failures. Speechreading can best be improved by constant practice in everyday life, rather than by repeated returns to the classroom. The student's progress depends largely upon himself, for the teacher can only chart the way. The student's intelligence, application, and determination are vital factors in achieving success.

It cannot be too strongly emphasized that a person with a hearing loss should frankly face his loss. The natural tendency is to ignore the hearing impairment or to attempt to conceal it. These efforts, even though partly successful for a time, lead to an increasing strain. Eventually, both social and business life will be affected.

A handicap in hearing can be successfully overcome by the efforts of the individual himself. Classroom instruction and guidance will provide the groundwork. Continual practice of speechreading in daily contacts will usually develop the skill to carry on a normal life comfortably.

AIDS TO COMMUNICATION

Anyone with a hearing loss may profitably consider the following suggestions for ease of communication.

1. Remember that hearing is the natural and normal way to understand speech. Therefore, select and get instruction in the use of the best possible hearing aid for your loss.

2. Be determined to master speechreading *now*. Don't forget that it can help you in every conversation.

3. Do not strain either to hear or to see speech. A combination of hearing and seeing enables you to understand most speakers readily. Actually, how you get it doesn't matter, just as long as you understand.

4. Avoid tension. Make every effort to relax.

5. Do not expect to get every word. Follow along with the speaker, and as you become familiar with the rhythm of his speech, key words will emerge to enable you to put two and two together.

6. Try to stage-manage the situation to your advantage. Since lighting is important, avoid facing a bright light, and try not to allow the speaker's face to be shadowed. Keep about six feet between you and the speaker so that you can more readily observe the entire situation.

7. Try to determine the topic under discussion. Friends can be coached to give a lead unobtrusively, such as "We are discussing the housing problem." This is particularly helpful in large conversational groups.

8. Maintain an active interest in people and events. Being abreast of national and world affairs, as well as of those of your community and intimate social circle, enables you to follow any discussions more readily.

9. Remember that conversation is a two-way affair. Do not monopolize it in an attempt to direct and control it.

10. Pay particular attention to your speech. A long-term hear-

ing loss, or even a sudden, profound loss, may cause a marked deterioration of voice and articulation. This condition must be corrected, for a pleasant, well-modulated voice is a great asset.

11. Cultivate those subtle traits of personality that do so much to win friends and influence people. A sincere, ready smile, an even disposition, and a genuine sympathetic interest in other people can do much to smooth your path.

12. Remember that the education of *your* public is your responsibility. Many people are embarrassed because they have no idea of how to talk with the wearer of a hearing aid or with a speechreader. Put them at ease, and assure them that quiet, natural speech is their greatest favor to you.

Suggested Readings

BRUHN, M. A. *The Muller-Walle Method of Lip-Reading.* Lynn, Mass.: The Nichols Press, 1929.

BUNGER, A. M. *Speech Reading – Jena Method.* Danville, Ill.: The Interstate Press, 1954.

EWING, I. R. *Lipreading and Hearing Aids.* Manchester, Eng.: Manchester University Press, 1944.

KINZIE, C. E., and R. KINZIE. *Lip-Reading for the Deafened Adult.* Philadelphia: The John C. Winston Company, 1931.

NITCHIE, E. B. *New Lessons in Lip Reading.* Philadelphia: J. B. Lippincott Company, 1950.

SORTINI, A. J. *Speechreading: A Guide for Laymen.* Washington, D.C.: Alexander Graham Bell Association for the Deaf, 1958.

STOWELL, A., E. E. SAMUELSON, and A. HELMAN. *Lip Reading for the Deafened Child.* New York: The Macmillan Company, 1928.

WHILDIN, O. A., and M. A. SCALLY. *Speech Reading for the Hard of Hearing Child.* Westminster, Md.: John William Eckenrode, 1939.

13

AUDITORY TRAINING

Raymond Carhart, Ph.D.

Satisfactory hearing depends upon the ability to recognize differences between sounds. From automobile horns to bird songs to human speech, the important noises in our world have distinctive character. It is not enough to receive these sounds; we must also be able to identify them. We must be aware of the special character of each.

The ability to distinguish sounds correctly is called *auditory discrimination.* In this chapter we are concerned with the nature of auditory discrimination, with the ways in which hearing losses interfere with normal identification of sounds, and with the methods of training which improve the ability to discriminate them.

Auditory Discrimination

We must clearly understand at the outset that *auditory discrimination is not identical with sensitivity of hearing.* The latter, as was pointed out in Chapters 2 and 7, dealing with the physiology of hearing and tests of hearing, is the capacity of the listener to hear faint sounds. While a sound must be heard before it can be distinguished from other sounds, the mere fact that a sound is audible does not ensure that it will be recognized accurately. We are concerned with auditory discrimination as a skill that is limited by the sensitivity of the ear, but that involves more than mere sensitivity.

The acoustic characteristics of sound furnish the clues by which the listener distinguishes one auditory experience from another. A pitch difference is heard when the distinction is one of frequency (number of vibrations per second). Similarly, changes in intensity produce variations in loudness. Likewise, the pattern of overtones (sound spectrum) imparts a special flavor, or quality, to each sound. Finally, the way these three basic aspects change from one instant

368

to another influences the impression that the listener receives. We sort sounds and tell them apart because they differ in frequency, in intensity, in overtone structure, and in pattern of change. Successful auditory discrimination occurs only when the hearer can and does take advantage of all four factors in identifying everyday sounds.

The auditory discriminations required in everyday life are of three main types. The simplest is the identification of important and highly distinctive noises. It is relatively easy to separate the siren from the automobile horn, the crash of breaking glass from the clap of thunder, the crying of a child from the barking of a dog. Distinguishing between sounds which are so highly dissimilar is known as *gross discrimination*.

The second type, usually called *simple speech discrimination*, is the recognition, under *favorable* listening conditions, of the sounds, or "phonetic elements," that are combined to make up human speech. Words are blends of vowels and consonants. We can understand spoken language only if we can distinguish enough vowels and enough consonants to recognize words and to interpret sentences. The normal listener has no difficulty in doing so, provided that he is in a relatively quiet place and is not too far from the speaker.

The third type, *difficult speech discrimination*, is the recognition of phonetic elements under *adverse* listening conditions. Two adverse conditions are particularly important. The first is a disturbing background noise. It is often difficult to understand spoken language because the background noise overrides, masks, and garbles some phonetic elements. Even normal listeners often have trouble in machine shops, in traffic, or in crowded restaurants. Another adverse condition occurs when the situation demands that every phonetic element be heard precisely. Unfamiliar words, personal names, and scientific terms require that the listener make exact discriminations because he cannot guess the words from their context. For example, in telephone conversations, by asking him to spell it, we often like to check the accuracy with which we have heard a stranger's name.

DEVELOPMENT OF AUDITORY DISCRIMINATION

We need to understand how the ability to distinguish sounds is developed by the child with normal hearing. It is well known that the newborn infant is frightened by loud noises, but we must remember that at first the baby does not recognize differences between sounds. *He must learn this recognition by stages.*

The baby begins his learning by isolating a few of the sounds most important in his life. For example, the clink of his bottle and the cooing of his mother begin to take on identity. He is building up his first gross discriminations. He is isolating a few noises on the basis of large differences, such as broad pattern of inflection and rhythm. Thus he distinguishes affection from disapproval long before he understands any of the words spoken to him.

After he has learned to follow broad "tunes," the baby masters finer and finer distinctions. Since speech is so frequently important to him, the infant soon reaches the stage of understanding whole phrases and single-word statements like "No." He is then ready to separate words from one another. The little events in his life help him by furnishing a multitude of experiences. These experiences clarify the meanings of common words. Even more important, these experiences are a continual urge toward the development of more complete auditory discrimination. They bring him sound patterns to which he must adjust. He unconsciously finds that his control of his world is increased as he learns to sort sounds more effectively.

Not far beyond infancy, life demands that the child recognize tenses and other subtle differences that depend on only one or two phonetic elements. Simultaneously, his discrimination for a wide variety of sounds other than speech has developed. Many children have learned by the age of three to make auditory discriminations which are sufficiently exact to meet the listening demands that the world imposes on the average adult. Of course, at this age children still have ahead of them the major task of building a vocabulary. Furthermore, special training in music or other fields may develop their skill in discrimination far beyond anything required in everyday life. The point we wish to stress here is that *the listening skill required for social adequacy is learned in early life.*

In fact, subsequent experience tends to fix habits of listening, so that *the capacity for mastering new sound discriminations diminishes* with age. It is common knowledge that a child will learn to speak fluently the language he hears, regardless of his race or nationality. By contrast, when an adult learns a new language, he finds that he has what native speakers call a "foreign accent." The fault is partly that he has fixed his habits of speech and partly that he has fixed his habits of listening. The latter interests us here. What happens is that he does not notice subtle differences in the phonetic elements and cadences of the two languages. He "hears" the elements in the new language as though they were identical with those of his native tongue. When he talks, he puts the old patterns in the new language. Unless he is taught to notice the subtle differences, he may go through life without even realizing that they exist. For example, some European languages, including Russian, do not employ the short "i" as in "pill" nor the long "ee" as in "peel"; but only a vowel sound halfway between the two is used. Those who speak these languages are not in the habit of distinguishing between the long and the short vowel either in listening or in speaking. They accept "peel" and "pill" as identical. We who are trained to notice the differences in length of this vowel are aware that the foreigner says "pill" wrong. The vowel is too long, and we laugh at him for saying that he took the "peel" the doctor gave him. When he speaks of the apple "pill" we also laugh, and perhaps we wonder at how he manages to interchange the two words every time. Actually he has not interchanged the words, but he has used the same intermediate word, which we, with our own habits of listening uncharitably interpret as always the wrong word. Yet, if this foreigner had also learned English as a child, he would have mastered the auditory distinctions of all three vowel sounds.

HEARING LOSS AND AUDITORY DISCRIMINATION

It is obvious that auditory discrimination may be seriously impaired by hearing loss. The effect depends upon the amount of loss and the stage in life at which it originates. A basic distinction must be made between the child who has never heard adequately and the person whose loss arises after auditory discrimination has been learned.

When the hearing impairment is present at birth or occurs very early in life, the youngster will not go through the normal stages in development of discrimination. An extreme case is the child with an early and severe hearing loss who may even acquire the habit of behaving as though he were completely deaf. Sounds loud enough to be audible for him occur so seldom that he never associates them with the important events in life. Instead of learning to assign meaning to the few sounds he hears, he may acquire the habit of disregarding them. Sound then assumes for him no more importance than the sensations you and I get from wearing comfortable clothes. We can turn our attention to these sensations, but we ordinarily are not conscious of them. Similarly, the child who habitually ignores sounds is no longer conscious of even loud sounds which could help him to adjust to people and things. He experiences the practical handicap of the completely deaf person, without having as severe a physical limitation. His extreme handicap can be overcome by teaching the child awareness of sound and developing the discriminations of which he is capable. As will be pointed out, a hearing aid can be a great help here.

A second type of child has good hearing for low-pitched tones but is deaf to notes of high frequency. Such a child is usually aware of noises because he can hear their low-frequency components. He is thus able to begin the process of learning auditory discrimination, but his hearing loss prevents his completing the process normally. He faces continual confusion because he misses the high-frequency elements which distinguish so many sounds, particularly some of the elements of speech. He is like a person who can see print on a page, but whose vision is too blurred to make out the letters. Unfortunately, such a child frequently finds his world not only confusing but also hostile. He may be unfairly labeled as a retarded, a queer, or an asocial child simply because his response to low-pitched sounds keeps people from realizing that he has a hearing loss. What he needs is auditory training and other special help that will reduce the confusion imposed by his impairment.

The third type of problem occurs in the youngster with partial, but relatively uniform, auditory deficiency. Such a child receives sound patterns in a fairly normal manner, provided that they are loud enough. His trouble is that his hearing is stimulated less often and less strongly than normally. Consequently, his auditory discriminations develop more slowly, and he learns to rely more heavily than usual upon senses other than hearing. This child must be vigorously encouraged to use the auditory channel as much as other people do, and a good hearing aid is often a great encouragement.

When a hearing loss occurs in late childhood or in adulthood, it often disturbs auditory discriminations which previously were entirely adequate. The effect of the hearing loss depends upon its type and amount, but in general, the listener can no longer perceive some of the sound clues that he previously used for discrimination. He must now base his judgments on a set of imperfect clues and distorted auditory patterns. Fortunately, a particular degree and contour of loss will be less disastrous at this age than it is to the child who must learn discrimination for the first time. Nevertheless, a substantial impairment in hearing may be very disturbing, especially if the person continues in his old "habits of listening" instead of learning to take fullest advantage of the clues that are still available. Even when a hearing aid restores sensitivity to the ear, some imperfections in discrimination usually remain. As has been pointed out in Chapter 11 on hearing aids, a severe loss of hearing, particularly if there is some sensory-neural impairment, cannot be *fully* compensated by even the best of modern hearing aids. Thus, whether he wears a hearing aid or not, the newly deafened person ordinarily needs a course of training to help him overcome his deficiencies. This need is particularly great if the loss has existed for a long time because *the confusions caused by imperfect hearing often lead to a progressive deterioration of the ability to discriminate.*

Auditory Training for Young Children

Auditory training is the process of teaching the child or adult who is hard of hearing to take full advantage of the sound clues which are still available to him.

THE NEED FOR AUDITORY TRAINING

Auditory training is vitally important for the child whose hearing loss existed at birth or occurred in infancy. Unless he has moderately good hearing in at least one ear, his prospects of utilizing sound without special instruction are poor. Fortunately, even most so-called "deaf" children have some residual hearing. When the remnant of hearing is small, auditory training can be used at least as an aid in developing command of language, in instructing the child to speak, and in encouraging better adjustment to the world of hearing people. The greater the residue, the more fully the child may be taught to make audition a useful tool in everyday life. Thus, to the degree that his residual hearing allows, auditory training helps the child build a firm foundation for his future adjustments in normal social situations.

SENSORY HABITS

We must realize that *sensory habits are as much a part of life as are muscular habits.* To be sure, we are more aware of muscular habits because we see their effects so repeatedly. But just as surely as the child learns good or bad table manners, he develops patterns of seeing and of hearing. As an illustration, we do not expect the city-bred boy to "see" the little clues that an Indian tracker uses, even though the boy's vision is as good as that of the Indian. In like manner, every child builds habits of audition. If his hearing is defective, he either learns faulty interpretations of sounds or learns to substitute other senses for the ear. In other words, since the child is faced with the problem of adjusting to his world, he seizes upon the sensory channels that serve him most effectively. Vision and touch tend to become his primary means of receiving communication. When hearing is faulty, sound assumes minor importance, and, as a consequence, development of speech is likely to be retarded and imperfect. Gestures tend to take the place of talking as the method for communication with other people. In this way and in many other ways the child's whole pattern of living is modified by his hearing loss.

To be sure, the process just described continues beyond early childhood. But the early years establish sensory habits and set the patterns for adjustment. Once the child develops faulty patterns, a double task faces anyone who would teach him to use his residual hearing effectively; for not only must the child be guided through the stages necessary to acquire auditory discrimination, but the guidance he is given must also break down the unfortunate sensory habits he has already acquired.

What has just been said points up a fact of supreme importance: *if there is any suspicion that a baby is hard of hearing, his early years must be filled with loud and varied sounds.* He must be given a special chance to learn to hear, and it is better to err on the side of overdoing than of neglect. More will be said on this point later. Here we need merely state that all the members of the infant's family must share in the responsibility for ensuring that he gets a "sound" start in life.

STEPS IN AUDITORY TRAINING

The four major stages in complete programs in auditory training for children are (1) the development of awareness of sound; (2) the development of gross discriminations; (3) the development of broad discriminations among simple speech patterns; and (4) the development of finer discriminations for speech. Each stage has its special purposes and methods.

Development of awareness of sound. The first requirement in auditory training is that the child learn to know when a sound is present. He must be taught to direct his attention to sound. He must be taught to realize that noises are meaningful. Obviously, this result can be gained only by presenting sounds to him. Care must be taken to guarantee that the sounds are loud enough to override his hearing loss. Care must also be taken to use sounds which he can relate to his own experience. An approach through play is particularly useful because it builds an enjoyment of sound. For example, one good method is to use marching games in which children beat on drums and triangles. However, not all sounds need be pleasurable. Loud sounds used in conjunction with disapproval and punishment are very helpful in penetrating his resistance to listening. In other words, the child should be surrounded with loud noises which are related to his everyday activities. Furthermore, when he shows by his reactions that he is aware of any sound, circumstances must be so arranged that this particular sound is repeated frequently. It can thus be made to serve as a wedge to introduce awareness of other sounds.

Development of gross discriminations. The next step is to teach the child that sounds differ from one another. He is trained to distinguish between highly dissimilar noises. To accomplish this the teacher employs a carefully selected set of noisemakers. Each noise-

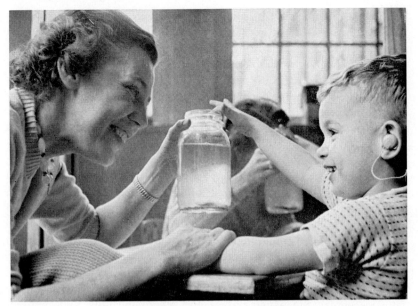

Fig. 13-1. Auditory and visual experiences are associated. (*Johns Hopkins University.*)

maker must produce a unique and reasonably loud sound. Examples of good noisemakers are bells, drums, cymbals, low-frequency whistles, and automobile horns. Each noisemaker should be an object that the child watches. The child then gets a chance to make the sounds himself. As soon as the child is fully familiar with the noisemakers, little games are played with them. The games may have many forms, but they are basically similar. A noisemaker is sounded while it is out of the child's sight. He then picks out the object that he thinks was used. If his choice is correct, the child is rewarded according to the rules of the game. If the choice is wrong, the noise is repeated while the child watches. He thus gets a chance to correct his misinterpretation.

Once the child has learned to identify highly dissimilar sounds by ear, the same procedures may be used to build finer discriminations. For example, several bells may be selected so that each has a distinctive pitch and quality. The child must then pick out the specific bell rung from among the whole group. A wide variety of games, exercises, and kinds of sound must be used to ensure repeated and diverse experience.

One point needs to be particularly stressed: the teacher must remember that even gross discriminations depend upon differences in frequency, in intensity, in sound composition, and in the sequences and patterns of these three acoustic elements. The training program and, for that matter, the testing program described in detail in Chapters 8 and 17, dealing with hard-of-hearing children, must be planned so as to stress each of these factors, both independently and in various combinations. One thus encourages a strong foundation on which later to build more exacting discriminations.

Development of broad discriminations among simple speech patterns. Once the child has learned that sounds differ from one another, he is ready to start learning to understand speech. Again, training must start by teaching him to make distinctions that are easy. We usually start by stressing differences in vowels. For example, the "ah" in "father" and the "ee" in "see" stand sharply apart from one another. These and other vowels may be contrasted, either alone or in simple words. Before long the simplest of the differences in consonants are also introduced.

Another approach is to start the training in speech discriminations with a few meaningful phrases. Here the goal is to have the child recognize the whole phrase and assign meaning to it without analyzing its parts. Each phrase must be closely related to his everyday experience. Typical phrases are: "Do you want a drink?" "Where is your doll?" "Show me the dog." When the child has learned to recognize and respond meaningfully to the initial group of phrases, new ones are added. The advantage of this method is that it reproduces the normal manner of learning. As the phrases become more familiar, the words begin to emerge and take on meaning. Understanding of speech grows naturally and with continual emphasis on the fact that speech is something that people use in getting along with one another.

Development of finer discriminations for speech. Auditory training is not complete until the child has learned to make distinctions as exact as his hearing loss allows. Thus, the final stage of auditory training aims toward building increasingly precise discriminations, particularly for speech. The methods used depend partly on the child's general maturity and partly on his past accomplishments in learning to hear effectively. Basically, however, three kinds of skill must be encouraged. First, the child needs repeated drills that encourage him to recognize the more subtle phonetic differences. Distinctions like those between "s" (sun) and "sh" (shun) and between "th" (thin) and "f" (fin) may be particularly hard to hear. Secondly, the child must be taught to know and understand a large vocabulary of spoken words. There must be variety in the words and phrases used for practice as well as opportunity to fix the meaning of words through diverse experiences. Finally, the child needs training in following connected speech; that is, he must learn to integrate his growing vocabulary so that he understands phrases and sentences quickly and accurately. Here the teacher finds stories, conversation periods, phonograph records, and other types of connected speech very helpful. Even if the child never reaches the stage where he can make difficult speech discriminations, he should deliberately and continually be encouraged to listen to speech. Normal patterns of speech will furnish a guide for the rhythm and intonation of the child's own speech, which in the case of very deaf children needs every possible help to make it intelligible.

THE HEARING AID IN AUDITORY TRAINING

The hard-of-hearing child needs to have sounds amplified. His ability to discriminate sounds is poor because sounds seldom are loud enough for him to hear them adequately. Hence, ordinary sounds must be made more intense for him. One method is to bring the sources of sound close to the child's ear. This method is especially valuable for very young children. A second method, which should be employed as early as feasible, is to use a modern hearing aid.

The child's first experiences with a hearing aid must be guided with care. For some children it is ordinarily best to start by using the instrument only during regular periods of auditory training. The hearing aid may be constructed to serve a single listener, but it is sometimes known as a "group hearing aid," since it may have enough earphones to be used by a whole class. A continuously variable tone control and an independent volume control for each earphone are usually included. Some instruments have several microphones, which allow sound to be picked up at the more important spots in the classroom. This type is convenient for the beginner to use in the classroom. The development of the inductance loop type of hearing aid has made it possible for the child to have more freedom of movement since he does not have to be wired to the teacher's microphone. In addition, a good classroom instrument reproduces sound more accurately than do most wearable hearing aids.

The primary reason for being so careful in introducing the child to amplified sound is that otherwise he may find the experience startling and frightening. He is likely to be disturbed by the sudden variety of auditory sensations that the instrument brings him. Furthermore, the hearing aid may be powerful enough to transmit sharp noises at levels that are uncomfortable to the child. Therefore, he should at first wear the earphones only for short periods, during which the sound is carefully supervised.

Once the child is adjusted to the hearing aid, a large part of his auditory training should be presented through the amplifying system.

Hearing aids are capable of amplifying to usable intensities sounds that originate some distance from the listener. They thereby widen the circle of auditory contacts that the hard-of-hearing child (or adult) has with his world. Hearing aids lessen the disability that the impairment imposes in everyday life. In consequence, *every acoustically handicapped child who can benefit from a hearing aid should be fitted with his own instrument as soon as he is ready for it.* We have already discussed, in Chapter 11, the practical questions of selecting the proper instrument and of using it effectively. Therefore, we need only mention here the primary considerations that determine the time when the child is ready for his own hearing aid.

Most important, the child's auditory training must have progressed to the point where the child notices sounds and is able to distinguish a reasonable number of them. In other words, his skill in discrimination must be sufficient for him to get some practical benefit from the instrument; otherwise, the child will gain so little from his hearing aid that he will come to dislike and resist it. If he does benefit from it, however, his everyday experiences with the instrument will supplement most helpfully his lessons in auditory training.

The child's general maturity and sense of responsibility help determine whether or not he is ready for an individual hearing aid. The instruments are expensive and delicate. It is practical to get a child his own instrument only after he has reached the stage when he may be expected to treat it with reasonable care. Among other things, he must be trustworthy about avoiding rough play while wearing his hearing aid.

The third consideration is that *the child must have a strong desire for his own instrument.* Effective use can come only if he wants to wear it. Naturally, wise teachers and parents will encourage the development of this desire.

Finally, we must remember that convenience in wearing an instrument is even more important to a youngster than it is to an adult. The size of the instrument is proportionately greater for the child. Therefore, the smaller and lighter the instrument the better, provided that quality of performance is not sacrificed. The child should be fitted with a specially designed jacket which carries his instrument snugly. The child can slip the jacket on in school and elsewhere when he wishes to use his hearing aid. He can slip the jacket off and quickly put it in a safe place when his play might endanger the instrument. Nevertheless, the child should wear the instrument as much as he possibly can and he should learn to protect it as he would eyeglasses.

AUDITORY TRAINING IN THE SCHOOL

Training children with acoustic handicaps to utilize their residual hearing effectively is a long and highly specialized task. The task can best be accomplished by teachers who have prepared themselves specifically for it. Such teachers are to be found in residential schools for the deaf and in public school systems that have programs for hard-of-hearing children. Parents of acoustically handicapped children should look to special schools and special teachers for formal education in auditory training. If necessary, parents must search out this training for their children.

AUDITORY TRAINING IN THE HOME

Special teachers are needed, but parents and other members of the home circle still have a vital responsibility in auditory training. This responsibility goes beyond cooperating fully with the school program. It springs from two facts that we dare not ignore.

In the first place, auditory training serves its purpose fully only if its lessons are carried into everyday life. The home is the site of so much of the child's experience that parents must be continually alert to make it a rich source of meaningful sounds. Under the guidance of the special teacher, intelligent parents can fix for the child the habit of relying upon sound as a major channel for adjustment to his world. The lessons of the school can thus be made the tools for living.

In the second place, it may not be practical for children to start formal auditory training until they are three or four years old. Like their companions with normal hearing, they spend their first years in the home. We have already pointed out that these years are the ones in which the child sets his basic habits of either utilizing hearing or ignoring sounds. The infant with an acoustic handicap will start on the wrong road unless his parents work continuously to bring him rich and varied sound experiences. As soon as they suspect a hearing loss, parents should seek expert advice. Detailed procedures for home training can thus be planned. Five general rules should be the foundation on which the procedures for home training are based:

1. Make a point of repeating and using in various ways any noises or vocal sounds to which the child responds. Make them an enjoyable part of his daily experiences.
2. Always talk aloud to the child when communicating with him.

Avoid the danger of relying on gestures without using speech. However, feel free to use gestures in combination with speech to make ideas clear.

3. Always speak distinctly and as close to the child as convenient. Speak loudly and naturally, but do not shout.

4. Make a special point of seeing that the child has a "speech period" each day. Take the child in your lap and talk six to eight inches from his ear. Tell him little stories, chat about picture books, and so on. In other words, have a little conversation period gauged to his abilities and interests.

5. Give the child full benefit of doubt. Continue the program even if he does not seem to respond. Remember that very few children are completely deaf, but that some children are slow in developing their first reactions to sound. Great is the tragedy of the youngster whose parents lacked the patience to make sound meaningful.

Auditory Training for Adults

Adults who have developed normal ability in auditory discrimination frequently find this ability impaired if they suffer hearing loss. But unless the loss is complete, the adult ordinarily retains much of his original skill. The task of auditory training of adults is primarily one of re-educating an impaired ability. The person must become fully aware of his limitations in discrimination and must get accustomed once more to hearing loud sounds, distinguishing speech from noise, localizing sounds, and so forth.

ASSESSMENT OF THE HANDICAP

The first step in the process of re-education is to discover the degree and type of the handicap. A series of tests is used to gather this information. It is ordinarily most convenient to start by determining how well the person can distinguish the various "phonetic elements" of spech. A good test for this purpose is one that presents isolated words that the listener must identify accurately. By noting the number and kinds of mistakes, we can define his deficiencies in speech discrimination. Only occasionally do we find someone whose recognition of speech is so poor that simpler tests must be used. When such a case is encountered, however, his ability to make gross discriminations must be determined by tests using highly distinctive noises and also broad differences in rhythm, in melody pattern, in pitch, and in loudness.

INDIVIDUALIZING THE PROGRAM

In any well-planned program, such as are now available in speech and hearing centers, auditory training is designed to meet the needs of each individual.

Each person listens to those sound patterns which are difficult for him to distinguish. He is then allowed to check the accuracy of his impressions. *The goal is to train him to take full advantage of the auditory clues that are still available to him.* The degree to which substitute clues may be used to restore successful discrimination is astonishing.

If the student requires a hearing aid, his program is built around his instrument. As a preliminary step, it is helpful to teach the student to listen to amplified sound. This experience helps to develop his tolerance for loud sound and gives him useful information and background to *help* him select the proper individual aid.

When his individual instrument has been chosen, the student should wear it during most of his practice. Auditory training must teach the person to interpret sound patterns as they are transmitted to him by his particular instrument. We foster the maximum utilization of residual hearing when we train the individual to use his hearing aid as efficiently as possible.

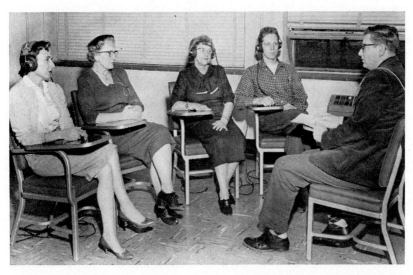

Fig. 13-2. Adults combine auditory training and speechreading. (*Central Institute for the Deaf.*)

Auditory training also includes practical instruction in the use and care of the hearing aid, as explained in Chapter 11. This training is not strictly "auditory," but it is important to the student.

STEPS IN AUDITORY TRAINING

The typical program designed to improve auditory discrimination in adults consists of several progressive stages.

As already pointed out, adults are victims of sensory habits. Patterns of auditory attention are fixed by experience. Because of these habits, we become less alert to subtle differences among sounds. If auditory training is to be effective for adults, this habitual inattention must be counteracted. *An attitude of critical listening* must be established at the outset.

There are various ways of encouraging the attitude of critical listening. One is to discuss with the student both his problem and the task ahead. Another method is to require him to report on a variety of listening assignments. Since discrimination can occur only as a person learns to identify differences in sound, a vital step is to re-establish an awareness of the differences once heard but now obscured by the hearing loss. Carefully planned drills in "listening" are required.

The first drills should contrast sound patterns which the student finds it moderately troublesome to distinguish from one another. For example, pairs of matched syllables like *mee–lee, moo–loo,* and *eel–eem,* are spoken aloud. The listener repeats what he hears. Whenever he makes an error, the pair is repeated for him several times. A similar type of exercise contrasts word pairs like *make–lake,* or *sail–same.* Obviously, the lessons must progress from simple distinctions to the more difficult ones.

Exercises which present single syllables and words should be used as soon as the student can differentiate contrasting pairs. One good method is to provide short, mimeographed lists of drill words. These words may be read aloud many times, each time in different order. Each listener has the list before him. He merely numbers the words in the order in which he thinks they are spoken. His paper is then corrected and the list is repeated so that he may re-examine the items he confused.

Skill in discrimination cannot be considered properly restored until sounds are recognized accurately and quickly on the first presentation. This level of mastery is required if hearing is to be adequate for everyday life, where most remarks are made only once. Consequently, the training program must develop *precise and rapid recognition* of phonetic elements. At this stage each drill item is presented a single time. Training materials may consist of word lists, sentences that are unrelated, anecdotes, brief descriptions, and other samples of connected speech. While the student must have frequent chances to check on the accuracy of his understanding, the emphasis is upon varied auditory experience.

Of course, as we have pointed out, some people have the misfortune to lose *completely* their ability to hear high frequencies and therefore can never relearn the *auditory* distinctions between certain pairs of sounds. Here, however, speechreading is of great assistance, and any intelligent course in auditory training should be accompanied by instruction and practice in the art of speechreading.

Sounds other than speech are important in practical situations. Therefore, the auditory training program must re-establish *recognition of significant noises.* Ordinarily, re-education of gross discrimination is not necessary. Consequently, simple noisemakers are not required. Instead we can use the subtle and complete patterns of environmental sound. Phonograph records, such as the sound-effect, records prepared for radio studios, are probably the best source for this type of material. With these records and a good phonograph, environmental sounds can be selected and reproduced at will. A personalized program of training can thus be maintained.

Life frequently demands that we make auditory discriminations under adverse circumstances. Therefore, the re-education of discriminatory skill requires practice in *listening under poor acoustical conditions.* The general aim is to transfer the newly acquired skills to difficult listening situations. Three types of situations most often require training in making the transfer.

The first situation is one in which background noise masks out, or obliterates, some of the auditory clues employed in discrimination. Some hard-of-hearing people find discrimination much more difficult in a noisy place than in a quiet one, and all benefit by special training while listening in noise. The advent of binaural hearing aids may make localization and discrimination in noise easier for some listeners. The single hearing aid worn at the ear permits the listener to take advantage of head movements in seeking out the source of a sound.

Drills like those described above are used, but the drills are given in the presence of background noise. The noise is produced by a phonograph or some other suitable source that is under the control of the instructor. Secondly, discrimination is sometimes poor when speech and other sounds come from a radio, a television set, a phonograph, or a public-address system. These sound reproducers lack perfect fidelity. The normal ear can tolerate their inaccuracy, but the impaired ear is often very sensitive to their imperfections. It follows that many hard-of-hearing people can benefit from auditory training in which words and sentences are presented through reproducing systems.

Lastly, many of the hard of hearing find that listening over a telephone presents a special difficulty. Those who use their unaided ear in telephoning may be able to hear the sounds but complain that the words seem "fuzzy." This group requires practice in listening over the telephone. The skill acquired by listening with one ear through a hearing aid does not automatically extend to telephone use with the other ear. Each ear may require practice separately.

By contrast, a person who must use his hearing aid for telephone conversations requires auditory training in which the telephone receiver is held against the hearing aid. Among other things, he must learn how to fit the two instruments together for most effective sound reception. This is true whether the conversation is transferred to the hearing aid acoustically by holding the receiver opening against the microphone of the hearing aid or, as in some modern hearing aids, by holding the receiver in the proper position in relation to a magnetic "telephone pickup" within the hearing aid.

LESSONS AND HOME PRACTICE

Programs in auditory re-education are best carried on under the guidance of a specialist in auditory training. The specialist has the responsibility for recognizing individual needs and arranging lessons to meet these needs. He may recommend private instruction, or he may advise group work. In either event, the lessons furnish the core of the program.

However, formal lessons in auditory training must be supplemented by home practice if ability in discrimination is to be most effectively restored. The lessons serve to give the student a clear understanding of the problems he faces. Furthermore, they furnish listening experiences designed to meet these special needs. However, they consume only a fraction of the time spent daily in listening. The wise student, therefore, seeks additional opportunities to improve his discriminatory skill. These additional opportunities are of two types. First, definite periods are set aside for home practice. The student enlists a relative or friend, who must have normal auditory ability and normal speech, to present the practice materials and check the accuracy of the discriminations made by the student. Second, the alert student will listen throughout each day for the sound distinctions he is learning in his lessons. He thus carries over his improving skill into life situations.

TRAINING IN THE USE OF A HEARING AID

Hearing aids should be incorporated at the earliest feasible moment in programs for auditory training. *The person who needs to wear an instrument must learn efficient discrimination of the sounds it brings him.* The methods outlined above are useful in accomplishing this end. Aside from the question of distinguishing differences between sounds, however, a person may face special problems in using a hearing aid. One such problem is difficulty in tolerating intense sounds.

The problem of *intolerance for strong sounds* has been discussed in Chapters 2, 7, and 11. Two of the facts mentioned there are important here. First, problems of tolerance can often be reduced or avoided by selecting a hearing aid of the proper power. Secondly, the level at which sound becomes intolerable is increased somewhat by experience and training. A person's ear may be unusually "tender" at first and therefore likely to become considerably "tougher" with a little practice. Sometimes it is necessary to select an instrument which at first is not fully tolerable in the presence of strong sounds. The program in auditory training is then adapted to help the student increase his tolerance limit. The basic procedure is to start by presenting practice materials to the hearing aid at intensities that are not disturbing. The intensity is then increased by small steps. Simultaneously, the use of a hearing aid in everyday life is limited at first to short periods and to specific situations. Finally, the instrument may be operated with a very low gain setting, or with a felt pad over the microphone, or with a plug of lamb's wool in the hole through the earmold. (The felt pad or the plug of wool also modifies the tone of the instrument by absorbing high frequencies, and neither should be used unless the lowest gain setting on the instrument gives more intensity than the wearer is at first willing to accept.) If practice is continued for a few weeks, the tolerance limit can often be raised considerably and to good advantage.

Some modern hearing aids include provision for adjusting the maximum power output to the user's needs. As a tender ear toughens with training and practice, the power output of such an aid can be adjusted accordingly. The ultimate adjustment will then be the one which provides the maximum amplification without discomfort.

Suggested Readings

EWING, I. R., and A. W. G. EWING. *The Handicap of Deafness.* New York: Longmans, Green & Company, 1938.

GOLDSTEIN, M. A. *The Acoustic Method*. St. Louis: The Laryngoscope Press, 1939.

HUDGINS, C. V. "Auditory Training: Its Possibilities and Limitations," *Volta Review*, 56: 339–349 (1954).

SILVERMAN, S. R. "Clinical and Educational Procedures for the Deaf," and "Clinical and Educational Procedure for the Hard of Hearing," in *Handbook of Speech Pathology*, L. E. Travis, ed. New York: Appleton-Century-Crofts, Inc., 1957, Chaps. 10 and 11.

——. "Training for Optimum Use of Hearing Aids," *The Laryngoscope*, 54: 29–36 (1944).

WEDENBERG, E. "Auditory Training of Deaf and Hard of Hearing Children," *Acta Oto-Laryngologica*, 1951, Supp. 94, pp. 1–129.

14

CONSERVATION
OF SPEECH

Raymond Carhart, Ph.D.

Speech is normally controlled by the ear.

Nowhere is this more clearly shown than in the way a baby learns to talk. At first the baby can only cry. Some weeks after his birth he begins cooing, gurgling, and laughing. He then seems to enjoy lying in his crib and entertaining himself by listening to his queer noises. Without realizing it, he is building connections between his ear and his voice. As he listens to his own randomly produced sounds, he is beginning to learn muscular control of his speech mechanism. Before long he passes into the "parrot" stage, in which he amuses himself by repeating noises over and over. He keeps himself happy by saying trains of syllables like "ba ba ba ba" or "da da da da." He is now on the brink of learning his first words, for his parents respond to some of the syllable trains in his babbling. For example, when he says "da da da da," his mother may get his doll. She may also say "doll" as she hands it to him. This is an important moment. His babbling has controlled another person. He has also heard that person say a syllable which is very close to the sounds he is making. On another occasion, his mother may say, "Do you want your doll?" as she hands him the toy. The child is likely to parrot her and say "da da da. . . ." His mother's pleased smile again rewards him. A few more experiences like this, and he will have learned to babble "da" whenever he wants his doll. He is now well on the road toward learning speech. All he needs is time: time for added experiences, time to learn new words through hearing them, and time to master vocal control by hearing his own speech.

The control which the ear exerts over speech is revealed differently by the adult. As was pointed out in Chapter 13, habits of hearing become so fixed that an older person has trouble mastering the pronunciations of a new language. His ear fails to distinguish new patterns from the ones to which he is accustomed. Erroneous impressions thus serve as the person's guide in speaking the new language. He talks with a foreign accent. For example, many Latin Americans have no need in their native Spanish to distinguish *b* and *v* except at the beginning of words. They consequently do not always use *b* and *v* correctly when they speak English.

Effect of Hearing Loss on Speech

Because it is natural for the ear to be the channel through which we learn to talk, a serious impairment in hearing will hinder a child's normal development of speech. Furthermore, because the ear serves as a guide to accurate control of the speech mechanism, degeneration of speech often follows hearing losses that occur later in life.

The most obvious example of the role played by hearing in acquisition of spoken language is furnished by the child who is born totally deaf. Unless special training is undertaken, such a child never learns to talk. He grows up mute. His deafness closes for him the door through which he would normally acquire both knowledge of speech and control of the speech organs.

The child who hears low frequencies well but is insensitive to middle- and high-pitched tones faces a different problem. It is likely to be years before this child's deficiency is discovered. Because he can hear low frequencies, he reacts to many of the sounds in his world. People, seeing his response, reason that his hearing is normal. They fail to realize how distorted and imperfect are his impressions of sound. Confusion is this child's lot. He misses the acoustic elements which give speech its distinctive character. One outcome of this confusion is slow and uncertain development of his use of language. Moreover, the child incorporates in his own speech only the imperfect distinctions which he perceives in the speech of others. The result is a mushy and slurred pattern of talking which may border on the unintelligible.

Any substantial loss of hearing which exists at birth or occurs soon thereafter will hinder both language development and the establishment of adequate speech habits. Two factors are responsible. First, the hearing loss reduces sharply the number of listening experiences that the child has and thus slows up the process of learning to talk. Secondly, losses of certain types make it impossible for the child to distinguish some of the elements in speech. No child will learn to pronounce distinctions he does not hear, unless, of course, he has special guidance.

Speech defects may arise as the result of hearing losses that begin after childhood. If the ear can no longer serve as a monitor when one talks, slow degeneration of speech results. The sharpness and precison of enunciation disintegrate. The melodies of speech become monotonous. Intonations lose their life. The quality of the voice becomes rigid. Finally, control over the loudness of the voice suffers.

THE NATURE OF SPEECH

We can understand better the problems in speech which grow out of auditory impairment if we survey briefly the three essential aspects of speech.

Phonetic elements. Syllables, words, and connected phrases are formed by various combinations of simple sounds, which are known as *phonetic elements*. The phonetic elements are the shortest units in human speech that can be recognized as having stable identity. In a general way, if we make allowances for the peculiarities of English spelling, the phonetic elements correspond to the letters of written language. However, the comparison is at best a rough one, since there are only twenty-six letters in the alphabet but about forty phonetic elements are used.

Phonetic elements are divided into three major classes: vowels, diphthongs, and consonants.

Vowels are relatively sustained and strong sounds. They are produced by initiating a tone in the voice box (larynx) and passing this tone through the mouth cavity, which is formed into a relatively open channel. Differences between vowels are achieved by shaping the mouth channel distinctively for each vowel. The tongue and the lips play a particularly important part in this shaping. Each vowel is actually a distinctive pattern of pure tones produced by the resonances of the various chambers of the mouth and nose. It is by means of this distinctive pattern that the listener identifies the vowel. Typical vowels (and their phonetic symbols) are those found in the following words: *seat* (i), *sit* (ɪ), *set* (ɛ), *sat* (æ), *saw* (ɔ), *soot* (ʊ), and *suit* (u).

Diphthongs are blends of two vowels. They are produced by shifting the mouth channel from one vowel position to another while the sound continues. Acoustically, the tone initiated by the voice box is "resonated" as for a vowel, but in this instance the distinctive feature is the glide from the initial pattern of resonance to the final one. Typical diphthongs are those appearing in the following words: *boy* (ɔɪ), *bay* (eɪ), *bough* (aʊ), and *buy* (aɪ).

Consonants are of various types. All, however, have as a common feature the fact that the mouth channel is either closed completely or is formed into a more restricted passage than is employed to produce vowels and diphthongs. Furthermore, each consonant is characterized by a particular shaping and use of the speech organs. The tongue, lips, and soft palate are the primary structures whose positions determine this shaping. Consonants fall into several major classes on the basis of their manner of production and their acoustic character. We shall review each class separately.

Semivowels and *glides* are quite similar to vowels and diphthongs. The primary distinction is that to produce semivowels and glides the mouth channel is more constricted. Consequently, the resonances of these sounds are distinctive but less intense. Words exemplifying these consonants are *rue* (r), *lieu* (l), *you* (j), and *woo* (w).

The *nasal consonants* are produced by completely blocking the mouth channel and allowing the tone from the voice box to escape through the nose. The sound patterns of the nasal consonants contain rather diffuse but definite resonances. These consonants are illustrated in the words *hum* (m), *hun* (n), and *hung*.

Most of the remaining consonants occur in pairs. One member of each pair is *voiced*, that is, it includes both the tone from the voice box and a second sound produced in the mouth. The other member of the pair is *voiceless*, that is, it consists only of the sound produced in the mouth. Typical pairs are *buy* (b) and *pie* (p), *vase* (v) and *face* (f), *zoo* (z), and *sue* (s).

Two major methods exist for initiating sounds in the mouth. One is to block completely the breath stream and then release it in a sudden gust which causes a pulse of noise. Consonants produced in this way are called *plosives*. The voiced plosives occur in *by* (b), *die* (d), and *guy* (g). Their voiceless counterparts occur in *pea* (p), *tea* (t), and *key* (k). By contrast, the fricative continuants are formed when the escaping breath stream produces a noise as it flows through an extremely constricted portion of the mouth channel. Acoustically, these consonants exhibit highly irregular sound patterns distributed over a wide pitch range. The voiced *fricatives* are exemplified in *vow* (v), *zoo* (z), *azure* (ʒ), and *thou* (ð). The voiceless fricatives are illustrated in *fin* (f), *sin* (s), *thin* (θ), and *him* (h).

Finally, a few blends of consonants have been incorporated as phonetic elements in English. These blends combine elements of their parent sounds, yet they have independent identity. Typical illustrations are found in *what* (hw), *check* (tʃ), are *just* (dʒ).

Articulatory defects. Speech deficiencies characterized by imperfect production of phonetic elements and transitions between them are called *articulatory defects.* Obviously, they may arise from many causes: physical deformity of the speech organs, disease, faulty habits, lazy enunciation, hearing loss, mental deficiency, and so on. Obviously, too, articulatory defects differ widely in severity and in type of error. Our present concern is limited to inadequacies arising because a hearing loss either prohibited the initial mastery of phonetic elements or removed the auditory control needed to maintain precise enunciation. In either event, since a prominent feature of the speech defect will be imperfect production of phonetic elements, an effective program of speech training must have as a major goal the elimination of articulatory errors.

Nonphonetic elements. Human speech possesses four aspects which are relatively unstandardized but which nevertheless contribute to the naturalness and acceptability of oral communication. These four aspects are *melody, quality, time,* and *force.* Each is a feature which, when properly used, helps to clarify meaning and add vitality.

The *melody* of speech is its "tune," or intonation pattern. Spoken language cannot escape having a melody. However, certain intonation patterns are conventionalized, and we expect them. An illustration is the rising inflection with which we designate a question. An unusual melody distracts the listener from the thought that is being expressed and thus may be considered a defect. For example, lack of variety, such as a monotonously pitched voice, imparts a lifelessness which reduces the effectiveness of speech.

Quality is the "flavor" of speech which distinguishes one voice from another. Quality is a very subtle feature which depends both upon physical conditions and upon habits of using the voice. Our interest in quality springs from the fact that an auditory impairment may lead to unfortunate habits, as, for example, in the strained and strident voice so often found in deaf children.

The *time* element of speech is its "rhythm." We have learned to expect and to accept certain rhythms as "natural." Deviations from acceptable rhythms create the impression of artificiality and, if extreme, may hinder understanding, as we saw in Dr. Pauls' discussion in Chapter 12 on stress and accent.

The element of *force* involves the emphasis given different syllables and words. Variations in force are achieved primarily by modifying loudness. Some patterns of emphasis are acceptable, whereas others are not.

In connected speech, the nonphonetic elements are completely blended and interwoven. We have already pointed out that proper blending helps clarify meaning and adds interest to spoken language. It follows that *a severe auditory impairment that makes it impossible for a person to hear the nonphonetic elements in his own speech may cause unnatural use of these elements and, hence, disturb the effectiveness of his oral communication.* The child with severe impairment will fail to learn proper control of melody, quality, time, and force. In the adult these same elements tend to degenerate slowly after he loses the power to hear them.

LOUDNESS OF THE VOICE

The speaker ordinarily adjusts the loudness of his voice to the situation in which he is talking. In fact, the adjustment is so natural that few people even realize it takes place. The speaker has unconsciously learned to raise his voice when background noise is strong or when the listener is at a little distance. We find that our voices are tired after conversing while riding on the bus. Our efforts to talk over the din of traffic lead us unconsciously to shout, and a half-hour of shouting tires the voice. By contrast, we unconsciously soften our voices in quiet surroundings. In other words, *we tend to maintain a favorable margin between the loudness of our speech and the background noise.* We thus achieve intelligibility without talking so that our listeners find our speech unpleasantly loud.

A person learns the proper balance between the loudness of his speech and his acoustic surroundings in the same way that he learns other features of acceptable speech, by the experience of hearing himself talk. Through his experience the ineffective levels of loudness are given up in favor of levels that result in successful communication.

A hearing loss disturbs the ability to adjust the level of one's voice to the needs of the moment. Two factors enter the picture. For one thing, the person with impaired hearing will miss much of the background noise. Thus, he has an imperfect gauge of the requirements of the moment. In the second place, the speaker with a hearing loss may receive a false impression of the loudness of his own voice. When the loss is of the sensory-neural type, his own voice sounds faint. Such a person has a tendency to talk loudly, regardless of the surrounding circumstances. In doing so his voice reaches a level where it seems of normal loudness to him. The reverse effect occurs when the loss is of the conductive type. Here the speaker's voice is transmitted effectively to his own ear by bone conduction. His voice seems to him so much stronger than other sounds that he often softens it until the balance between his voice and the background noise is more to his satisfaction. Such a person tends to talk more faintly than he should, and, as a consequence, he is hard to understand.

Speech Training for Deaf Children

As we have already pointed out, the child who suffers an early and complete hearing loss will remain a mute unless special methods of education are used with him. The difficulty and laboriousness of the educational task are tremendous. It is necessary to teach the child to put his speech mechanism to use. One must also build his vocabulary and the other basic skills of language. Ordinarily, when the training program begins, the child will have no adequate concept of either speech or language.

We discussed earlier the manner in which the child with normal hearing learns speech and language. The deaf child must be guided through a similar series of stages. However, two differences exist. First, successive stages cannot be attained as early in his life. Secondly, since the auditory channel for learning is closed to the deaf child, substitute means must be used to stimulate the development of his language skills. The substitute means are less effective than hearing in accomplishing the goal, and the process is therefore extremely laborious.

There are three major channels which may be substituted for the ear: vision, the sense of touch, and the internal senses of movement and position. The reader will realize immediately that any superior program of training will interweave stimulation through these three channels and, of course, the auditory channel. For convenience, however, the discussion that follows considers each separately.

VISUAL CLUES

Visual clues offer the deaf child his main approach to the experience of communication. He not only learns to interpret gestures; he also sees the facial activity that is the visible aspect of speech. By proper guidance, he can be taught to attend to these facial activities as meaningful signals of the wishes and intentions of others. He can thus be started on the road to speechreading and mastery of language. An invention called "Visible Speech" seemed for a time to offer rich possibilities for training the deaf to speak properly. In this method a pattern of light and dark bands is formed on a moving, phosphorescent screen in response to the sounds of the voice. The pattern moves steadily from right to left. The height of the bright bands above the base line is determined by the frequency of the funda-

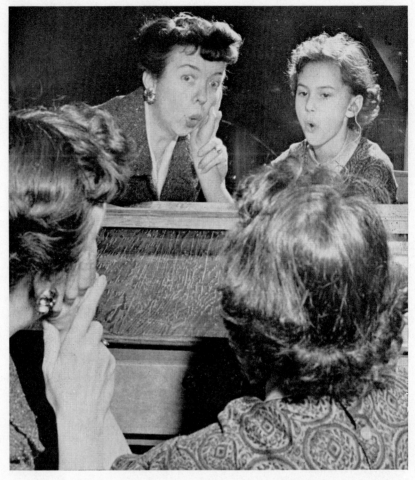

Fig. 14-1. Speech instruction for a severely hard-of-hearing child. The instructor uses vision, touch, and hearing. The mirror helps the child to monitor her articulation. (*Central Institute for the Deaf.*)

mental voice sound and of the formants that give it the particular vowel qualities. It is possible to learn to read this form of visible, running frequency-analysis of speech, but the method has not proved to be of any real assistance in teaching deaf children to talk.

TACTILE CLUES

Through the sense of *touch*, the deaf child learns that the visible movements of speech are accompanied by a modulated flow of the breath and by vibration. Although he cannot hear the sounds produced as the breath is modulated by the larynx, tongue, and lips, the deaf child can be made aware of many tactile clues which will help him understand the nature of the process. For example, the skilled teacher places the child's hand in front of her mouth as she articulates plosive consonants (such as *p* or *b*). The child is trained to feel the momentary gust of air escaping from the mouth as the plosive is released. Similarly, a hand placed on the cheek receives vibratory sensations when vowels are produced. The nasal consonants produce agitation that can be felt on the nose, and all voiced sounds give rise to vibration that can be felt at the Adam's apple (larynx). These various tactile clues are among those used, not only to make the child aware of major phases in speech production but also to teach him to control his own speech mechanism. By alternately feeling the effects produced as the teacher speaks and then attempting to achieve the same effects with his own speech organs, the child learns techniques of sound production and enunciation. Some techniques use sounding boards, including pianos, and diaphragms which are caused to vibrate by speech and music. Progress is usually slow and the end result is seldom speech that is completely natural. A level of intelligibility is obtainable, however, which allows the child the freedom of direct communication with those who hear. The gains in social adequacy and in independence more than repay the effort.

It has been suggested that speech could be analyzed by the method of "Visible Speech" and the resulting pattern delivered to the sense of touch instead of being made visible. Such a method of training the voice has not actually been tried, however, as far as we are aware.

KINESTHETIC CLUES

In the final analysis, the deaf child must control his speech primarily through the sensations he receives from effects occurring within his own body. These internal sensations are called *kinesthetic* clues. They are of various types, such as feelings of jaw movement, tongue movement, position of the lip, position of the soft palate, nasal vibrations, and laryngeal vibration. During the initial stages of training, the teacher may even manipulate the child's organs of speech so that they execute patterns of movement that the child must learn. The purpose is to get the child to feel the kinesthetic clues that characterize each movement. Furthermore, as the child is required to control his own speech through vision and touch, kinesthetic sensations will also occur. With the passing of time he learns to rely upon these kinesthetic sensations to tell him what he is doing. Thus, whereas the person with normal hearing judges the adequacy of his speech by the way it *sounds,* the deaf child must base the same judgment on the way it *feels.*

From what has been said, it is clear that teaching a deaf child to talk is an exacting task. The teacher must know both the principles of speech and the limitations of deaf children. The teacher must be adept at using visual, tactile, and kinesthetic clues to make the child try to speak. For these reasons, development of speech in deaf children can be best accomplished by teachers specializing in education of the deaf and the hard of hearing.

Parents and friends have three major responsibilities in encouraging the development of speech in a deaf child. The first responsibility is to seek out a competent teacher and place the child under her guidance. The second responsibility is to speak naturally, but with the addition of clarifying gestures, in the presence of the child. The parents thus keep before the child the fact that human communication is accompanied by activity of the structures in the face and neck. The third responsibility, once the child has begun to talk, is to respond positively to every effort he makes to speak. Even though the effort is imperfect, it is vital (if the speech can be understood at all) that parents and friends react appropriately. When they do so, the child soon learns to rely upon his speech efforts as a means of controlling other people and of adapting to his social environment. Thus, and only thus, will speech be made a functional tool in the child's everyday life.

Speech Training for Hard-of-Hearing Children

When a child possesses a reasonable amount of residual hearing, his requirements for speech training are ordinarily different from what they would be if he were deaf. For one thing, the fact that he has some usable hearing means that he will probably acquire patterns of speech spontaneously. However, these patterns will be faulty and imperfect. Thus, one of his needs is *re-education* designed to eliminate his faults. Furthermore, since he will have some understanding of language and its use, he needs encouragement toward fuller language development rather than the building of language skill from its very beginning.

It is important for two reasons that speech training start as early in the child's life as possible. In the first place, the period in life most favorable to the development of speech habits is thus utilized constructively. Moreover, early training will minimize the work required to counteract the faulty habits of speech, since these habits will be less firmly fixed than if training is delayed.

SPECIAL METHODS

Speech training for the hard-of-hearing child requires special methods that utilize both the child's residual hearing and his other sensory channels. Visual clues are particularly important. As in the case of the deaf child, these clues add awareness of speech activities. Furthermore, many of the phonetic elements that are particularly difficult to hear involve movements of the jaw and lips that are relatively easy to see. Visual clues thus offer opportunity for stressing the phase of enunciatory skill that the child particularly needs to learn. Attempts are still being made to translate the acoustic information in speech into a form in which it may be perceived by the eye, but the results in teaching the deaf by such methods have not been very encouraging.

Both the sense of touch and kinesthetic clues are important in the total training process, but these need not be used so copiously as with the deaf child. However, they can profitably be employed to help the child master articulatory movements that are difficult for him and to give him nonauditory means for controlling this everyday speech.

Auditory clues must be used to the fullest extent possible in teaching the hard-of-hearing child to talk better. Advantage can thus be taken of a natural bond between the ear and the voice. The child is helped to learn habits for controlling his own speech through the auditory experience he receives from it.

Obviously, the way in which auditory clues are best used in speech training is an individual matter. Each child has unique potentialities and special needs that depend upon the details of his hearing loss. However, the general rule that must be met is to *bring sound to the child in the form that is most usable to him*. Here the principles discussed in the chapter on auditory training apply. Speaking close to the child's ear is often a practical means of presenting useful auditory stimulation. Moreover, the semiportable hearing aid is an excellent tool in the hands of a skilled teacher. Such an instrument allows the speech of both the teacher and the child himself to be amplified. Drill material of all types (from isolated sounds to connected passages) may be used. Sometimes drills are presented through the instrument by the teacher. The pupil then repeats the drills. At other times, the child speaks the drills without previous example. Throughout the whole process the child's attention is directed to the auditory features of the errors he makes and the successes he achieves. The ear is thus made a functional channel to mastery of speech.

When the child begins to wear his own hearing aid, he has an additional advantage. The instrument will bring to him with greater clarity the patterns of speech he is using in life situations. He can thus rely more heavily upon his ear to guide his speech performance. The child who is properly prepared for this stage is encouraged to make his successful efforts habitual.

The reader will observe that instruction in speech and auditory training have much in common. Actually, it is profitable to combine the two. Furthermore, as with all phases of education for those with impaired hearing, the speech training that we have been discussing is most effective when carried on in a special school or by a qualified teacher of the acoustically handicapped.

HELP OF PARENTS AND FRIENDS

Parents and friends can encourage speech development in the hard-of-hearing child. The first rule is to *see that the child gets plenty of auditory stimulation,* particularly by talking to him at close range or through a hearing aid. The second rule is to ensure that he realizes the communicative importance of speech. This result can be gained in part by using questions, comments, and explanations whenever possible during the everyday activities in which he participates. However, it also requires that the parents respond positively to any speech efforts the child himself makes in the initial stages of his training program, thus giving him the experience of controlling others through speech. In the later stages of the program, parents and teachers should *require as precise speech from the child as his accomplishment warrants.* At this stage, response to his speech efforts should be withheld whenever these efforts are inadequate. Here the guidance of the teacher is necessary in order to ensure that the parents require a fair level of performance; otherwise the child's progress may be frustrated by a feeling of failure when he is trying his hardest and doing his best.

Preservation of Adequate Speech

As we have already pointed out, the occurrence of a substantial loss of hearing may cause deterioration in speech. Such a situation exists when the auditory impairment does not occur until after normal patterns of speech have been firmly established. Thus, it is a situation that affects only older children and adults. Furthermore, the deterioration in speech is neither instantaneous nor complete.

SPEECH INSURANCE

The facts just mentioned call for a special type of training based on the concept of *speech insurance*. Stated differently, the person we are discussing enters the ranks of the hard of hearing with normal habits of speech. The main educational task is to teach him to *retain* these habits in order to conserve the skill he already has. *If training can be started soon enough after the hearing loss occurs, no deterioration in speech need result.* The technique is to give the person substitute channels for controlling his speech efforts, since his ear no longer serves as a fully effective monitor when he talks.

Only under two circumstances is it necessary to combine speech re-education with the program of speech insurance. Sometimes the hearing loss has existed long enough so that deterioration in speech is evident, and sometimes the person has a speech defect that is independent of the hearing loss. In either event, faulty habits must be broken down. They must be replaced by adequate habits, and at the same time the substitute channels of control must be learned.

When the hearing loss is complete (or nearly so), speech insurance must depend mainly on learning effective use of kinesthetic clues. To this end, the person with extreme loss must first become acquainted with the nature of the speech process. He must understand the activity that he wishes to control. He must learn to preserve the phonetic elements of speech by becoming fully aware of the kinesthetic peculiarities of each element. Second, he must develop awareness of the bodily sensations associated with proper control of melody, quality, rhythm, and emphasis. In the third place, he must maintain physical alertness, facial expressiveness, and spontaneous gestures. Naturalness in speaking depends in part upon abandoning oneself to the act of communication. Finally, the person must learn to maintain effective control of the loudness of his voice.

PROBLEMS OF PARTIAL HEARING LOSS

Successful mastery of control of loudness is particularly difficult. However, two measures allow a reasonable solution to the difficulty. The person must first master the ability to talk at each of four or five general levels of loudness. He must learn to shift at will from one level to another. These levels, which are under kinesthetic control, must range from soft speech to very loud speech. Second, the person must study and classify typical sound environments. With the help of his instructor, he can learn what level of background noise he is most likely to encounter in each type of situation. He can then

meet the requirements of loudness with reasonable success by speaking at the level (of the five he has learned) that is ordinarily demanded by the situation at hand. Furthermore, an alert talker will
notice when his listeners are having difficulty responding to his speech
and will raise his voice to the next level. He thus avoids relying
rigidly on a set of rules in situations where it happens that the rules
do not apply.

When the hearing loss is partial, both the need for speech insurance and the techniques necessary to achieve it depend upon the
degree and pattern of the hearing loss. The primary requisite is to
retain insofar as possible control of speech by the ear. *Here a good
hearing aid can be of great help,* since it may raise to a usable level
many elements of the wearer's own speech that are inaudible to him
without the instrument.

The task of speech conservation then divides itself into two
phases. To the degree that components of speech remain inaudible
even while the hearing aid is being worn, the person must be taught
kinesthetic control of speech. Second, if some components that are
made audible by the instrument are reproduced somewhat "un-
naturally," he will require auditory training in interpreting his own
speech. For example, when wearing a hearing aid, the person must
learn to make allowances for changes in the way phonetic elements
sound through his instrument. Otherwise, he may modify his articulation to satisfy his own unschooled ear and thus achieve an enunciation that is less effective for his listeners. Another example involves
the loudness of speech. A peculiar situation often exists because the
wearer's own voice seems extremely loud to him through the hearing
aid. The balance between his own voice and the background noise
is entirely different without the aid from what it is when he is using
the instrument. This difference will work to his disadvantage unless he is taught to accept a balance that he does not particularly
like but that is most acceptable to the listener.

PROGRESSIVE HEARING LOSS

Special considerations enter the picture when the hearing loss
has been diagnosed as one which is progressive. The auditory impairment may not at the moment be sufficient to endanger the
patterns of speech. However, the future outlook may demand that
a program of speech conservation be begun immediately. A full
system of kinesthetic control over speech should be built while
the patterns of speech are still good and while it is still easy for the
person to understand instructions from the teacher. The person can

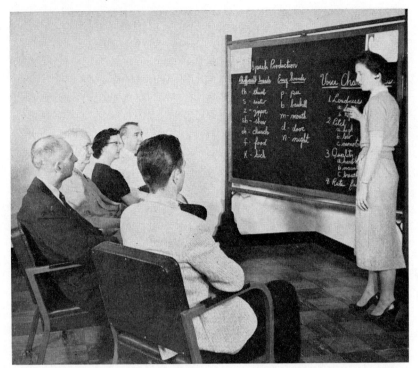

Fig. 14-2. A class in speech conservation and improvement. The instructor analyzes the factors that influence the intelligibility and quality of speech. (*Veterans Administration.*)

thus be prepared to apply kinesthetic control when his hearing drops to the point where this control becomes necessary.

Training in the preservation of speech is best obtained from teachers who have been specifically prepared for their type of work. Such teachers are to be found in schools offering special work for hard-of-hearing children. They are also to be found in hearing clinics, aural rehabilitation centers, and similar organizations. Children needing guidance in speech conservation can often get help through schools, while both adults and children have access to hearing clinics and to the organizations enumerated in Chapter 20.

Family and friends can help the person who is fighting the threat of speech deterioration. As with other problems, the first step is to find a qualified teacher and enlist her participation. The second step is to cooperate fully with the teacher. The cooperation can be extensive, since the person in training can profit from much drill at home. The student needs the help of either a relative or a friend. Following specific instructions from the teacher, this assistant, who must have both normal hearing and normal speech, serves as a monitor who corrects errors made by the student as he works on his drills. And finally, members of the student's immediate social circle can build favorable morale by taking a positive and sympathetic attitude toward his misfortune and toward his efforts.

Suggested Readings

FAIRBANKS, G. *Voice and Articulation Drillbook.* New York: Harper & Brothers, 1940.

GRAY, G. W., and C. M. WISE. *The Bases of Speech.* 3d ed. New York: Harper & Brothers, 1959.

TRAVIS, L. E., ed. *Handbook of Speech Pathology.* New York: Appleton-Century-Crofts, Inc., 1957.

PART 5

EDUCATION AND PSYCHOLOGY

15

FROM ARISTOTLE
TO BELL

S. R. Silverman, Ph.D.

The evolution of the present social point of view toward deafness has been marked by a growing recognition of its problems and by an increasing collective effort to do something practical toward their solution. We need go no further than the pages of this book for a forceful illustration of the variety of talents that are now cooperating in the attack. The removal of professional barriers, which now permits the physician, the researcher, the educator, the sociologist, the psychologist, the physicist, the audiologist, parents, and laymen to work together with mutual understanding, is one of the most promising developments of recent years. It forecasts a progressively broader and more intelligent base of social awareness of the entire question.

The development of an increasingly enlightened social attitude toward deafness, however, is no exception to the general rule that man's struggle toward enlightenment is slow, faltering, and, in many instances, haphazard. This development might be traced in the history of the education of the deaf, but only fragmentary bits of information are available prior to the sixteenth century. Some of the bits are indirect and inferred, and it is difficult to trace any complete structure of systematic thought.

In the pre-Christian era, however, Aristotle and, later, Pliny the Elder observed that there was some relationship between congenital deafness and dumbness, but neither one elaborated the relationship. It is still questionable whether Aristotle assumed a common organic basis for deafness and dumbness, but he placed strong emphasis on sound (speech) as the primary vehicle for conveying thought and therefore as the chief medium for education. Aristotle presumably believed, therefore, that since the deaf could neither give utterance to speech nor comprehend it from others, they were relatively incapable of instruction; and, furthermore, that the deaf were less capable of instruction than the blind. At any rate, Aristotle made no clear statement that dumbness is a consequence of deafness (of the congenital type) and that speech is an acquired skill whose patterns are learned through the ear. Of course, hearing is the normal channel through which speech is most readily perceived and consequently imitated. Note the stress on the *normal* channel, for we have also learned that it is possible for the deaf to acquire speech through touch, sight, and the sense of movement. Many deaf receive information through the use of manual alphabets and the language of signs.

The idea that deafness and muteness depend on a common organic abnormality and that the deaf were poor educational prospects persisted through medieval times. It is probable that the derogatory use of "dumbness" in our modern slang, suggesting an inferior intellect, has its roots in the supposed mental incapacity of the deaf. And it was inevitable that the notion of the limited mental capacity of the deaf should exercise a powerful influence on their legal and civil status. Roman law classified the deaf and dumb with the mentally incompetent, and the Justinian Code (sixth century A.D.) excluded the deaf and dumb from the rights (entering into contracts, and so on) and obligations (witnessing in a court of law) of citizenship. In justice to Justinian's Code, it must be said that a sharp differentiation was made between deaf-mutes and those whose deafness was acquired and who had learned speech and writing. Although the Code did not prohibit marriage for the deaf, its influence later caused medieval law to deny to the congenitally deaf and dumb the highly cherished right of primogeniture.

Although information concerning the attitude of religious institutions toward deafness during this early period is comparatively meager, fragments of evidence from church literature indicate that the church shared the prevailing notions of the times. Mosaic Law, through its Code of Holiness in the sixth century B.C., exhorted the faithful not to curse the deaf since their deafness was presumably willed by the Lord. In the second century B.C. the rabbis of the Talmud classified the deaf with fools and children. Although the rabbis were perfectly correct in calling attention to individual differences, their pronouncements reflect an inadequate understanding of deafness. It is strange that Jeremiah, usually recognized as the most forward-looking social philosopher among the prophets, made no mention of the deaf.

Similarly, the Christian Church looked with disdain on the intellectual capabilities of the deaf, although it did permit marriage by a ceremony conducted in the language of signs. We perceive a glimmer of enlightenment, however, in Bede's references (about the seventh century A.D.) to the feat of Bishop John of York in teaching a deaf-and-dumb youth to speak intelligibly. This accomplishment, however, is chronicled in the nature of a miracle, and the educational method is left to our imaginations. Nevertheless, the mere recording of the incident is a first, admittedly feeble, attempt, conscious or otherwise, to dispel the fog of misunderstanding in which deafness was enshrouded.

It was not until the middle of the sixteenth century that the mists began to lift. At that time an intellectually versatile Italian physician, Girolamo Cardano of Padua, in referring to the work of Rudolphus Agricola of Gröningen, proposed a set of principles that promised a more hopeful educational, and hence social, outlook for the deaf. He stated, in essence, that the deaf could be taught to comprehend written symbols or combinations of symbols by associating them with the object or picture of the object they were intended to represent. To this day, the association of meaningful language with experience is the keystone of techniques for teaching the deaf. The significance of Cardano's contribution lies not so much in his statement of basic principles of teaching as in his implicit rejection of the notion that the deaf cannot be educated and consequently are doomed to social inadequacy. It would not be too extravagant to attribute to Cardano the concept of an educational Magna Carta for the deaf.

Cardano's pronouncements initiated a series of serious, although sporadic, attempts to implement his principles. It is reasonable to credit these heartening developments in part also to the liberation of humanistic forces by the Renaissance and to the subsequent popularization of education in the vernacular induced by the Reformation. As early as 1555 we find oral education of deaf children of the nobility carried on by a Spanish monk, Pedro Ponce de Leon, in a convent of Valladolid. It was in Spain, too, that the first book exclusively on the deaf, by Juan Pablo Bonet, appeared in 1620. Bonet's pupils were taught articulation and language supplemented by a manual alphabet and the language of signs. Other works in many tongues dealing with the education and intellectual and spiritual status of the deaf appeared soon after. John Bulwer, John Wallis, William Holder, and George Dalgarno carried on in the British Isles; Jan Baptiste Van Helmont and John Conrad Amman in Holland; St. Francis de Sales in Switzerland; Ernaud and Pereire in France; and Otto Lasius and Arnoldi (among a host of others) in Germany.

In contrast to Aristotle's views comparing the intellectual capabilities of the deaf and blind, the beginning of enlightenment is best typified by a quotation from Dalgarno's *Didascalocophus,* published at Oxford in 1680:

Taking it for granted, That Deaf people are equal, in the faculties
of apprehension, and memory, not only to the Blind; but even to those
that have all their senses: and having formerly shewn; that these
faculties can as easily receive, and retain, the Images of things by the
conveiance of Figures, thro the Eye, as of Sounds thro the ear: It will
follow, That the Deaf man is, not only, as capable, but also as soon
capable of Instruction in Letters, as the blind man. And if we compare
them, as to their intrinsick powers, has the advantage of him too;
insomuch as he has a more distinct and perfect perception, of external
Objects, then the other. . . . I conceive, there might be successful
addresses made to a Dumb child, even in his cradle. . . .

Note the emphasis on equality with others and the suggestion that the
deaf could be taught even in early childhood.

Two individuals, however, tower above all others in their contributions to advancing the cause of the deaf in the latter part of the
eighteenth century—Abbé Charles Michel de l'Épée in France and
Samuel Heinicke in Germany. De l'Épée found a fruitful outlet for his
religious emotions, as many clergymen have since his time, in promoting the well-being of the deaf through education. It is to his everlasting
credit that he founded the first public school for the deaf in 1775 in
Paris. Heinicke, his contemporary in Germany, founded the first public school for the deaf in Germany and the first recognized by any
government. De l'Épée and Heinicke disagreed about the merits of
signs and "oralism" as methods of instruction, De l'Épée favoring signs
and Heinicke writing prolifically on the advantages of speech and of
speechreading. So widespread was the influence of these two men
that the pattern of their controversy was reproduced subsequently in
many countries, the United States included. Our purpose here, however, is not to evaluate the merits of their contentions but to stress their
extremely important contributions to the liberalization of the social
point of view toward deafness. By the end of the eighteenth century
it had been convincingly demonstrated that the deaf were capable of
instruction, and it was also clearly recognized that it was the moral and
legal obligation of society to see that instruction was provided, even
though the development of free public schools was slow. Such recognition was indeed a landmark of social progress.

The moral and intellectual advancement of the social attitude
toward deafness in Europe naturally exerted its influence in the United
States. Although there had been scattered instances of instruction of
the deaf, of attempts to found permanent schools, and of mention of
the deaf in the literature, it was not until 1817 that the first permanent
public school for the deaf in the United States was founded, at
Hartford, Connecticut. The establishment of this school was given its

chief impetus by a young divinity student, Thomas Hopkins Gallaudet, who was sent abroad by a group of citizens to observe European methods in the education of the deaf. On visiting England he was disappointed in the help he received from the Braidwoods, who were said to be obtaining good results using the oral approach to deaf children. It appears that the Braidwoods, British educators of the deaf, were secretive about their methods.

Gallaudet therefore crossed the Channel to France and enlisted the services of Laurent Clerc, a French teacher of the deaf trained in the manual approach of De l'Épée, whom he succeeded in bringing to Hartford. Incidentally, Clerc, who was introduced to Gallaudet by Abbé Roch-Ambroise Sicard, De l'Épée's successor, was deaf himself and hence was the first deaf teacher of the deaf in the United States. The school at Hartford, called the American Asylum for the Education and Instruction of the Deaf and Dumb (now known as the American School for the Deaf), had to depend upon private funds for support, but in a relatively short time public assistance was made available. It was the forerunner of the great system of state-supported schools for the deaf which we have in the United States today. Later in the nineteenth century and early in the twentieth century outstanding private and denominational schools were also established and were notable for their encouragement of oral methods of instruction.

Thanks to the indefatigable efforts of such trail blazers as Thomas Hopkins Gallaudet, for whom the federally sponsored college for the deaf in Washington, D.C., is named; Edward Miner Gallaudet, who carried on his father's work; Sarah Fuller, who promoted the day school for the deaf; Alexander Graham Bell and his father, Melville, who among other accomplishments elevated speech to the status of a science; Caroline Yale, who implemented many of the Bells' principles; and Max A. Goldstein, founder of the Central Institute for the Deaf, who drove home the needs of the deaf to the medical profession and who developed methods for training residual hearing, the great vision of universality of educational opportunity for the deaf has been transformed into reality. The ever-expanding opportunities for the deaf in publicly supported residential and day schools and in parochial and private institutions attest the wisdom of these great workers in the cause of the deaf. It is because of their foresight and energy that no deaf child need be denied an opportunity for education.

The happy combination of talents brought to bear on the problem of increasing the opportunities for the deaf is best epitomized in the person of Alexander Graham Bell. As we shall see in Chapter 20, by establishing a bureau of information on deafness he opened new vistas in the teaching of speech to the deaf; and, of course, his invention of the telephone laid a firm foundation for the electrical transmission of sound. The writers of this book, consciously or otherwise, take inspiration and stimulation from his sympathetic understanding, his spirit of incisive inquiry, and his inventive genius. It was fitting that 1947 (the date of the first edition of this book), the hundredth anniversary of the birth of Alexander Graham Bell, should witness the emergence of the art and science of audiology, which in broad terms seeks the answer to the question, "How can we do a better job for the deaf and the hard of hearing?" There is no doubt that Bell is still with us as we seek more and better answers to this basic question.

As the schools for the deaf became more widespread and adequate, it was inevitable that the social point of view toward deafness should become proportionately more enlightened. The alumni of these schools were beginning to demonstrate how seriously the deaf had previously been underestimated. They have taken the initiative in promoting broad and intensive studies now underway dealing with the psychiatric and vocational needs of the deaf. The schools themselves are tending to become purely educational institutions, subject to boards of education and not to administrators of almshouses or to penal authorities.

Society now understands that the deaf not only can be educated but can also, with proper guidance and assistance, become economically and socially productive men and women. Agencies for vocational rehabilitation and guidance, emphasizing special training for adults in cooperation with schools and industry, have been established to facilitate the economic and social adjustment not only of the deaf but of the hard of hearing as well. And paralleling the enlarging educational and economic opportunities for the deaf, the unnecessary legal restrictions upon them have gradually been removed.

The progressive development of the education of the deaf generally reflected the popularization and liberalization of general education, particularly with respect to the spread of opportunity for education, the improvement of teacher training, and the application of better teaching techniques. The process has also worked in reverse. Educators of the hearing have consciously or otherwise borrowed from teachers of the deaf—especially the principle of "learning by doing." It is heartening to note also that recognized universities are increasingly introducing curricula dealing with educational, psychological, sociological, and physiological problems of deafness.

Academic interest in problems of deafness is illustrated by recent significant international gatherings, such as the International Conference on Audiology, held in St. Louis, Missouri, in May, 1957; the International Congress on Modern Educational Treatment of Deafness held in Manchester, England, in July, 1958; and the Fourth Congress of the International Society of Audiology held in Padua, Italy in October, 1958.

Although man has traveled a long, tortuous road from the pre-Christian era in evolving an enlightened understanding of the social problems of deafness, a large portion of society still looks upon the deaf and the hard of hearing as queer, dependent, and, sometimes, ridiculous. We are all familiar with the cheap humor of which they are often the target. Since their handicap is not as visible as that of the blind and the crippled, the deaf often find themselves in embarrassing and humiliating situations because others do not understand their special problems.

The answer of the deaf to such misunderstanding is to continue their social and economic achievements as self-respecting and productive individuals. Our social action for the deaf, therefore, should not aim for special privileges for them but should constantly strive to provide opportunity without discrimination for the deaf to help themselves. They deserve no less from an enlightened society.

Suggested Readings

American Annals of the Deaf, Vol. 103, March, 1958. A special issue containing the contributions to the Institute on Personal, Social and Vocational Adjustment to Total Deafness.

BÉKÉSY, G. VON, and W. A. ROSENBLITH. "The Early History of Hearing—Observations and Theories," *Journal of the Acoustical Society of America*, 20: 727–748 (1948).

Authors' Summary: "The debris of broken systems and exploded dogmas form a great mound, a Monte Testaccio of the shards and remnants of old vessels which once held human beliefs. If you take the trouble to climb to the top of it, you will widen your horizon, and in these days of specialized knowledge your horizon is not likely to be any too wide." Oliver Wendell Holmes, 1882.

BEST, H. *Deafness and the Deaf in the United States.* New York: The Macmillan Company, 1943.

BOATNER, M. T. *Voice of the Deaf: A Biography of Edward Miner Gallaudet.* Washington, D.C.: Public Affairs Press, 1959.

A sympathetic treatment of the life of the man associated with the founding and nurturing of Gallaudet College. Chapter 13 is particularly interesting because it discusses Gallaudet's relations with Alexander Graham Bell.

FARRAR, A. *Arnold's Education of the Deaf.* 2d ed. Derby: Francis Carter, 1923.

GOLDSTEIN, M. A. *Problems of the Deaf.* St. Louis: The Laryngoscope Press, 1933. Essentially a collection of scientific essays on a variety of topics pertinent to deafness, including an excellent historical chapter.

HODGSON, K. W. *The Deaf and Their Problems.* New York: Philosophical Library, 1954.

A historical study in special education by a British author including the growth of teaching systems and social attitudes toward deafness.

International Conference on Audiology. Special issue of *The Laryngoscope*, Vol. 68, March, 1958.

Proceedings of the International Conference on Audiology, St. Louis, May, 1957, on the themes of assessment of auditory function, the physiology of audition, and the relation of hearing loss to noise-exposure.

16

DEAF CHILDREN

S. R. Silverman, Ph.D.,

H. S. Lane, Ph.D., and

D. G. Doehring, Ph.D.

The approximately 25,000 deaf children of school age in the United States present a problem somewhat different from that of the more numerous hard-of-hearing children to be discussed in Chapter 17. Most deaf children either are born deaf or lose their hearing before patterns of language and speech have been established. By "deaf" children we here mean those who do not have sufficient residual hearing to enable them to understand speech successfully, even with a hearing aid, without special instruction. And even those children who lose their hearing after patterns of language and speech have been firmly established suffer more deterioration of speech than do hard-of-hearing children. On the other hand, a congenitally deaf child is not dumb. His mechanism for speech is normal, but he has simply never been taught to speak.

In their formative years children learn speech and language, both reception and expression, primarily through the ear. Sectional pronunciations and accents learned as children are likely to be retained throughout life. The New Englander who uses the broad *a* in "park," as distinguished from the Midwesterner who rolls the *r* in the same word, is merely imitating what he has heard as a youth in his section of the country. In the same sense our use and understanding of language naturally depend at first upon hearing. The two-year-old deaf child has no useful verbal language, whereas the hearing child of the same age has begun to develop a meaningful spoken and hearing vocabulary. Hence, means of communication with the deaf child must be developed through systematic and, in many instances, laborious procedures.

The detection and diagnosis of deafness and other abnormalities of communication have been discussed in Chapter 8, but it is important to keep clearly in mind the kind of child we are talking about when we refer to the "deaf child."

A great deal of unnecessary confusion among the laity and well-intentioned professional workers alike has surrounded the precise classification of hard-of-hearing and deaf children and unfortunately has frequently obfuscated discussions of their problems. The confusion seems to grow out of the differences in frameworks of reference to which classification and nomenclature are related. For example, some workers classify the child who develops speech and language prior to onset of deafness as "hard of hearing" even though he may not be able to hear pure tones or speech at any intensity. This child, it is argued, unlike the congenitally profoundly deaf child who has not acquired speech naturally, behaves as a hard-of-hearing child in that his speech is relatively natural or "normal" and, therefore, he should be classified as "hard of hearing." It is obvious that a not too precise educational standard has guided the labeling if not the definition of the child. If, however, we consider the same child from a purely physiological standpoint, it is grossly misleading to term him "hard of hearing" when for all practical purposes he hears nothing at all.

The situation is complicated further by the use of terms that suggest not only physiological communication and educational factors but also gradations of hearing loss and time of onset. To this category belong such terms as *deaf and dumb, mute, deaf-mute, semideaf, semimute, deafened, partially deaf,* and others. These terms are of little value from the physiological, communicative, or educational points of view, and it would be well to eliminate them from general usage. (See also Chapter 4.)

For purposes of our chapter we need to define the deaf child in terms of his educational and psychological potential. For some, the significant dimension would be the child's ability to talk. In England, for example, under the School Health Regulations, children are described as (1) deaf, and (2) partially deaf. The former are those who have no "naturally" acquired speech when they are admitted to school, the latter are those who have begun to talk naturally (however imperfectly) before being admitted to school. According to this scheme children with defective hearing are classified in three grades:

Grade   I: Children who are found to have defects of hearing (which in most cases are amenable to medical treatment) but who do not need hearing aids or special educational treatment.
Grade II: Children who have some naturally acquired ability to talk but need special educational treatment, on either a part-

time or a full-time basis. Many of these children need hearing aids.

Grade III: Deaf children who are without naturally acquired speech
when admitted to school. Many of these children are not
totally deaf and can be helped by hearing aids in learning
to talk and to speak distinctly.[1]

For others, the important dimension is the hearing loss expressed
by the child's ability to respond to various environmental sounds,
speech, and pure tones. Itard, in the early nineteenth century, classified children according to their responses—to bells, drums, and flutes;
Urbantschitsch some years later used a harmonica with a six-octave
range (E^{-1}—e^4) and an intensity regulator for the same purpose. Both
of these workers also used speech stimuli, and Urbantschitsch's classification is fairly representative of the categories that emerge from these
approaches—(1) total deafness, (2) tone-hearing, (3) vowel-hearing,
(4) word-hearing, and (5) sentence-hearing. Others have translated
this dimension to hearing for pure tones on the decibel scale by such
schemes as are described in Chapters 4, 9, and 17.

Of course, the time of onset of deafness affects the psychological
and educational developmental patterns and should be borne in mind
in labeling and classifying a child. The important points on the "time-
of-onset" dimension for the profoundly deaf are the age range from
three to five years and the time when adulthood is reached. As we
have said, children who are deaf before the age of three are not likely
to retain normal patterns of speech and language. Obviously, from the
age of three to five years, the later a child has lost his hearing the more
apt he is to retain "natural" patterns of communication by speech.

In 1937 the Committee on Nomenclature of the Conference of
Executives of American Schools for the Deaf recognized the importance of ability to speak, ability to hear (as shown by their use of the
word "functional"), and time of onset in proposing the following classification and definitions:

> 1. THE DEAF: Those in whom the sense of hearing is nonfunc-
> tional for the ordinary purposes of life. This general group is made
> up of two distinct classes based entirely on the time of the loss of
> hearing. *a. The congenitally deaf:* Those who were born deaf. *b. The
> adventitiously deaf:* Those who were born with normal hearing but in
> whom the sense of hearing becomes nonfunctional later through illness
> or accident.
> 2. THE HARD OF HEARING: Those in whom the sense of hearing,
> although defective, is functional with or without a hearing aid.

[1] I. R. Ewing and A. W. G. Ewing, *Speech and the Deaf Child* (Washington,
D.C.: The Volta Bureau, 1954).

Some object vigorously to the restricting influence of the definitions and classifications of impaired hearing contained in these proposals of the Conference of Executives. They maintain that the continuing increase of fundamental clinical and therapeutic audiological knowledge precludes any "static categorization." For example, study of the thresholds of tolerance for speech and for pure tones has suggested that there is a useful portion of the auditory area even beyond the range of classical audiometry. Some individuals who have heretofore been termed "totally deaf" as a result of audiometric tests may be reached by auditory stimulation using proper amplification. And it may prove to be more fruitful to classify the person with a physical disability on some psychological scale of behavior that expresses how he lives with his disability.

We are aware that delimiting definitions are hazardous and we recognize that each child's capabilities must be assessed individually by the best methods available to us so that we are not restricted by the tyranny of classification. Nevertheless, we need some orientation as to the kind of child we are writing about. This chapter will therefore be concerned with the child who, when we first encounter him, has not developed the expressive and receptive skills of communication before the onset of his deafness. He cannot talk and he cannot understand the speech of others as does a normally hearing child of the same age. We shall also include the child who has acquired some of these skills of communication before the onset of his deafness but whose incompetence in language still calls for special educational techniques. For convenience, we shall refer to both of them as deaf children.

Magnitude of the Problem

If we examine the results of mass testing surveys among school children we find a range from 2 to 21 per cent reported as having defective hearing. This great variability in reports of hearing impairment is undoubtedly due to differences in definitions of hearing impairment; in techniques, apparatus, and conditions of testing; and in the socioeconomic status and climate of the communities in which the surveys were carried out. *Our best estimate is that 5 per cent of school-age children have hearing levels outside the range of normal* (see Chapters 7 and 9), *and that from one to two of every ten in this group require special educational attention.*[2] The others are likely to respond to medi-

---

[2] According to the January 2, 1959, issue of the *U.S. News & World Report,* the estimated total kindergarten and grade school enrollment in the United States at the end of 1958 was 31,255,000. The high school enrollment was 9,810,000. These estimates were derived from figures of the United States Census Bureau.

cal care or their hearing loss is not apt to reach the handicapping stage. How most of these hard-of-hearing children are handled we shall discuss in the following chapter.

As we have described them, how many deaf children are there in the United States? This is difficult to state precisely because the enrollment in our schools for the deaf is likely to include children who are hard of hearing or aphasic and is not likely to include all the children of preschool age and deaf children who are in schools for the hearing or in other kinds of schools. Our guiding figure is the reported enrollment of 24,279 [3] children in all schools for the deaf in 1957–1958, a formidable even if not quite accurate figure.

The Goals of Education of the Deaf

How we go about educating deaf children is obviously related to the goals we have set for them, and these goals are in turn determined by what we consider to be the over-all potential of the deaf—educational, psychological, and social. Or, otherwise said, some of the sharp differences of opinion concerning the most desirable arrangements and methods for the education of deaf children really have their roots in fundamental differences of opinion as to the long-range outlook for them.

The overwhelming amount of literature on the subject (a bibliography would probably exceed two thousand titles), ranging from school papers and convention resolutions to lengthy sections of books, reveals an intense polemicism that rests mainly on a nonexperimental empirical foundation. Of course, there are many shades of opinion, but stated views and observed practices suggest what we may term three "schools of thought." We are aware that we may be indulging in caricature and that "it all depends on the individual child," but we believe that a sorting out of views is desirable if we are to understand the rationale for particular views on the education of deaf children.

One group appears to stress the limitations, especially the social limitations, of deafness. It is concerned about the exclusion of the deaf from certain types of desirable employment, the effect on the deaf of insurance practices and legislation, the implication of what amounts to minority status in certain educational and social contexts, the impact of isolation from other deaf people, the difficult if not impossible task for some of learning speech and speechreading, and the misunderstandings of the general public concerning the abilities and aspirations of the deaf. This group would suit the method of communication to the child, and its view is best summarized by the following statement:

[3] See *American Annals of the Deaf,* Vol. 103, January, 1958.

The aim of the education of the deaf child should be to make him a well-integrated, happy deaf individual, and not a pale imitation of a hearing person. Let us aim to produce happy, well-adjusted deaf *individuals,* each different from the other, each with his own personality. If a child cannot learn to read lips well or cannot speak well, far better develop other modes of expression and communication, writing and gesturing, than make him feel ashamed and frustrated because he cannot acquire the very difficult art of speech and lip reading. Our aim must be a well-balanced, happy *deaf* person and not an imitation of a hearing one.[4]

A second group emphasizes the great possibilities of the deaf, as yet untapped, particularly for education and for participation in a world of hearing people. It stresses the importance of early education and the great possibilities of auditory training, and it is apt to emphasize the objective of "normalization." In essence, there is "one world" in which the deaf person must function and that is a world of hearing and speaking people. There is no separate world for the deaf.

A third school of thought points to the record of economic, academic, and social achievement of deaf persons *among the deaf and the hearing* as a strong, tangible justification for the belief that forward-looking, proper, and early fundamental training enables the deaf child to make the fullest use of his capabilities. Yet it is apparent, at least in our present state of knowledge, that there are situations in which the deaf will always be marginal and our approach to them should be influenced accordingly. Realism urges us to spare parents and the child himself the psychological distress of failure to achieve the "normalcy" that was set up as an attainable goal.

At any rate, until more facts are available to fill the gaps now occupied by opinion, a rational attitude points to the recognition that deafness imposes certain unavoidable limitations that must be accepted. At the same time, proper education in its broadest sense strives to relate the deaf person to the world about him in a psychologically satisfying way.

We now turn to consideration of what we judge to be a "proper education." It is both convenient and logical to organize our discussion around the following topics:

1. Organization and Administration of the Education of the Deaf in the United States: The Rise of the Preschool Movement
2. Mental Ability of Deaf Children
    a. Educational Achievement
    b. Language Development

[4] W. G. Hardy, *Children with Impaired Hearing* (Children's Bureau Publication No. 326; Washington, D.C.: Government Printing Office, 1952), p. 15.

    c. Other Aspects of Mental Ability
3. The Skills of Communication
    a. Speech
    b. Auditory Training
    c. Speechreading
    d. Language

Because there is universal agreement among educators of the deaf that every deaf child should be given an opportunity to communicate by speech, our attention shall be directed solely to this approach, which is called *oralism*. Some educators also advocate supplementing or, if indicated, supplanting oral instruction with other forms of communication. One of these other forms is the *manual alphabet*, which is a method of forming the letters from A to Z by certain fixed positions of the fingers of one hand. This is a form of "writing" in the air. The *language of signs* is another form of communication. This is a system of conventional gestures of the hands and arms that by and large are suggestive of the shape, form, or thought which they represent. The combined method, which attempts to provide speech communication, the manual alphabet, and the language of signs, depends upon the aptitude of the child and the context of the communication. For example, the language of signs and the manual alphabet are frequently employed in public assemblies. The combined method is usually employed in public residential schools.

As we have seen in Chapter 15, the "oral-manual" controversy has deep historical roots. In our own country the influence of De l'Épée through Laurent Clerc and Thomas Hopkins Gallaudet established the tradition of manualism early in the nineteenth century, and it was not until well after the middle of that century that oralism began to take hold. At the present time 60 per cent [5] of children enrolled in schools for the deaf are taught by the oral method of communication. The remainder are taught manually or by some combination of manual and oral methods. Although all organizations of educators of the deaf are on record officially as advocating an opportunity for all deaf children to learn to speak and to speech-read, the fact that 40 per cent of the deaf children are not taught by *exclusively* oral methods shows that there is significant (and often heated) difference of opinion as to what properly constitutes a fair opportunity. The criteria for transferring a child from an oral to a manual class, presumably because he shows no aptitude for oralism, are frequently vague and nebulous. Some educators make the transfer during the child's first year in school; others may wait until the child has been in school for three or four years; and

[5] See *American Annals of the Deaf*, Vol. 103, January, 1958.

still others provide oral instruction throughout but permit association in the dormitory with manually taught children. The latter plan obviously makes the oral instruction less effective because the speaking child must adjust himself to the child who cannot talk, and valuable practice in oral communication is lost.

Those who advocate some manualism generally contend that too often the results of exclusively oral teaching are unsatisfactory and that the deaf child cannot make himself understood to an untrained listener. Furthermore, it is argued, many children do not have the aptitude to benefit from oral instruction and the time spent in this type of instruction could more profitably be used in concentrating on the child's "mental" development rather than on his means of communication. Also, some advocates of manualism feel that the deaf prefer to associate with other deaf and therefore have little or no need for oral communication.

The fundamental assumption of the oralists (advocates of oral instruction for the deaf), on the other hand, is that training in speech and in speechreading gives an easier adjustment to a world in which speech is the chief medium of communication. It does not confine the deaf man or woman to association with those who know the manual alphabet or to those who are willing to resort to pad and pencil. An employer is more inclined to favor a deaf man to whom he can give oral instruction over a man of equal ability with whom he must communicate by gestures or in writing. It is not always possible, especially in smaller communities, for the deaf to find employment or social companionship among other deaf people. Oralists feel that, in the main, orally trained children have done well and are likely to do better as more teachers are adequately trained in the methods of oral instruction.

The oral-manual controversy is not yet settled. There are no completely convincing scientific data on which to base an objective conclusion, and no useful purpose is served by laboring the arguments.

The Education of the Deaf

Perhaps the most significant fact about the education of the deaf in the United States is that it is universally available to all deaf children of school age. Of course, the quality of education may vary, but it is important that no child need be denied an opportunity for it. Where are these opportunities available?

Of 24,279 children enrolled in schools for the deaf in the academic year 1957–1958, 14,654 attended public residential schools for the deaf. These schools, open to qualified children without charge, are supported either directly or indirectly by state tax funds. Most of the public residential schools are supported by legislative appropriation and hence come under the control of state authorities. The educational services of the remaining schools are purchased by the states on a per diem or per capita basis and are controlled by their own boards. Examples of the first group are the Indiana and Illinois Schools for the Deaf; in the second group we find such schools as the Lexington (New York) and the Clarke (Massachusetts) Schools for the Deaf.

Other tax-supported institutions for the deaf are public day schools and classes. A day school is usually large enough to be a separate entity; for example, Horace Mann School, Roxbury, Massachusetts. Day classes are usually groups within a larger school unit and there may be as few as one in a school or as many as ten; for example, La Crosse, Wisconsin. In 1957–1958, 1872 children were being educated in public day schools and 5279 were in public day classes. The remaining children, 2259, were being educated in denominational or private schools, such as Lutheran School (Detroit) and Central Institute for the Deaf (St. Louis). The latter schools may be either day or residential. There were 215 children in schools and classes for the multiple handicapped. The number of children in each class ranges generally from five to ten. Some deaf children have been absorbed into classes for the hearing. Deaf individuals attend high schools and colleges for the hearing. Most public residential schools provide education at the secondary level, and higher education exclusively for the deaf is available at Gallaudet College, Washington, D.C.

Until we have more evidence to support the point of view of either the day or the residential school, we must study each child's situation thoroughly to determine what educational placement is likely to be most fruitful for him. This points up the crucial need for early diagnosis and careful assessment. In addition to information aboult a child's hearing, among the significant points to be considered are the etiology of the deafness, the child's age at its onset, his physical development, his behavioral development, his social maturity, his home environment, and the insight of his parents.

THE RISE OF THE PRESCHOOL MOVEMENT

The encouraging progress in the assessment of hearing of young children has stressed the value of preschool programs for deaf children. The period from birth to the age of five is particularly critical for the learning and over-all development of children, whether hearing or deaf. Since the young deaf child is denied many of the normal experiences that lead to better socialization, it is all the more essential that he be given help and opportunity for his best development as

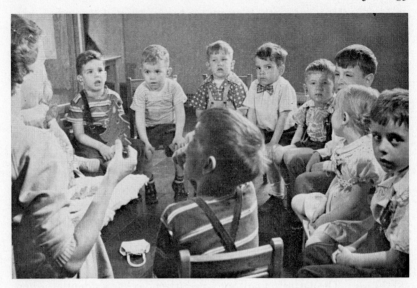

Fig. 16-1. Getting an early educational start—a preschool class. (*Johns Hopkins University.*)

early in life as possible. This means not just a sensible program for developing the skills of communication which so greatly contribute to socialization, but also a regime that removes wherever possible the barrier which tends to isolate the deaf child from the world about him, from the world of his home, his parents, his sisters and brothers, and other children. Formal and informal intercommunications (by whatever means) tend to lessen the child's feeling of apartness and hence to make him feel wanted and significant.

The child is thus motivated to communicate and it is the task of the parent and the teacher to show him the usefulness of speech as a tool of communication. "These situations," according to the prominent British educators of the deaf, Professor and Mrs. Ewing, "do not happen enough by themselves; they must be anticipated and contrived frequently and deliberately" by all who are in close contact with the child.

Although it is not generally mandatory for tax-supported schools to provide preschool classes for deaf children, the need is beginning to be recognized. In the academic year 1957–1958, of 14,654 children enrolled in public residential schools for the deaf in the United States, 813 were under the age of six; of 7151 children in public day schools and classes, 1060 were of preschool age; and of the 2259 children in denominational and private schools, 834 were under the age of six.

The proportions reflect the initiative of private groups in promoting programs for preschool deaf children.

It is appropriate, in discussing the young deaf child, to mention the increasing amount of information and guidance for parents of deaf children. Although here and there an effort may be misguided, the proliferation of parent institutes and clinics, and of correspondence courses, reading lists, and literary output is one of the most constructive and forward-looking developments in the education of the deaf. One parent put it succinctly: ". . . the tough thing about deafness is likely to be social isolation, social adjustment. There is no one in the world, and there never can be anyone, as important in determining any child's social adjustment as that child's own parents and his own family at home. For that reason parents are important."

For the parents of very young deaf children there are now correspondence courses which offer guidance, practical suggestions, and information concerning the home care of the child before the nursery school years. Probably the first such correspondence course was established by the Wright Oral School in New York City; but the best known at the present time is operated by the John Tracy Clinic in Los Angeles. Intelligent and cooperative parents have found these courses most helpful in giving them specific step-by-step procedures in beginning speechreading and a good psychological approach to the deaf child. Other procedures include the development of visual discrimination by matching colors and pictures and the comparison of objects varying in size and shape; practice in discriminating odors and tastes; exercises in the imitation of bodily movements; and the use of materials that will aid the child in better muscular coordination. Training of this type is continued in the nursery school on a more extensive and advanced scale. Such a correspondence course is particularly useful for those who are too remote to obtain information and advice in person from one of the well-established schools for the deaf. Children instructed by the parents who have followed a correspondence course of this type are better prepared to benefit immediately from a nursery school.

Most of these commendable efforts in orientation and guidance have been directed at parents of children of preschool age. This is natural, since the initial shock of the discovery of deafness must be intelligently cushioned, and crucial and immediate decisions must be made about the child's future. Even though we are here discussing children of preschool age, it should be realized that the placement of a child in a satisfactory educational situation in no way decreases the need for the guidance of parents. This was forcefully driven home to us in a survey made of the parents of present and former pupils at Central

Institute for the Deaf. Parents of teen-agers and young adults wanted an opportunity to share information and experiences about such problems as choices of occupation, marriage with the deaf or hearing, the genetics of deafness, and the choice of companions for the deaf. In short, social adjustment is just as much a problem for the deaf youth as it is for the preschool child, and it is essential that parent institutes and clinics concerned with their problems be fostered also.

Mental Ability of Deaf Children

When dealing with an ability of any sort, we are concerned simply with what a person can do. We judge the degree of a person's ability for a certain type of activity by observing how well he performs that activity. The term "mental ability" refers to the performance of certain types of activity that are relatively complicated, such as reasoning and problem solving. These types of mental activity are performed most efficiently by the use of language, and it is therefore not surprising that most judgments of mental ability involve an estimate of a person's facility in using language.

As we have implied, the fundamental observable difference between a deaf child and a hearing child is simply that the deaf child cannot hear sounds of any kind. Consequently, the deaf child lacks any ability that depends solely upon the hearing of sounds, such as the ability to hear the doorbell ringing. In learning to use language, the hearing child listens to the voices of others and to his own voice. The deaf child needs special instructions so that he may substitute other modes of perception during the learning of language. This instruction usually begins after the age at which a hearing child would have learned to speak and to understand speech, and therefore the deaf child does not become competent in the use of language until long after the hearing child.

In teaching language to a deaf child we teach him to understand speech or the manual alphabet and/or the language of signs, and to use language expressively either in speech or in writing. When this training has been successful, the mental ability of the deaf child usually appears to be normal. Many deaf children have graduated from college and gone on to successful careers in the business or professional world. Before language training has been completed, however, the mental ability of the deaf child may appear to be below normal as a result of his language handicap. In assessing his mental ability at this stage, therefore, we should choose tests that do not require the use of language.

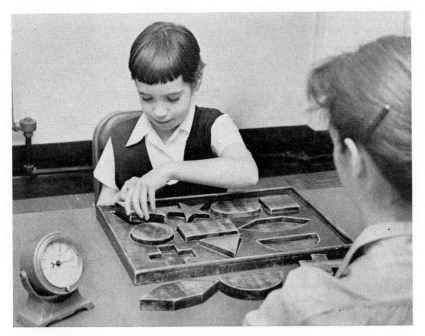

Fig. 16-2. A form board is used to test mental ability. (*Central Institute for the Deaf.*)

INTELLIGENCE

Mental ability can be assessed by means of intelligence tests which may or may not test language skills. On such tests the child's ability is evaluated by comparing his performance with that of the "standardization group" for his age. This group usually consists of children who have had normal educational opportunities and who do not possess any serious organic or mental defect. On an intelligence test where the average score of the standardization group for a given age is 100, a child of that age who scores well above 100 will be considered above normal in mental ability, and a child who scores well below 100 will be considered below normal in mental ability.

The intelligence tests used for estimating the mental ability of deaf children are called *nonlanguage, nonverbal,* or *performance* tests. Care must be exercised in selecting a test that is nonverbal both as to the instructions given by the examiner and as to the responses of the child tested. For example, pantomime instructions may need to be standardized and substituted for "Watch me carefully and do as I do" or "Put the blocks in the box quickly." Individual tests are preferable to group tests to ensure better rapport, to observe the attention of the child, and to stress the importance of speed on tests that are timed. Some of the most widely used of these tests are the Grace Arthur Scale, the Nebraska Test of Learning Aptitude, the Randall's Island Performance Series, and the performance subtests of the Wechsler Intelligence Scale for Children.[6] For the types of performance measured by these tests, deaf children fall within the normal range of ability.

Great care should be taken in interpreting scores of nonlanguage tests. The examiner should have some knowledge of the background of the child's deafness. As explained in Chapter 4, deafness in children may result from injury, disease, or hereditary factors. The causal agent may affect other parts of the body as well as the hearing mechanism. Such concomitant defects may seriously handicap a child's performance on a nonlanguage intelligence test. For example, a child with defective vision would be hampered in any task requiring precise visual discrimination and a child with defective muscular coordination would be handicapped in any task requiring skillful use of the hands. In some cases, such as a cerebral-palsied and deaf child, a precise estimate of mental ability may not be possible.

The examiner should have information about other evaluations of the child. Frequently deaf children have been seen at various clinics and tests have been administered. There is great overlapping of test items among the various performance tests, and scores can be influenced by previous experience or familiarity with test items.

The problem of the mentally deficient who are deaf or hard-of-hearing is difficult to solve. There is no general pattern of arrangement for educational placement for them and at present the management of their problem is far from satisfactory.

EDUCATIONAL ACHIEVEMENT

When the deaf child enters school he is usually without speech or an understanding of language. It takes approximately three years to prepare the child for the first grade and a total of from ten to twelve years to complete the eight elementary grades. The deaf child therefore becomes retarded as a result of his difficulty in the acquisition of language.

Educational progress can be measured by the use of educational achievement tests. These tests measure the child's level of attainment in school subjects, such as reading, arithmetic, language skills, and social studies, by comparing his performance with that of a representa-

[6] Stanley Berlinsky, "Measurement of the Intelligence and Personality of the Deaf: A review of the literature," *Journal of Speech and Hearing Disorders,* 17: 39–55 (1952).

tive group of children of his own age. These tests should be administered annually beginning at the second-grade level. These are group tests of the same type as those given to hearing children in elementary schools. The examiner must be certain that the child understands test directions, and visual signals must be given to start and stop the test. Such tests measure the amount of retardation and the rate of progress annually for each school subject included in the equivalent forms of the battery of tests.

Deaf children are usually found to be retarded by two years or more in educational achievement. Their performance tends to follow a very consistent pattern. In the achievement of *concrete* skills, such as grammar, punctuation, capitalization, spelling, and arithmetical computation, they approach a normal level of achievement. In the achievement of abstract skills, such as the comprehension of the meaning of words and paragraphs or the solving of arithmetic problems, they tend to be considerably below normal. This appears to be a direct consequence of their retardation in the language skills.

The rate of progress for deaf children varies from the norms of hearing children. For example, it takes a deaf child approximately two years to complete the second grade and one and a half years to cover third-grade material. This plateau in learning is discouraging to parents and children.

Educational achievement scores are influenced by the age at which the deaf child enters school, the amount of recreational reading, the amount and use of residual hearing, and the opportunities for problem solving.

LANGUAGE DEVELOPMENT

In teaching the deaf child we are greatly concerned with language training, and as this training progresses we expect an increase in the mental abilities that involve language. It would be very helpful if we had some measure of a deaf child's attainments in language, in order that we might better assess the results of our training. Unfortunately, there is at present no well-established test of language development that is applicable to deaf children. Several tests that are now being standardized may eventually serve this purpose.

Equally helpful would be a test of the *ability to learn* language. This would be of particular value in deciding whether a child's handicap is purely auditory (a peripheral deafness) or whether there is a central handicap in addition. The methods of teaching that are most efficient and appropriate for the child with peripheral deafness are quite beyond the abilities of the child with the aphasic type of handicap. At present we still rely chiefly on close observation, clinical ex-

perience, and the results of actual trial of one method of instruction
or the other.

The deaf child can learn, although with difficulty, to make use
of written language in a normal manner, but in face-to-face communication with other persons it is hard for him to overcome completely
the handicap imposed by his lack of hearing. Even though he can
understand words that are spoken to him, he may be unaware of the
emotional content of the speech, since this must often be judged solely
on the basis of the tone of voice used by the speaker. The deaf child
is restricted to judgments based on facial expressions, and he may thus
react inappropriately in many social situations. Another social handicap
is a difficulty in the production of intelligible speech. This may make
it difficult for him to participate in social situations with hearing people.
The ability to communicate adequately in social situations is not
measured by intelligence or achievement tests, but it is certainly an
important aspect of mental ability, and it is the responsibility of the
educator to develop this ability as fully as possible.

The mental growth of a child depends largely on the formation
of concepts about himself and his environment. The deaf child is
handicapped in forming any concepts that make use of sounds. His
concept of an "angry dog" may be distorted by the fact that he cannot
hear the growling of an angry dog, and his concept of the passage of
time never includes the sounds made by a clock. It is important for us
to study the nature of deafness itself and its effect on the behavior of
the person as a whole and not merely as a cause of inability to communicate verbally. At the present time investigations of factors that
influence the adjustment of persons with impaired hearing give little
insight into how deafness affects personality.

The Skills of Communication

It is obvious that the skills of speech, of understanding speech
(speechreading and "hearing"), and of language are interrelated in
their development. For convenience, however, and without slighting
the interrelationships, we shall consider separately the following topics
(treated generally in Chapters 12, 13, and 14): speech, auditory training, speechreading, and language.

Studies of the speech of deaf children have, by and large, dealt
with differences between the speech of the deaf and of normally hear-

ing subjects. By a technique of kymographic recording, Dr. C. V. Hudgins, at Clarke School for the Deaf, found the following abnormalities in the speech of the deaf: slow and labored speech, usually accompanied by high chest pressure with the expenditure of excessive amounts of breath; prolonged vowels with consequent distortion; abnormalities of rhythm; excessive nasality of both vowels and consonants; and imperfect joining of consonants with the consequent addition of superfluous syllables between abutting pairs.

We gain a substantial insight into the speech of the deaf from the investigation of Dr. Hudgins and F. C. Numbers, who departed from the usual approach of comparing the speech of the deaf and of the hearing and studied the relation between errors of articulation and rhythm and the intelligibility of the speech of deaf school children. Ten sentences spoken by deaf children were recorded and then were analyzed by a group of auditors. They found two general types of error: errors of articulation involving both consonants and vowels, and errors of rhythm.

Consonant errors were classified into seven general types, as follows: failure to distinguish between voice and breath consonants; consonant substitutions; excessive nasality; malarticulation of compound consonants; malarticulation of abutting consonants; omission of arresting consonants; and omission of releasing consonants.

The vowel errors were vowel substitutions; malarticulation of diphthongs; diphthongization of vowels; neutralization of vowels; and nasalization of vowels.

In general, our experimental and empirical evidence indicates that the deaf child who lacks an adequate auditory monitor is likely to develop, at least under present methods of instruction, a breathy, nasalized vocal quality, abnormal temporal patterns, and some surprisingly consistent errors of articulation. These observations do not imply that deaf children cannot be taught to speak intelligibly. Many do. They do, however, show where there is the greatest opportunity to improve our methods of teaching speech to deaf children.

Fundamental attitude. As we have indicated previously, all educators of the deaf endorse the proposition that all deaf children shall have an opportunity to learn to speak. But the implementation of this notion in everyday practice reveals fundamental differences in attitudes.

For some educators, speech is a subject to be taught like a foreign language to those who can "benefit" from it. Practice and atmosphere are not aimed at vitalizing speech for the child. Rather, speech is viewed as an eminently desirable but not essential skill to cultivate. For others (including ourselves), a corollary to the proposition of universality of opportunity to learn speech is inescapable: speech is a basic

means of communication and hence is a vital mechanism of adjustment
to the communicating world about us. Therefore, we set the stage for
the child *everywhere*—in the home, on the playground, in the schoolroom—from the moment we learn that he is deaf, so that speech eventually becomes meaningful, significant, and purposeful for him at all
times. We believe that parents, counselors, teachers, and all others who
are responsible for the child's development should share this attitude.
Only constant practice and actual use of speech will develop fully the
deaf child's latent ability to communicate by speech. The absence of
a "living speech environment" may account for some of the so-called
oral failures in schools for the deaf.

   The multisensory approach.   Obviously the teacher must use all
available sensory channels for teaching speech to a deaf child: the
visual, the auditory, the tactile, and the kinesthetic.

   When we consider the use to which we put the visual system in
teaching speech we tend to think primarily of speechreading. The
child learns to watch with purpose the movements of the lips and the
expressions of the faces of those about him and to imitate, however
imperfectly, these movements in attempts to express himself. This
really is the initial technique with deaf infants. In addition to speechreading, well-known uses of vision include systems of orthography,
color codes that differentiate the manner of production of phonetic
elements, models and diagrams that show position and movement of
the mechanisms of speech, and acoustic translators of various sorts that
display speech patterns visually and can carry information to the eye
about time, frequency, and intensity.

   We know that the literature even of the nineteenth century (Urbantschitsch, 1897) mentions the desirability of using the auditory
system to aid in teaching speech to the deaf. But today we are better
able to exploit this possibility because of the development of modern
wearable as well as group hearing aids designed to deliver speech to
the auditory area that the child still possesses. For the kind of child
whom we are here discussing the auditory area is greatly restricted,
but, as we have seen in Chapter 13, even a limited perception of stress
patterns can help a child achieve better rhythmic and voice quality and
better understand speech.

   The tactile or vibratory sense is most commonly used by placing
the child's fingertips or hands in contact with his own or the teacher's
face or head during speech or during phonation. We have mentioned
that some techniques use sounding boards, including pianos, and diaphragms which are caused to vibrate by speech and music. Surprisingly
good differential sensitivity of the thoracic region of severely deaf
children has been demonstrated. It has been suggested that transla-

tion of speech to the sense of touch by the principle of frequency analysis used in the visible-speech machine is possible. The argument is that the visible-speech instrument has shown how much and what kind of information must be transmitted to identify the words that are spoken. But rather than vision, the sense of touch is to be used. It is too early to assess the results of this approach, but it is unlikely, on general principles, that it will be any more successful than visible speech itself. (See Chapter 14.)

The kinesthetic sense is used in "getting the feel" of certain articulatory and vocal movements and in tongue and lip exercises. Some teachers employ rhythmic gross-muscle movements to reinforce kinesthetically the utterance of connected speech and of suitable nonsense syllables.

Many techniques to teach speech to the deaf are in common use. One reason for their variety is the wide difference of opinion concerning the relative emphasis that should be placed on each sensory pathway. Some believe that speech is better learned if attention is concentrated on one sense at a time and the others are deliberately excluded. The opposite view favors mutual reinforcement of the senses and a coordinated sensory input. In support of this view, it has been shown that a small fragment of hearing may be trained to supplement vision usefully in a visual-auditory presentation. In others words, the eye and the ear together perceive speech better than either one alone. Hence, it is argued, the bisensory approach is likely to produce better speech. The counterargument is that, at least in the early stages, speechreading should be excluded from auditory training because the speechreading is likely to divert the child from full use of his hearing. Shutting the eyes of the child while he is learning to differentiate vibrations has also been suggested.

In developing techniques, it is desirable for the teacher to analyze the speech skill she is trying to cultivate and to select the combination of sensory channels best suited to stimulate the child. For example, the perception of the phonetic element p is best accomplished through vision reinforced by feeling, and vowel differentiation is greatly aided by a combination of auditory, visual, and tactile stimulation. We believe that the sum of reinforced multisensory stimulation is greater than any of its parts. It is, in fact, "the nearest approach to the normal than can be made by the deaf child."

Systems of orthography. Students of speech are aware of the irrationality of our symbols for discrete units of speech. The letters of our alphabet bear no consistent relation to the sounds they represent. Furthermore, most of our symbols represent more than one sound and most of our sounds are represented by more than one symbol. This

CONSONANT SOUNDS

h——

wh   w——

p   b   m

t   d   n   l   r——

k   g̍   ng
ck
c

f   v
ph

t̍h   t̎h

s̍   z
c(e)   s̎
c(i)
c(y)

sh   zh   y——

ch   j   x = ks   qu = kwh
tch   g̎—
          —ge
          dge

Fig. 16-3(a). **The Northampton Consonant Chart.** In the consonant chart the left-hand column is occupied by the English breath consonants; the second column by the voiced forms of the same sounds; the third by the nasal sounds. The horizontal arrangement classifies these sounds according to formation. A dash following a letter indicates that the sound is initial in a word or syllable.

situation has led teachers of the deaf to devise systems of orthography that carry more information about speech units than do the unrelated letters of the alphabet.

The Bells created their system of visible speech in 1894. In this system consonants are represented by four fundamental curves that

VOWEL SOUNDS

$\overset{1}{\text{oo}}$	$\overset{2}{\text{oo}}$	o—e	aw	—o—
(r) u—e		oa	au	
(r) ew		$\overset{2}{\text{—o}}$	o(r)	
		ow		

ee	—i—	a—e	$\overset{}{\text{—e—}}$	—a—
—e	—y	ai	$\overset{2}{\text{ea}}$	
$\overset{1}{\text{ea}}$		ay		
e—e				

a(r)	—u—	ur
	—a	er
		ir

a—e	i—e	o—e	ou	oi	u—e
ai	igh	oa	$\overset{1}{\text{ow}}$	oy	ew
ay	–y	$\overset{2}{\text{—o}}$			
		ow			

Fig. 16-3(b). **The Northampton Vowel Chart.** In the vowel chart the upper line contains the back round vowels (those modified chiefly by the back of the tongue and the rounded aperture of the lips). The second line contains the front vowels (those modified chiefly by the front of the tongue). Remaining vowels are in the third line. The lowest line contains all the diphthongal sounds. Although ā and ō appear in the rows to which their radical (long component) parts belong, they are repeated here because their compound nature makes them diphthongs also.

An attempt is also made in these charts to teach the simple rules of pronunciation. For illustration, *a-e* (representing *ā*) when contrasted with *-a-* (representing *ă*), is easily made intelligible by the introduction of the same consonants in both sets of blanks: *rate, rat; hate, hat*, etc. Children will not find diacritical marks over the words in their books or in other material, but if they are familiar with the principles of pronunciation represented here, they will know that final *e* modifies the sound of the vowel preceding it, making *a, ā; e, ē; i, ī; o, ō*. The secondary spellings under each sound generally indicate frequently occurring variations of spellings for those sounds. Numbers above the sounds differentiate pronunciations for similar spellings. In this way words are made to pronounce themselves to the eye of the child. Eventually, the children learn the diacritical marks of the dictionary. (*Adapted from Caroline A. Yale, Formation and Development of English Elementary Sounds, Northampton, Mass., 1925, Gazette Printing Company.*)

relate to the "articulators," i.e., to the back of the tongue, the top of the tongue, the point of the tongue, and the lips. The insertion of a short "voice" line in the bow of the curve changes a voiceless consonant to a voiced consonant. For example, ꝗ (which is *k*) becomes ꝗ (which is *g*). There is also a system for modifying the fundamental symbols to represent the vowels. This system is described in the Bells' book, entitled *The Mechanism of Speech*.

The Northampton charts, originated at Clarke School for the Deaf and popular with many teachers of the deaf, are arranged to give more phonetic significance to letters of the English alphabet. The charts do this by arranging the symbols in columns and rows according to the method of production of the sounds. Thus the consonants *p*, *b*, and *m* are in the same row because the lips are initially shut in the production of all three. They are in different columns because *p* is voiceless, *b* is voiced, and *m* is nasal. This arrangement shows the differences and similarities among sounds that are described by Dr. Carhart in Chapter 14. The multiplicity of letters and combinations of letters that represent the same sound is handled by arranging second-ary spellings under the primary symbol, which is the one that occurs most frequently in English usage. Thus *a-e* is the primary symbol for the diphthong in "cake." Here the dash represents any consonant. A secondary spelling under *a-e* is *ay*, as in "say."

The diacritical system used in our dictionaries assumes familiarity with the pronounciation of common key words. Where one letter may represent more than one sound, a differentiating symbol is used; thus *e* as in "be" is ē, and *e* as in "bed" is ĕ.

Phoneticians and linguists generally use the International Phonetic Alphabet, which has a single standard symbol for each sound and adds new symbols to the Roman alphabet to provide the necessary extra symbols.

Dr. A. Zaliouk, Director of the Institute for the Deaf (in Haifa, Israel), has devised a "visual-tactile system of phonetic symbolization" for teaching speech to the deaf. This uses two categories of symbols, static and dynamic. The static symbols represent the hard palate, the tongue, the teeth, and the lips, all of which participate in various "ar-ticulatory positions." The dynamic symbols indicate movement.

There have been other attempts, too numerous to mention, that have sought through shorthand or other means to convey phonetic in-formation by a logical and consistent system of symbols. An ideal sys-tem of orthography would convey information on how to articulate, use the ordinary alphabet, be within the grasp of children, and be free of ambiguities. Obviously these criteria are in conflict and some compromises must be made. For example, if we were looking primarily for symbols to convey information on how to articulate, we would probably choose the system of Bell or of Zaliouk. The Northampton charts, with their secondary spellings, represent the letters and combinations of letters used most frequently in the English language, and hence should show how to pronounce the written word. On the other hand, because there are so many secondary spellings and exceptions, the learned combinations may be confusing out of the context of the chart. The diacritical markings of the dictionary are obviously useful, but everyday printed English does not carry these marks. One of the drawbacks of the International Phonetic Alphabet is that some of its symbols are not letters of the alphabet. Some teachers prefer to start children with the Northampton charts and then to teach the diacritical marks when children reach the appropriate academic level. These comments on the various systems are by no means exhaustive, but they may be useful as a guide in choosing a system of phonetic symbolization.

Units of speech. The various approaches to teaching articulation to the deaf may properly be placed on a continuum ranging from an elemental, analytical method to a patterned or "natural" approach. The former would emphasize the development of individual elements out of speech contexts and the latter would begin with words and phrases "as it is natural for hearing children to do." The elementalists argue that in the absence of an appropriate auditory monitor, the kinesthesia of each phonetic element must be fixed before precise articulation can be achieved, lest fluency be attained only at the expense of good articulation. The "naturalists" contend that we must take advantage of the spontaneous articulation, temporal patterns, and voice qualities of young children. These generally are not isolated elements, and the naturalists believe that precision *can* be achieved within the framework of natural spontaneous vocal output without sacrificing fluency.

Most present-day practice lies between these two extremes. It regards the syllable as the basic unit. The syllable is probably the simplest possible utterance in speech. Individual sounds cannot be uttered without somehow making a syllable. As Stetson, a great phonetician, expressed it, "when teachers and demonstrators give what they think are 'separate sounds' they are actually uttering syllables; the vowels and on occasion the liquids and nasals constitute separate syllables, as in 'oh, a, rr . . . , ll . . . ,' long drawn out fricatives, ss . . . etc., become vowel substitutes, and other consonants are given with a brief vowel, as in 'buh, puh' . . . ." Of course, individual sounds may be corrected but they should not be considered learned until they are articulated properly in the kinds of syllables in which they are likely to occur. Furthermore, speech rhythm, which contributes to intelligibility, is primarily a matter of grouping, accentuating, and phrasing syllables. The babbled syllable and the building of connected rhythmic speech from syllabic units are used in many methods for the development of speech.

In studies of the development of sounds in young normal-hearing children it has been shown that by the tenth month practically all of the different sounds have appeared. Yet it is curious that even though a child may have produced *l* and *r* during his infantile babbling, he frequently cannot at the age of two or three produce these sounds correctly in English words. Apparently he finds it difficult to use the phonetic elements of his babbling as the phonemes of his language. This relearning comes about by perceptive development, both auditory and kinesthetic, and in the case of the deaf child by whatever sensory channels are available.

Evaluation of speech. Frequent critical evaluation of the *intelligibility* of the speech of deaf children is important, both as a guide to modifying existing methods of teaching and, particularly, as an objective assessment of the oral method. Evaluations can be made periodically during the school career of a deaf child, during which he is exposed to formal training in speech by one method or another. Other long-range procedures could be designed to discover how intelligible the speech of deaf pupils continues to be after they have graduated from schools for the deaf.

A child's improvement in speech intelligibility may be evaluated by periodic tests, but the available tests are not as objective or as valid as our corresponding tests of many other skills or of a child's mastery of subject matter. In one popular procedure a child reads a selection and auditors indicate the extent to which the selection has been understood. Or carefully selected word samples are read and scored by the auditors. Although this may yield a limited but fairly reasonable appraisal of the child's speech mechanics, it does not simulate the pattern of usual oral intercourse which takes place without benefit of a printed or written visual aid. What is being evaluated is a form of *oral reading* and not speech in broad social terms. The translation of the child's *own* thoughts into intelligible speech is an ability neglected by this type of evaluation.

The use of memorized material without visual aid is subject to similar criticism, since the thoughts expressed usually are not the child's own; or, if they are, they have been memorized. This furnishes the child an advantage which he does not have in a normal social situation. The interview, in which the child is stimulated to talk freely, may yield a fairly accurate appraisal of speech if it is conducted skillfully. Very often in an interview, however, the child may correctly anticipate the questions; furthermore, the technique fails to appraise the child's ability to initiate speech. The use of speech recordings for periodic evaluation has considerable value. However, the limitations of read or memorized selections or the question-and-answer type of sample should be kept in mind. Of course, it would help to capture for study the casual conversation of children.

The outcomes of speech teaching which are most important in the long run are those that reveal the extent to which the benefits of the child's training in speech persist after he has left school. Unfortunately, we have no satisfactory evidence in this area, and the information that comes to us is frequently biased and invariably anecdotal. Good follow-up studies are a task which zealous oralists might profitably undertake.

Our discussion of teaching speech to the deaf suggests the following guides to practice:

1. An environment must be created or maintained for the child in which speech is experienced as a vitally significant and successful means of communication. Oralism is as much an atmosphere and an attitude as it is a "method" of teaching.

2. Spontaneity of speech should be encouraged, but formal instruction is necessary at the appropriate stage in a child's development. Good speech in deaf children does not come of itself.

3. The proper combination of the visual, auditory, tactile, and kinesthetic pathways should be exploited rationally and vigorously.

4. The syllable is a suitable unit for the development of articulation and of desirable temporal patterns in speech. Through its use, adequate coordination of parts of the speech mechanism is more likely to be achieved.

5. A functional system of orthography is essential.

6. Judicious correction of poor articulation, including individual phonetic elements, and of undesirable rhythm and voice quality is necessary. The acceptance of poor speech encourages its use. The teacher is the only monitor of the child's speech and she must let him know how he can improve it.

7. Periodic and long-range evaluations of the social effectiveness of the speech of the deaf, even though it be informal, is useful both for diagnosis and for educational planning.

Auditory training. The great advance in electroacoustic instrumentation of the past three decades, both for testing hearing and for amplifying sound, has generated a sustained and substantial interest in auditory training. We must remind ourselves that in this chapter we are concerned with children who have a severely restricted auditory area. The auditory area that remains to them, if any, lies at high sound pressure levels near the threshold of pain (see Chapter 2). These levels can be reached for communication only by means of powerful, well-designed hearing aids. Both group hearing aids and individual hearing aids have been described in Chapters 10 and 11. There we have pointed out the necessity for proper limitation of acoustic output and the advantages and limitations of compression amplification in "packaging" speech for effective delivery to the child's restricted auditory area. At best, however, the auditory information that the child receives is limited, and auditory training is necessary if he is to make full use of it.

Several objectives of auditory training are within reach of deaf children:

IMPROVEMENT IN SPEECH PERCEPTION. These children are not likely to achieve much auditory discrimination for speech, certainly not enough to understand ordinary language through hearing alone. However, they can be taught to appreciate temporal patterns of speech and also to improve their control of the intensity and, in some instances, the pitch of their own voices. Refined appreciation of phrasing and stress patterns may be expected to improve the child's ability to attain the "rhythmic grouping" which can contribute greatly to the intelligibility of his own speech. Auditory training improves speech perception, particularly when it is combined with speech-reading. Failure of improvement in communication by speech after a regime of auditory training may often be due to the fact that the training was not begun early enough. It should begin in the first year of life.

IMPROVEMENT IN LANGUAGE SKILLS. Although there is no definitive experimental evidence to indicate that auditory training improves language skills, it seems likely that the information carried by stressing and phrasing, not easily discerned by speechreading, adds to the meaning and significance of connected language. Vocabulary, particularly words with auditory associations, may be enriched. For example, if a child reads, "The baby cried," the word "cried," which has auditory connotations, has limited meaning for him even though he is able to draw a line between it and the word "baby" in his workbook and he has seen a picture of a baby crying. On the other hand, a recording of the cry of a baby played over an amplifying system, even though not perceived precisely, should enrich the meaning of the word "cry."

IMPROVEMENT IN PSYCHOLOGICAL COUPLING TO THE HEARING WORLD. Again, convincing experimental evidence is lacking. Nevertheless, consider the deaf child at a ball game. A thrilling play is made on the diamond that evokes a spontaneous outburst of yelling from the crowd. The child sees the hands clap and wave, the spectators rise from their seats, the mouths open, but he has not caught the full emotional impact of the moment because its basic richness lies in the yelling of the crowd and the accompanying noises. This is an auditory experience. If the child could perceive just the presence of these noises, however distorted, through a hearing aid he would be a richer sharer in the group experience. Not to be overlooked are the esthetic appreciations which may result from auditory exposure to the rhythm of music. Many deaf children who have been trained to appreciate rhythmic cadences seem to enjoy dancing and eurythmics.

Although it is likely that the future will reveal additional and greater values of auditory training, our statements of objectives within reach suggest that we must be cautious of the extravagant claims sometimes made for the use of hearing aids by deaf children, particularly the claim that if they are equipped from infancy with a hearing aid they do not need special education.

Dr. Carhart, in Chapter 13, has delineated the fundamental steps in auditory training for children.

Despite the unsolved problems that are still with us, there is no longer any question about the usefulness of the auditory system in the education of deaf children. Out of our experience grow the following guides for practice in auditory training:

1. Most deaf children have a small but useful portion of the auditory area that lies above the range of usual audiometry. Consequently, many children who have been termed "totally deaf" as a result of audiometric tests actually can hear properly amplified sound. Audiograms may not tell the whole story of a child's ability to appreciate speech by his hearing. Formal auditory training is essential, however, to teach the deaf child to make use of this remnant of hearing. The hearing aid alone is not enough.

2. Auditory training tends to be more effective, through mutual reinforcement, when hearing is combined with vision and/or touch. There are, of course, times when hearing alone is used in tests to assess a child's progress.

3. The techniques of auditory training should be geared to a child's auditory capabilities. This requires frequent assessment of his hearing.

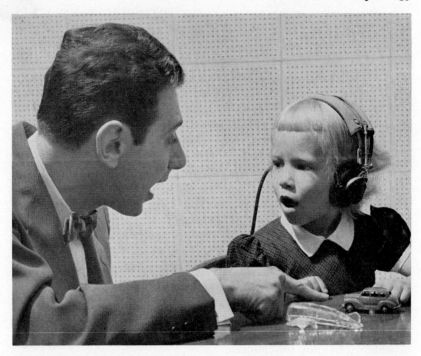

Fig. 16-4. Combining the auditory and visual approaches to teaching speech. (*Central Institute for the Deaf.*)

4. Auditory training, even without a hearing aid, should be begun as soon as it is determined that a child is deaf.

5. By teaching children to discriminate, even though grossly, various environmental sounds, and, within the limits of their hearing, by teaching them to understand speech by hearing, formal techniques aim to make hearing aids acceptable to children by giving them experiences that are meaningful.

6. Informally and wherever practical, the child should have the benefit of amplified sound in all of his classroom work, either by a group or a wearable hearing aid, at home and also at play.

7. Children should be taught as early as possible the use, the management, and the care of their own hearing aids.

SPEECHREADING

As we have said repeatedly, children with normal hearing learn oral language primarily by hearing, which is reinforced by other sensory experience. The sounds are later associated with the visual symbols, the movements of the talker's face, that partly represent language. This is speechreading. The deaf child is denied the possibility of learning this by association with auditory language, and is forced to learn his visual speechreading language directly. The extent to which he is able to do this may depend upon a number of factors, some of which are exceedingly complex and difficult to analyze. One group of factors concerns the speaker. These include his distance and position and how well his face is illuminated. They include the character of his speech, his precision of articulation, how fast he talks, his use of sectional expressions, the mobility of his face, and the familiarity of the speechreader with the particular speaker. Then there are factors concerning the language material, such as the vocabulary and the language structure. Finally, there is the speechreader himself, his vision, his intelligence, his general information, and his ability to synthesize from contextual clues, his ability to recognize discrete units of speech, his ability to associate his own "feel" for speech with the speech he sees on the face, and the fundamental structure of his personality which may determine his attitude toward speechreading.

Speechreading is further complicated by the ambiguities that result from hidden movements, such as *h* and *k*, from homophenous words (words that look alike on the lips, such as "smell" and "spell"), and from the difficulty of appreciating patterns of stress, intonation, and phrasing.

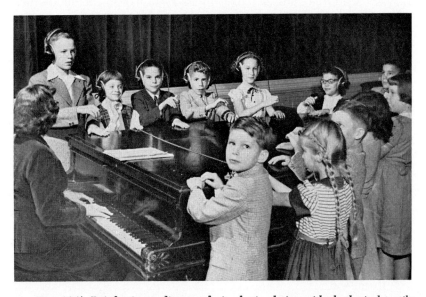

Fig. 16-5. Reinforcing auditory and visual stimulation with rhythmical tactile impressions from the piano. This procedure helps the fluency of speech. (*Central Institute for the Deaf.*)

Numerous attempts have been made to assess the role of these factors in speechreading with a view to diagnosis of difficulties, to evaluation of progress and of methods of instruction, and to prediction of performance.

Among the possible factors that may be related to skill in speechreading, and which have been investigated, are intelligence, reading ability, and rhythmic skills. These studies have led to no generalizations in which we have confidence. One of the major problems in studying these relations is the adequacy of tests of speechreading. The test constructers are faced with formidable variables that are unique to the population to be tested. Among these are the degree and kind of hearing loss, the time of onset of impaired hearing, the language ability of the subjects, the standardization of the test material itself and particularly of the manner of its presentation, and the difficulty of establishing norms for a heterogeneous population. Furthermore, the validation of the tests appears to rely solely on teacher ratings, a fact which introduces new problems.

Instruction in speechreading for deaf children is usually not a thing apart. In the beginning, even before the child enters school, he is encouraged to watch the face of the talker. The deaf child is not as aware as the hearing child that he can get information, in its broadest sense, by watching the movements of the face. When formal instruction is begun, the child is taught to associate movements of the lips, jaws, and tongue with objects, feelings, and actions. The objective here is not merely the enlargement of speechreading vocabulary but cultivation of the idea that watching the face of the talker is useful. Finally, speechreading pervades every act of speech perception of the child and becomes an increasingly useful tool of communication as it is practiced in purposeful situations.

The inadequacy of our formal tools for assessment of the ability to speech-read need not deter us from suggesting the following guides to practice in developing this valuable skill in deaf children:

1. An atmosphere of oral communication must be created and maintained. Speechreading must be shown to serve a purpose.

2. Even if the child is not expected to understand every word of a spoken message, he should be talked to and he should be encouraged to take advantage of situational clues.

3. Speechreading should be reinforced by other sensory clues whenever practical.

LANGUAGE

In our discussion of the skills of communication to this point we have, in a sense, considered the development of the skills of talking

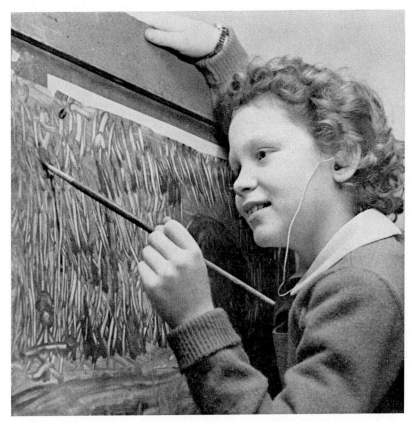

Fig. 16-6. Art is an excellent medium of expression for deaf children. (*Central Institute for the Deaf.*)

and "listening," namely, speech, auditory training, and speechreading. We now turn to the message itself, the stuff of oral communication. This is language. The "ear-to-voice link" is essential for talking and listening. It is the basis of a child's attachment of meaning, in speaking, in writing, in listening, and in reading, to words and combination of words. The absence of hearing is catastrophic for the "natural" and complex development of association of language with experience.

It is the task of the teacher, nevertheless, to develop language in deaf children although they do not have full use of the sensory channel that is considered essential for the growth of language. In the performance of this task she needs to be aware of the unique problems created by the total absence of hearing or by the severe distortions of auditory verbal experience. Among the major problems for the child

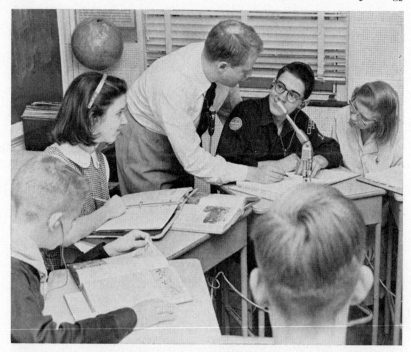

Fig. 16-7. A class in social studies. Note the Y-cord hearing aid on the student and the "necktie" microphone on the instructor. (*Central Institute for the Deaf.*)

are vocabulary, multiple meanings of words, the verbalization of abstractions, and the complexity of the structure of language.

VOCABULARY. It is difficult to determine when a child really "knows" a word. Is it in his spoken, written, reading, or listening vocabulary? This accounts for differences in the estimates of the functional vocabulary of children. At any rate, it is interesting that one representative study shows that hearing children "know" 272 words at the age of two, 1540 at four, and 2562 at six.[7] Compare this with zero words that the deaf child is likely to know when he enters school, even at the age of three or, more frequently, at six.

MULTIPLE MEANINGS. Single words in our language may have many meanings that are eventually clarified for hearing children, chiefly by the repeated auditory experience that is denied the deaf child. An average of almost four meanings per recurring word was found by count in twelve commonly used arithmetic textbooks. For

[7] M. E. Smith, "An Investigation of the Development of the Sentence and the Extent of Vocabulary of Young Children." *University of Iowa Studies in Child Welfare,* Vol. III, No. 5, 1936.

example, the word "over" could mean "above" (the number over 5 is the quotient); "across" (over the Arctic Ocean); "again" (do your work over); "at an end" (the show is over); "more than" (over half the children); "besides" (left over); "during" (over a period of two years); "present" (turn the meeting over to); "on the other side" (turn the card "over"); "by means of" (over the radio).

VERBALIZATION OF ABSTRACTIONS. Of course, hearing children and, for that matter, adults may experience difficulty in attaching words to abstract concepts, but the deaf child is in particular need of formal and informal but nonetheless deliberate instruction in the meaning of such relatively simple abstractions as *hope* and *want*.

COMPLEXITY OF STRUCTURE. Smith has shown that by the age of five the spoken sentence of the average child has reached five words in length. For the superior child it is about ten words long. This increase in length is inevitably accompanied by the use of complex syntactical relations that clarify and enrich meaning. These involve such grammatical concepts as pronouns, connectives, tense, person, and word order, as well as relations among clauses and among phrases of various sorts. If the hearing child reaches these levels of complexity at the age of five, we are again struck by the extent of the language gap between the deaf and the hearing. It was found by the Heiders at Clarke School, after their thorough comparison of sentence structure in the written compositions of deaf and hearing children, that the "whole picture indicates a simpler style [for the deaf] involving relatively rigid unrelated language units which follow each other with little overlapping structure or meaning."

In general, the deaf appear to be comparatively deficient in the flexible manipulation of our language to make the best use of it as a tool of communication. This may be due to their educational retardation, which has been variously estimated as ranging from two to five years; it may be due to the methods of teaching language, or, in addition to these, to the idea suggested by the Heiders that "the difference between the deaf and the hearing cannot be fully expressed in quantitative terms as the degree of retardation and that they represent differences not merely of skill in the use of language forms but in the whole thought structure."

METHODS OF INSTRUCTION IN LANGUAGE. Methods of instruction of the deaf in language can be divided conveniently into two major approaches: the natural method, sometimes known as the synthetic, informal, or mother method; and the grammatical method, sometimes referred to as the logical, systematic, formal, analytical, or artificial method.

Historically, the grammatical method preceded the natural

method. It was based on the notion that after memorization of classifications of words and their conjugations and declensions, they could be used as building blocks for connected language. This approach evolved into a multiplicity of "systems" that were created primarily to provide a systematic set of visible symbols to guide deaf children in the use of language. We shall briefly describe the more popular ones.

1. *The Barry Five-Slate System.* The assumption underlying this system, developed by Katherine E. Barry (1899) at the Colorado School for the Deaf, is that ability to analyze the relations among parts of sentences is necessary to the "clear thinking" essential to an understanding of language. Five slates or columns are visible on the walls of the schoolroom. The subject of a sentence goes on the first slate, the verb on the second, the object of the verb on the third, the preposition on the fourth, and the object of the preposition on the fifth. Children then learn the rationale of the verbalization of their actions according to the visual aid afforded by the slates. This system, many believe, tends to stultify idiomatic expression and actually may result in ungrammatical, stilted language.

2. *Wing's Symbols.* This system, devised in 1883 by George Wing of the Minnesota School for the Deaf, is based on a set of symbols, mostly numbers and letters, representing the functions of different parts of speech in a sentence. These symbols are placed over the word, phrase, or clause in order to demonstrate the form, function, and position of the parts of a sentence, rather than just to illustrate parts of speech. For example, *1* stands for the noun, *2* for a possessive, and *0* for the object. Advocates of the system believe that it is of great value as a corrective tool throughout the child's career and that it encourages correct grammatical usage.

3. *The Fitzgerald Key.* This system, first published in 1926, was developed by Edith Fitzgerald (1937), a congenitally deaf person, when she was head teacher at the Virginia School. Miss Fitzgerald advocated developing "natural" language but felt that this could be aided by developing the child's power of reasoning, judgment, and discrimination about language. This is accomplished by a set of key words and symbols related to language that was developed as it was needed by the children. There are six symbols, one each for verbs, infinitives, present participles, connectives, pronouns, and adjectives. For example, the symbol for a verb is $=$. Among the advantages of the method are its comprehensiveness, its flexibility, and the possibilities for self-correction.

The basic feature of the grammatical systems is the emphasis on getting the child to *analyze* functional relations among discrete units of language and, by repetition and visual aids, to impart to him an understanding of language principles, including how the arrangement of words affects the meaning of a sentence.

One of the early advocates of the natural method was D. Greenberger, who headed what is now the Lexington School for the Deaf in New York City. He felt that language was best learned by supplying it to children in the situations in which they had need for it. Practice was geared to actual and natural situations. A leading advocate of this approach is Dr. Mildred Groht, who suggests that prior to the time a language principle is to be introduced formally it should be used in natural situations through speechreading and writing. It is then drilled on in various ways that are interesting and purposeful for the child. In essence, the teacher creates situations which provide many and varied contacts with the principles of language. The method is claimed to be more consistent with the laws of learning of language by hearing children than is a formal, analytical method.

Until we gain more insight into how the deaf child conceptualizes, the teacher of language will need to use all the knowledge and ingenuity at her command to combine the best features of a grammatical method with the obvious excellent possibilities of the natural method. She will use such commonly accepted techniques as general conversation, composition, news items, trips, action work, topical essays, experience stories, letters, and descriptions of places, events, and persons. The child's progress in acquiring language will be governed only by the extent to which the teacher uses her own ingenuity, flexibility, and knowledge of how children grow and develop. Perhaps she may find some help in the following guides to practice:

1. Language teaching should be related to significant and meaningful experiences of children.

2. Language should constantly be made to serve a purpose for the child.

3. All sensory channels should be used to teach language.

4. Teachers need to be alert to the ideas that are developing in children so that they may provide the children with language with which to express them.

5. Children need many varied contacts with the same language in order to make it theirs.

6. Many children need formal, systematic aids to the acquisition of language. Many shun language when they feel insecure in its use.

7. Schools and homes should create an atmosphere where language is used and where books are read regularly.

In general, curriculums, textbooks, and other teaching materials of schools for the deaf resemble those used in schools for the hearing, with appropriate adaptations for difficulties of verbal communication. There are also the usual provisions for instruction in art, physical education, and vocational subjects. Special textbooks for the deaf in reading and in content subjects have practically disappeared from the educational scene.

The outlook for the aphasic child, discussed in Chapters 4 and 8, who may or may not have a hearing loss and who may be mistaken for a mentally retarded child, is encouraging. According to Mildred McGinnis, who has had many years of experience with this type of child at Central Institute for the Deaf, temper tantrums and extreme negativism often characterize the behavior of aphasic children. The quality of their voices in crying and babbling and their responses to some environmental sounds indicate that they can actually hear. A poor memory span for speech is characteristic. This poor memory for speech and lack of understanding of language prevent the aphasic child from profiting by the usual methods of instruction for the deaf. When placed in a school for the deaf, he is often classified as mentally retarded; in some schools he may be transferred to the manual department; and from still other schools he may be sent to an institution for the feeble-minded.

Associations through every sensory channel must be employed in developing an aphasic child's understanding. Behavior improves with understanding, and the child begins to use his hearing when speech becomes meaningful. Given normal intelligence, early diagnosis, and education begun at least by the age of four, rehabilitation is possible sooner for him than for a deaf child.

Problems of Parents

In concluding our chapter on deaf children it is fitting to return to the problems of parents.

When parents become aware that their child is deaf, their initial reaction is one of profound grief. It is not pleasant to hear that one's child is deaf and that it is hopeless to expect a restoration of his hearing. Unfortunately, some parents refuse far too long to face the fact squarely. They begin a pilgrimage from one doctor to another, always hoping for a miracle and still not heeding advice about the necessity for special education. Instead, they may squander funds and waste valuable nursery school years grasping for any and every "cure" they read about, from airplane rides to surgery.

Other parents surround the deaf child with an overwhelming, protective "love" as soon as deafness is recognized. They want to do everything for the child to compensate for his deprivation; they dress him, feed him, and amuse him, and shield him from contacts with other children. He is thereby deprived of opportunities for normal development, and his education is delayed.

Sooner or later all parents realize, as many do at the very first, that special education is necessary; but here they are naturally bewildered. "My child is deaf, but what do I do next?" Otologists, educators, and audiologists can help the parent make the educational arrangements best suited to the child's needs. Children differ, schools differ, communities differ. No single answer is correct for all deaf children in all places. We have outlined some of the principles of education for the deaf child, but the actual choice of a particular school is often a difficult problem.

Finally, however, a school for the deaf child is selected, and now comes the "long pull" for the parents, the extended period of learning how to work most effectively with the school throughout their child's educational career. Parents are more apt to enter willingly on this third and important stage of their evolving attitude if they realize that their earlier grief and bewilderment have been recognized, sympathetically understood, and met with kind, clear, but not too insistent, counsel. Here a heavy responsibility lies upon the school: first, to recognize the nature of the strong emotions that surround the relationship of the parents with their deaf child; secondly, to develop home cooperation by sending constructive and informative reports and by encouraging the parents to make frequent visits to the classroom.

Parents must seize upon every opportunity at home for the child to employ and practice the speech and the speechreading that he has learned at school. They can assist materially in the developing and correcting of the child's speech, in enriching his vocabulary, and in translating his experiences into meaningful language. If the child is at a residential school, contacts with home should be maintained by letters and photographs. News from home is very essential to the deaf child's happiness. Reports from the teachers and at least an annual visit keep the parents informed concerning the child's progress.

As the deaf child reaches adolescence, his basic needs are the same as those of other children. He must soon be ready to earn money, to make decisions, to associate with the opposite sex, and to compete socially with the hearing. The schools and the home must prepare the deaf child for this broader environment.

Teachers, parents, and school executives must again cooperate in the selection of a school for further education or for vocational training after the boy or girl is graduated from the school for the deaf. Once more, many variables affect the decision: the age of the child, his intelligence, his academic record, his interests and skills, schools available to him, and the vocational opportunities in his community. Generally speaking, a small school for hearing children in the home community is the best selection. Parents should also make a sincere effort to help the deaf child make friends in his home community.

When the parents are able to observe the fruits of their long labors, they experience the comforting satisfaction that their efforts, augmenting those of the school, have played a tremendously significant role in the happy adjustment of their child. And on the part of the school, no Pollyanna philosophy but an attitude of realistic understanding of the parents' problem has facilitated the arduously long process of adjustment. Parents should not overlook their debt to the teachers, whose wisdom, patience, and understanding have made possible the deaf child's development and growth.

Suggested Readings

BARKER, R. G., B. A. WRIGHT, L. MYERSON, and M. R. GONICK. "Adjustment to Physical Handicap and Illness: A Survey of the Social Psychology of Physique and Disability." Bulletin 55. New York: Social Science Research Council, 1953.
   Contains a critical analysis of investigations dealing with psychological adjustment of the deaf and hard of hearing.
BERLINSKY, S. "Measurement of the Intelligence and Personality of the Deaf: A Review of the Literature," *Journal of Speech and Hearing Disorders,* XVII (1952), 39–55.
EWING, A. W. G., ed. *Educational Guidance and the Deaf Child.* Washington, D.C.: The Volta Bureau, 1957.
   A summary of experiments at Manchester University in England relating to the education of deaf children from infancy through school age.
EWING, I. R., and A. W. G. EWING. *Speech and the Deaf Child.* Washington, D.C.: The Volta Bureau, 1954.
   An analysis of the principles guiding instruction in speech for the deaf.
GROHT, M. *Natural Language for Deaf Children.* Washington, D.C.: The Volta Bureau, 1958.
   Exposition of the "natural method" of teaching language to deaf children by a prominent teacher.
HAYCOCK, G. S. *The Teaching of Speech.* Washington, D.C.: The Volta Bureau, 1942.

A systematic set of procedures for teaching speech to the deaf. Contains helpful suggestions for correcting faulty speech.

HEIDER, F. K., and G. M. HEIDER. "A Comparison of Sentence Structure of Deaf and Hearing Children," in *Psychological Monographs,* No. 232. Studies in the Psychology of the Deaf. Columbus: American Psychological Association, 1940, pp. 42–103.
An investigation that analyzes the differences in structural features of language between deaf and hearing children.

HUDGINS, C. V., and F. C. NUMBERS. "An Investigation of the Intelligibility of Speech of the Deaf," *Genetic Psychology Monographs,* 25: 289–392 (1942).
An analysis of errors of articulation and temporal patterns in the speech of deaf children.

LACK, A. *The Teaching of Language to Deaf Children.* London: Oxford University Press, 1955.
Systematic step-by-step procedures for teaching language to deaf children. Contains many specific suggestions for correlating spoken and written language.

LASSMAN, G. *Language for the Preschool Deaf Child.* New York: Grune & Stratton, Inc., 1951.
Helpful suggestion for fostering language in the very young deaf child. Good for parents and teachers.

MCGINNIS, M. S., F. R. KLEFFNER, and R. GOLDSTEIN. "Teaching Aphasic Children," *Volta Review,* 58: 239–244 (1956).
Principles and techniques used at Central Institute for the Deaf for teaching aphasic children.

SILVERMAN, S. R. "Clinical and Educational Procedures for the Deaf," in *Handbook of Speech Pathology,* L. Travis, ed. New York: Appleton-Century-Crofts, Inc., 1957, Chap. 10.
A comprehensive exposition of the education of the deaf in the United States. Contains an extensive bibliography.

SMITH, M. E. "An Investigation of the Development of the Sentence and the Extent of Vocabulary of Young Children." *University of Iowa Studies in Child Welfare,* Vol. III, No. 5, 1936.

STRENG, A. "On Improving the Teaching of Language," *American Annals of the Deaf,* 103: 553–563 (1958).
Suggestions for teachers in improving the teaching of language to the deaf based on principles from the psychology of learning and from linguistics.

TERVOORT, B. T. "Acoustic and Visual Language Communicating Systems," *Volta Review,* 60: 374–380 (1958).
An exposition of the linguistic grammatical and syntactical problems of the deaf child from the point of view of a linguist.

WEDENBERG, E. "Auditory Training of Deaf and Hard-of-Hearing Children," *Acta Oto-Laryngologica,* 1951, Supp. 94, 1–129.
A set of suggested principles to guide auditory training in deaf and hard-of-hearing children and an investigation of the application of these principles.

YALE, C. A. *Formation and Development of Elementary English Sounds.* Northampton, Mass.: Gazette Printing Co., 1925.
A description and principles of the Northampton charts.

ZALIOUK, A. "A Visual-Tactile System of Phonetical Symbolization," *Journal of Speech and Hearing Disorders,* 19: 190–207 (1954).

17

HARD-OF-HEARING CHILDREN

S. R. Silverman, Ph.D.

This chapter deals with children whose hearing impairments are mild enough for them to learn without great difficulty to communicate by speech and hearing. The distinction between these hard-of-hearing children and those whom we have called the deaf is not always entirely clear. The reason is that individual children may differ greatly in the use that they are able to make of the remainder of their hearing. It is not simply a matter of the hearing level for speech but also of such different factors as the age of onset, of the severity and the exact type of hearing loss, the intelligence of the child, the amount of training that the child has had, and, particularly, the age at which the training was begun. It is a matter also of the attitude of parents and their degree of understanding of the significance of the hearing impairment.

Even within the broad group of the hard of hearing there is a wide range of the ability to make use of hearing for communication by speech. As we have seen in Chapter 9, the relatively mild hearing losses with hearing levels for speech of less than 30 db cause only a little handicap, except perhaps for faint speech or for hearing at a distance. At the other extreme, with hearing levels for speech of 60 db or thereabouts and particularly if the hearing loss was congenital or of early onset, the child may require painstaking instruction to learn to hear adequately, even with a hearing aid, and to understand and use language. Furthermore, the impairment of hearing is often not merely a loss of sensitivity that may be overcome by amplification, but may involve also a loss of ability to discriminate between certain sounds. Such a failure of discrimination is common when there is a great loss of sensitivity for the high frequencies.

Just as there are gradations in the usefulness of hearing, so there

452

are gradations in the quality and intelligibility of the speech of hard-of-hearing children. Many hard-of-hearing children speak so well that the lay observer notices no abnormality, whereas the severely impaired may be almost unintelligible to those who are not accustomed to this type of speech.

Many investigators have sought to define the relations of these various factors of hearing impairment: intelligence, personality, emotional stability, social behavior, and the like. Our best generalization from their studies is that it is impossible to draw a *single* composite picture of the hard-of-hearing child. There is too much variation, both in the severity of the hearing impairment and in the many other pertinent factors. The personality structure of a child with hearing impairment is determined by many factors other than his difficulty in hearing.

In this chapter we shall describe the hard-of-hearing child particularly in terms of his ability to understand speech, his ability to progress in school, and the extent to which these abilities are affected by his hearing loss. In making generalizations about the significance of various degrees of hearing impairment we shall assume that the hearing loss occurred before the child acquired speech and learned to use language. Obviously, if speech and language are acquired before the hearing loss occurs, the handicap imposed by the loss is much less severe. Hence the age of onset of the hearing impairment is an important factor.

Hard-of-hearing children may be usefully divided into five classes, depending on their hearing levels for speech. These levels may be estimated quite accurately, as pointed out in Chapter 9, by averaging the hearing levels for pure tones at 500, 1000, and 2000 cps.

> Class 1: Hearing level for speech better than 30 db. These children may have difficulty in hearing faint or distant speech but are likely to "get along" in school and to have normal speech.
> Class 2: Hearing level for speech between 30 and 45 db. These children usually understand conversational speech at a distance of three to five feet without great difficulty. They may have some defects in the articulation of their own speech and they may have difficulty in hearing adequately in school if the talker's voice is faint or if his face is not visible to them.
> Class 3: Hearing level for speech between 45 and 60 db. These children understand conversational speech only if it is loud, and they have considerable difficulty in group and classroom discussions. Their language and, especially, their vocabularies may be limited, and abnormalities of articulation and voice production are obvious.
> Class 4: Hearing level for speech between 60 and 80 db. These children may hear the sound of a loud voice about one foot from the

ear and they may identify some environmental noises and may distinguish vowels, but, even with hearing aids, they have difficulty with consonants. The quality of their voices is not entirely normal and they must be taught both speech and language. Many, but not all, children in this class should be considered "deaf" for educational purposes until or unless the combination of an adequate hearing aid and sufficient auditory training makes them only "hard of hearing."

Class 5: Hearing level for speech 80 db or worse. These children are deaf, even though they may hear some very loud sounds. They never can rely on the auditory channel as a primary avenue of communication. Their speech and their language must both be developed through careful and extensive training.

The hearing levels that mark the divisions of these classes are substantially the same as those formulated by the Committee on Hearing of the National Research Council and presented in Chapter 9. It will be noted that a hearing level of 80 rather than 90 decibels is here chosen as the level dividing the fifth from the fourth class. This choice agrees well with a more recent definition of "100 per cent hearing impairment" for medicolegal purposes and discussed in Chapter 9. The scale given by the Committee on Hearing also subdivides what is here the first class into "normal" and "near normal." For the purposes of the present chapter, however, we have grouped all of these children together because they are all likely to "get along" in school and to have normal speech.

The Significance of the Problem

The problem of the hard-of-hearing child is one of serious social significance.

Specifically, the community should feel a concern for the unfortunate financial and social effects of the retardation in school of children whose handicap has been neglected or not recognized. The average annual cost per capita for school children in the United States is approximately $340. Obviously, the repetition of grades is costly, and, in the long run, it is only a grossly superficial remedy which leaves the root of the problem quite untouched.

To those public school authorities and taxpayers who view with alarm the financial outlay necessary for a really constructive program for the hard-of-hearing child we may point out that the saving from avoiding repetition of grades offsets a large part of the cost of the program. In addition, we must reckon the cost of truancy and various forms of antisocial behavior which characterizes the child who becomes bored with the schoolwork in which it is so difficult for him to participate.

But the financial aspects of the problem must in no way obscure the solemn moral obligation of every American community to provide for each child the opportunity to develop according to his maximum potentialities. This is the fundamental principle of our system of democratic education, and the community that shirks responsibility for an adequate program for the physically handicapped child stands guilty of its violation.

In the smaller community of the schoolroom itself the teacher is often not aware that the learning or behavior difficulty of a hard-of-hearing child is due to his impaired hearing and not to lack of mental ability or to some fault in her methods of teaching. Failure to understand the basic cause of the child's difficulties frequently leads to fruitless remedial measures that are time consuming for both the child and his classmates. And when by good fortune the teacher recognizes the child's hearing impairment, her lack of special training and information and the requirements of other children in the room make quite impossible any adequate solution of the child's particular problem.

In the narrower confines of the family circle, too, the hard-of-hearing child presents a problem that requires wholesome and sympathetic understanding. Apparent inattention to the spoken word is often interpreted as sheer naughtiness. The misdirected punishment often results in tensions within the family which would be avoided if the parents were only aware of their child's handicap. Furthermore, repetition of grades in school delays the day when the child can become a self-supporting individual. In many families the prolonged dependence is a serious problem.

The desirability of testing hearing losses early by various methods of screening audiometry and individual hearing tests, as well as the possibility of conserving hearing by proper diagnosis and by treatment of the medical conditions that are so disclosed, has been discussed in Chapters 4 and 7. In detecting hearing losses in children, informal procedures and simple intelligent observation can be of great value. Both teachers and parents should be informed of the clues in a child's behavior that suggest the possibility of a hearing loss. The symptoms include inattention, frequent requests for repetition of spoken words, cupping the hand to the ear, cocking the head, difficulty in copying dictation, indifference to music, abnormalities of speech, reluctance to participate in activities that require oral communication, such as dramatics, failure to follow oral directions, daydreaming, and poor scholarship. Not to be overlooked are truancy, lying, stealing, extreme introversion, and other forms of a typical behavior that frequently serve as compensations for the child who feels socially inadequate and wishes to attract attention to himself. Of course, such behavior may also depend on a host of other conditions. We merely note that the possibility of hearing impairment as a cause should not be overlooked by teachers or laymen. Medical indications, such as earache, bad tonsils, frequent colds, and so on, have already been discussed in Chapter 4.

Educational Needs and Procedures

The educational needs of the hard-of-hearing child are different from those of the deaf child discussed in the preceding chapter. The hard-of-hearing child can learn to talk and to understand speech and to learn language by more nearly natural means and relying primarily on his sense of hearing. Furthermore, if his difficulties are recognized and if he is given proper assistance, his needs may well be met in a special class for the hard of hearing within the public school system, or even in the regular classroom itself. The assignment to a particular class will depend both upon his hearing level and on the availability of special help. The aim should be to educate him with normal-hearing children wherever this is practical.

The particular needs of hard-of-hearing children may be summarized as follows, according to their classification by hearing level for speech:

Class 1: Better than 30 db. These children should be given the benefit of favorable seating in regular classrooms and may be assisted by special instruction in speechreading.

Class 2: 30 to 45 db. These children should wear hearing aids and be given training in their use. They should be taught speechreading and also be given the benefit of speech correction and conservation of speech. They should also have the advantage of favorable seating in classrooms.

Class 3: 45 to 60 db. Hearing aids and auditory training, special training in speech, and special language work are all essential. With such assistance and with favorable seating, some children can continue in regular classes. Others may derive more benefit from special classes.

Class 4: 60 to 80 db. These children should be taught by means of educational procedures for the deaf child which were described in the preceding chapter, with special emphasis on speech, on auditory training, and on language. After a period of such instruction it is possible that these children may enter classes in regular schools.

Class 5: Worse than 80 db. These are deaf children who require the special educational procedures described in the preceding chapter. Some of these children, however, eventually enter high schools for the hearing.

In Chapters 12, 13, and 14 Dr. Pauls and Dr. Carhart have acquainted us with the principles and techniques of speechreading, auditory training, speech correction, and conservation of speech that are suitable for hard-of-hearing children. Special help in these aids to communication may be available through a special class, an itinerant teacher, or a speech-and-hearing center of a hospital or university, or in one of the chapters of the American Hearing Society.

Guidance

Certainly we must not overlook the need for psychological, educational, and vocational guidance which should avert or eliminate the atypical forms of behavior that frequently characterize the hard-of-hearing child. He must be made to understand that speechreading lessons and his hearing aid are as necessary as geography, arithmetic, or any other school activity. In fact, they may be more so. He should be particularly encouraged to join in extracurricular and community activities, such as scouting, athletics, Hi-Y, 4-H, church functions, and other wholesome pastimes of youth. Success in any of these activities should do much to avert extreme introversion and preoccupation with the impairment of hearing. Of course, extreme cases should be referred for psychiatric study. Vocational plans for the child should take into account the existence of hearing impairment. Obviously, we would not suggest preparation for any calling which demands a high degree of accuracy in oral communication. We are too well aware of the psychological distress which inevitably accompanies a trying occupational situation. Bookkeeping, for example, would be preferable to stenography. On the other hand, vocational guidance should stress the child's assets and not his liabilities. There are many occupations at all levels in which hearing impairment is not a barrier to success.

Throughout our discussion we have implied, and it is well now to stress, that, although the welfare of the hard-of-hearing child should be entrusted to specially trained personnel, all remedial measures should be carried out within the framework of the regular school and health system. It is psychologically and educationally desirable that the child should not be prevented from associating with children who hear normally. True, he must be segregated for speechreading lessons and auditory training, but these activities should be considered part of his school program. In fact, we suggest that academic credit be given for participation in such classes, since, for the hard-of-hearing child, they involve the development of communication skills as important as composition or public speaking. They should be so recognized and integrated with the curriculum. When the child is convinced that he is a normal boy or girl with a particular need that has been recognized, he has hurdled the chief obstacle to his eventual adjustment.

In summary, the management of hard-of-hearing children requires

1. Public information about hearing impairment
2. Case-finding through appropriate screening programs in clinics for babies and in schools
3. Complete medical diagnosis of hearing difficulties
4. Appropriate medical and surgical treatment
5. Thorough assessment of hearing after all indicated medical and surgical procedures have been completed, with particular attention to educational needs
6. Special educational measures that include auditory training, speechreading, speech correction and conservation of speech, vocational planning, and psychological guidance

Suggested Readings

HARDY, W. G. *Children with Impaired Hearing.* Children's Bureau Publication No. 326. Washington, D.C.: Government Printing Office, 1952.

A comprehensive statement on the modern management of children with impaired hearing particularly from the public health point of view.

JORDAN, R. C. Moderator. "Symposium: Deafness in Children—Knowledge and Practice," *Transactions of the American Academy of Ophthalmology and Otolaryngology,* 61: 706–727 (1957).

The subtitles are "Evaluation of Hearing in Preschool Children," "Problems of Testing and Managing Children with Communication Difficulties," "Otosurgical Developments and the Hard of Hearing Child," and "Nonmedical Care of Children with Hearing Impairment."

SILVERMAN, S. R. "Clinical and Educational Procedures for the Hard of Hearing," in *Handbook of Speech Pathology,* L. Travis, ed. New York: Appleton-Century-Crofts, Inc., 1957, Chap. 11.

18

THE PSYCHOLOGY OF THE HARD-OF-HEARING AND THE DEAFENED ADULT

D. A. Ramsdell, Ph.D.

Anyone who has closely observed an adult soon after he has lost his hearing has noted that he becomes discouraged and struggles with feelings of depression. Sometimes he even becomes suspicious of friends and family. In order to understand the psychology of the deaf, it is necessary to understand why this personality change occurs and why it does not occur with equal severity in children who are born deaf or in those who become blind.

That loss of hearing does tend to result in this peculiar and serious personality change has long been known, but the reason for the change is not obvious. The depression is usually more serious than we should expect from the loss of easy two-way communication, particularly if we recall that the adult has already learned to talk, to read, and to write before the onset of deafness. Nor is the depression prevented by prompt instruction in speechreading, although this assistance to communication is both desirable and helpful.

A study of the reactions of soldiers who lost their hearing in World War II has shown that the loss of communication is not the deaf man's only or most serious loss. Deafness produces a psychological impairment more basic and more severe than the difficulty in communication. The characteristic depression is caused by this more subtle impairment. Recognition and understanding of the cause are necessary if the depression is to be overcome and not attributed, as is so often the case, to a character weakness in the deafened. Fortunately, an understanding of the psychological factors involved is, in itself, a powerful means of overcoming the depression.

This chapter is written in the hope that it will help those adults

459

who have suffered permanent impairment of hearing to understand the psychological problems involved and thereby overcome their depressive reactions, and that it will provide the families of the deafened with a clearer insight into the difficulties that deafness entails so that they, too, can help.

Before the person with normal hearing can attempt to understand the problem of deafness, he must make a conscious effort to imagine what it is like to become suddenly and totally deaf, cut off in a world of silence from the familiar sounds of everyday living. Most of us take normal hearing completely for granted because we hear without conscious effort. We do not even have to open an "earlid" in order to listen, nor do we have an "earlid" to close if we wish to experience for a moment what deafness is like.

One way to gain some idea of the deaf person's experience is to imagine what it would be like to start home in a silent world after your day's work. The outside door makes no noise as you close it after you and step out on the sidewalk. A heavy rain is falling silently. Five o'clock traffic is jamming the street; people are crowding past you, but you hear no sound. Newsboys in front of the building are arguing angrily over something, but you can only see the exaggerated movement of their lips as they shout at each other. Cars suddenly swerve to the curb and stop. Everyone turns to look behind you, startled by a sound that you have not heard. An ambulance rushes silently past. Everything moves with the unreality of pantomime. When you reach home, you see your family's smiles of greeting, you see their lips move, but the rich experience of hearing the tone and rhythm of their familiar voices is lost. They, too, are like actors on a silent stage. If you can imagine such a silent world, you know something of how the deaf man feels, in close visual contact with his family and his surroundings but forced to substitute sight for hearing.

The loss of any sense organ imposes limitations, but the nature and severity of those limitations depend upon the particular sense organ affected. The most obvious limitation of the deaf man is that he cannot hear the spoken word. He may partially compensate, to be sure, by learning speechreading and, if he has sufficient residual hearing, by using a hearing aid. But if he depends on speechreading, he is definitely limited to clearly visible conversation directed to him. The deaf man's participation in the feelings and observations of others is restricted to those who deliberately address him. Without the full range of normal hearing, he misses the little asides that add immeasurably to the savor and zest of general conversation. He also misses the snatches of talk normally overheard as we ride the subway or bus or walk on a crowded street. Until these casual contacts are lost, it is impossible to realize how enormously they contribute to the feeling of group participation. The social handicap to communication with those around him therefore remains for the deaf man, even though it may seem to be partially overcome by speechreading or by the use of a hearing aid.

Because a blind man must also substitute one sense for another, blindness and deafness are popularly classed together. What we fail to realize is that the psychological effects of deafness are fundamentally different from those of blindness. The similarity between the two impairments is superficial, and the tendency to evaluate the effects of deafness in the terms used for blindness has retarded an understanding of the psychology of the deafened.

The Three Psychological Levels of Hearing

To understand the psychological changes which accompany the loss of hearing, it is necessary first to comprehend how normal hearing operates. In order to make the explanation as simple as possible, we shall discuss normal hearing as though it occurred on three levels:

1. At the social level, as we all realize, hearing is used to comprehend language. Words are symbols for objects around us and for activities. The word "tree" symbolizes the tree growing in the yard; the word "gallop" symbolizes the rapid gait of a horse. Since language is symbolic in its nature, we shall call this level of auditory function the *symbolic* level.

2. Sound also serves as a direct sign or signal of events to which we make constant adjustments in daily living. At this level it is not the word "bee" (which is a symbol for the actual bee itself), but the sound of its angry buzz that makes us jump. We stop our car, not because someone says "policeman" (the symbol for the officer), but because we hear the shrill sound of his whistle. This level of auditory function we shall call the *signal*, or *warning*, level.

3. Finally, and most basically, sound serves neither as symbol nor as warning but simply as *the auditory background* of all daily living. At this level we react to such sounds as the tick of a clock, the distant roar of traffic, vague echoes of people moving in other rooms in the house, without being aware that we do hear them. These incidental noises maintain our feeling of being part of a living world and contribute to our own sense of being alive. We are not conscious of the important role which these background sounds play in our comfortable merging of ourselves with the life around us, because we are not aware that we hear them. Nor is the deaf man aware that he

has lost these sounds; he only knows that *he feels as if the world were dead*. The real importance of this third level of hearing is the creation of a *background of feeling*, which the psychologist calls an "affective tone."

It was the constant reiteration, by hard-of-hearing patients at Deshon Army Hospital, of the statement that the world seemed dead which led to the investigation of this third level of hearing and of the psychological effect of its loss upon the deaf. This third level has not generally been recognized, although it is psychologically the most fundamental of the auditory functions. It relates us to the world at a very primitive level, somewhere below the level of clear consciousness and perception. The loss of this feeling of relationship with the world is the major cause of the well-recognized feeling of "deadness" and also of the depression that permeates the suddenly deafened and, to a less degree, those in whom deafness develops gradually. This level of hearing we shall designate as the *primitive* level.

The concept of levels of hearing has been chosen as the organizing principle of this chapter because this approach allows us to isolate and discuss the diverse but related auditory processes, together with their special implications for the deaf. "Hearing" is, of course, a combination of all these processes. At any given moment all are going on simultaneously. We hear on all the three levels at once. We hear the symbols of language, the signal of the ringing of the telephone, and we react to the background of sounds which we do not consciously discriminate and of which we are not aware. These diverse processes, however, vary independently, sometimes with a predominance of one, sometimes of another, but there is usually an interweaving contribution from each in the total pattern of hearing.

We shall begin our analysis of the psychological problems of the deaf at the most basic, least objective, and least structured level (the *primitive* level) and then explain the other two levels in the order of their objectivity—second, the *warning* level, and third, the *symbolic* level. Although such an approach may seem to be working backward, the reverse is true. Impairment or loss at the primitive "affective" level is most fundamentally and intimately connected with the emotional difficulties of the deaf.

HEARING AT THE PRIMITIVE LEVEL

At the primitive level of hearing, we react to the changing background sounds of the world around us *without being aware that we hear them*. This primitive function of hearing relates us to a world that is constantly in change, but it relates us to it in such a way that we are not conscious of the relationship, nor of the feeling it establishes of being part of our environment.

When we are at a concert listening to someone sing, we are not aware of the constantly changing pattern of sounds from the audience around us, the little noises of body movement, of breathing, of creaking seats, because our attention is on the singer. We are, however, reacting to these background sounds without realizing it. This constant reaction establishes in us states of feeling that are the foundation for our conscious experiences, a foundation which gives us the conviction that the world in which we live is also alive and moving. This process is a difficult one to describe, yet one so fundamental to an understanding of the primitive level of hearing that it must be labored in order to be made clear.

While we are focusing our attention on the singer at the concert, we do not consciously hear the background sounds from the audience or from the city outside. At any given moment, however, one of these background sounds may vary and attract our attention. The woman beside us may change the rhythm of her breathing by coughing. A horn on a car outside may become stuck and blow until we are aware of it. But the moment we become aware of such a background sound, it is no longer on the primitive level. As soon as we identify a sound, give it "thing" character, we are hearing on one of the other levels.

The most distinctive feature of these background sounds is that they are constantly changing because the world around us is in a state of constant activity. In the natural world there is constant motion: the wind blows; rain falls; animals move. In man's mechanical world, the same constant motion occurs. The pattern of environmental sound from this continued activity changes with each moment and with the different times of day.

In the human body there is also constant change and activity. Even in our deepest sleep we breathe, we digest our food, our hearts beat, and the brain continues its activity. We have then two patterns of change always in motion, the pattern of environmental change in the world around us and the pattern of change in the human body. By far the most efficient and indispensable mechanism for "coupling" the constant activity of the human organism to nature's activity is the primitive function of hearing.

We as living organisms are not and can never be completely independent of our environment. We live in our environment in different degrees of security, and since the security is never complete, we must maintain a readiness to react, to withdraw, or to approach as need arises. The primitive function of hearing maintains this readiness to react by keeping us constantly informed of events about us which do not make enough noise to challenge our attention. *The feeling state established by the primitive function of hearing is therefore characterized by this readiness to react as well as by the comfortable sense of being part of a living, active world.*

We must remember that this "coupling" of the individual with the world is not a conscious process. It is even less conscious than beating time to martial music without realizing that our feet are moving. That this "coupling" does exist, that it establishes an unconscious feeling of aliveness in us, is demonstrated by the overwhelming feeling of deadness in the deafened. It is possible to maintain some degree of coupling with the environment through other senses than hearing, but none of the others is so effective—as the characteristic depression of the deaf indicates.

THE DEPRESSION OF THE DEAF

Observation of hundreds of patients has convinced this author that the answer to their persistent question, "Why do I feel so depressed, so caught in a dead world?" is to be found in the destruction of the sound-coupling which connects the individual at an unconscious level with the aliveness and activity of the world. Undoubtedly the loss of conversation makes the deaf man feel isolated from those around him, but the basic emotional upset is caused by the loss of hearing at the primitive level.

The depressive reaction is much the same whether the impairment in hearing has been sudden or gradual. Soldier patients who had suddenly become deaf were, however, so bewildered by their unexpected depression that they attempted to describe it. All of them were conscious of an undefined feeling of loss. Many of them felt vaguely sad and insecure. One of them stated that it was almost impossible to believe in the passage of time since he couldn't hear a clock tick. Several fell asleep every time they turned off the hearing aids that brought them some sound from the world around them. Even those who faced the practical difficulties of deafness in a realistic manner still suffered from the same undefined but permeating depression.

One reason for the overwhelming nature of the depression is that, until it is pointed out to him, *the deafened person is not aware of the loss he has suffered* at the primitive level of hearing or of its effect upon his feeling state. He is unaware of the loss because he is unaware that there is such a thing as this primitive level of hearing in the first place. Frequently, he attributes his depression to a lack of character, and often he feels that if he were man enough, he could shake it off. Bewilderment and self-accusation heighten the burden he has to bear.

An extremely important step toward relieving the characteristic depression is taken when the deaf person realizes the reason for his emotional state. The realization itself makes his depression more objective and thereby makes it possible for him to cope with it without bewilderment or self-blame. As long as he is blind to its cause, he suffers from the same vague feelings of discomfort that characterize the early stages of a disease before the symptoms have yet developed clearly. Diagnosis does not instantly remove a disease, but it makes the proper treatment possible. Similarly, knowing the cause of depression does not remove it, but fortunately *the mere understanding of the reason for a feeling state does much psychologically to relieve its intensity.*

The nature of the impairment of deafness at the primitive level and its consequent loss of coupling involve the deaf in a double threat. We have just described the aspect of experience where its chief characteristic was that of feeling. But hearing at this low level also operates as a signal. It not only gives a quality of life to the present; it also serves as an indicator of what is to come. Even these undifferentiated feelings contain some reference to the future and serve to orient us unconsciously to meet it. They maintain in us a readiness to react to our environment. Without this orientation we suffer from a vague sense of insecurity which may be described in the words of a patient who said, "When I went deaf I lost my way of acting."

If the impairment of hearing is severe, the loss of the primitive hearing sense and its effect upon "feeling tone" are permanent and absolute unless a hearing aid can bring *some* sound from the outer world. When compensation for the loss in the primitive function is the objective, it is not essential that the hearing aid transmit sounds in their true character or speech which is intelligible, since the basic function operates with undifferentiated sounds. From a psychological point of view the use of a hearing aid is advisable even when it only serves to couple the individual to a world of sound patterns.

A type of compensation for severe loss in the primitive function has been developed independently and unconsciously by many recently deafened individuals. They substitute continuous muscular movement for the missing sensation of movement in the world. This continuous muscular activity is an overcompensation for the loss of those involuntary shifts in muscular tension which are the normal response to sounds heard at the primitive level. It is a good idea to make this muscular activity purposeful by keeping busy at something. Practical suggestions made later in the chapter will help the deaf person to substitute a satisfying activity for purposeless movement, such as pacing the floor.

SOUNDS AS SIGNS AND WARNINGS

So far, major emphasis has been placed on the hearing of background sounds. Obviously, however, hearing at a higher level plays an even more important part in biological adjustment and survival. At this level, sound serves as a sign or signal and conveys factual knowledge about objects and activities within the range of hearing: there is a fan operating; someone is washing dishes; someone is coming up the stairs. Many of our adjustments are initiated by sounds of low intensity, that is, sounds that arise at a distance. The horn of the approaching automobile warns us far enough in advance to avoid an accident. The eye can see distant objects, but hearing has the advantage of being able to warn us of approaching events that are not directly in our line of vision. Because sound waves can bend around corners and travel through darkness, the ear can warn us of many things that we cannot see. A lack of hearing leaves us uninformed of events outside the visual field. At a given moment, we can see only a *fraction* of what it is possible to observe, whereas we can receive *all* the possible sound signals simultaneously and without interruption, except, of course, as one sound may drown out another. A pedestrian cannot watch at the same time the automobile approaching him from the right and the truck approaching him from the left, but he can *hear* them simultaneously.

Hearing informs us of the events taking place around us, and it can also tell us something about the direction from which a sound comes. We can thus locate the event in which we are interested. Not only do we need advance notice that an automobile is approaching, but we need to know from what direction it is bearing down upon us. Localization of the source of sound is most accurate in the horizontal plane when we distinguish right from left. Discrimination is less accurate between front and back and still less accurate between up and down. Both ears are needed to perceive the direction from which sound comes, but in locating the source of a sound we are helped greatly by many additional clues and associations. The nature of the noise often restricts the number of possible directions from which it may come. An airplane in flight, for example, is always above, but an automobile is on the ground. If you know in which direction the nearby river lies, you will never be confused as to whether the sound of a boat whistle is coming from in front of or behind you, although you might be completely uncertain about the direction of a pure musical tone of unknown source.

The only noticeable handicap imposed by deafness in one ear is in the localization of the sources of sounds. For hearing language and background noises, one ear is almost as good as two. The man with one-sided deafness does not, however, suffer a complete loss of localization, since, as we have just mentioned, the principal cues for distance and some of the cues for direction do not depend upon binaural hearing. The accuracy of localization depends largely upon the recognition of the type of noise and its possible source. This substitute procedure, however, is not always accurate or quick enough in an emergency. The man with one-sided deafness is still liable to the right-left confusion that rarely occurs in a person with two normal ears.

Compensation for loss of hearing is easier at this warning level where sound is a sign or a signal than it is at the primitive level. Loss at this utilitarian level does not cause so basic an emotional upset. It does result in a feeling of insecurity because we are not able to hear warning signals or are uncertain as to their source. Practical readjustments can be learned to help the individual meet the everyday demands of his environment. When the capacity to locate moving objects by their sounds is reduced or inadequate, a trained visual awareness will compensate to a considerable degree. A careful study of the conditions to be expected in certain situations, such as crossing a busy street, will give a feeling of security which approaches that of the hearing person.

AESTHETIC EXPERIENCE

In addition to its function as signal or warning for biological survival, hearing contributes at the second level to our aesthetic experience. We listen to music and the sounds of nature for the pleasure that we derive from the sounds themselves. All people do not possess an equal need for this type of aesthetic auditory experience, nor do they suffer equally from the loss of the aesthetic experience of sound.

Just as there are differences in the degree of need, so there are differences in the kind of experiences sought. Some of us need visual, others need auditory, and others (apparently) do not need any aesthetic experience at all. If the loss of hearing occurs in someone with a pronounced aesthetic need in the auditory field, the absence of musical experience is felt as an impoverishment, and the lack is interpreted unconsciously as a lack in one's self.

In individuals with a pronounced aesthetic auditory need, this lack sometimes assumes acute proportions. A musician of this author's acquaintance who had a severe impairment declared that she would gladly sacrifice a year of her life if she could only once hear a symphony again. Such acute need is unusual, however, and occurs most often in those who have reinforced their natural auditory need by an occupation in the field of music.

Probably those who satisfy an aesthetic auditory need through the varied and multitudinous sounds of nature outnumber those who have found the answer to their need in music. The sounds of nature are available to everyone, whereas music is not. The sound of the sea, the singing of birds, the patter of rain furnish many people aesthetic experiences as poignant as those received through music. The silence of the natural world deadens it for them and superimposes upon the self the same lack felt by music lovers.

A hearing aid for those with some residual hearing, or even the vibratory sense by which the totally deaf can appreciate the rhythm of music, may enable a person with an auditory aesthetic need to capture enough of the desired sounds and rhythms to stimulate his imagination to re-create familiar and beloved auditory images either from music or from the natural world and thus satisfy his need in part.

SOUNDS AS SYMBOLS

Animals as well as men depend on sound for warning; they also recognize the meaning of particular sounds, such as the trickle of water, the snapping of twigs, or the call of a mate. Man, however, can use ordered sounds as symbols for things not immediately present and even for abstract ideas. The use of sound as language sets human society apart as unique and different from animal societies. By the use of spoken language, man's sphere of influencing and being influenced is enormously increased and made more complex.

Hearing in its symbolic, linguistic function enriches human life in *three* ways: (1) Language makes possible the communication of experiences through a medium that is flexible and manifold almost to the degree to which experience itself is complex. (2) Language clarifies and organizes our thoughts by supplying a grammatical, syntactical, and logical framework and thus makes possible man's higher-order knowledge. (3) In the growing child, language serves to formalize and to bind those social prohibitions and permissions which make up the moral code: the *voice* of conscience, not a forbidding *glance*, directs our moral behavior.

Loss of hearing does not impair each of these three functions to an equal degree. The degree of hearing loss and the time of its onset are important in determining the effect of the impairment upon the personality. The adult who suffers a sudden and severe hearing loss is plunged into a world where sensory deficits form his principal handicap. The organizing of thought and the formulation of moral permissions and prohibitions have already been established; once established, they continue even with total deafness. The framework for higher-order knowledge and the moral code are not affected.

CONGENITAL DEAFNESS

So far we have considered only the problems of the adult who either suddenly or gradually loses his hearing. The psychological effects of deafness are somewhat different in the child who is born deaf or who becomes deaf before he has learned the structure of language. His failure to learn to talk spontaneously or to be able to communicate any but the simplest ideas without intensive and special training has been considered in Chapter 16. Fortunately, the greater difficulties in relation to communication are partly offset by a less devastating effect of the absence of the primitive auditory function. The child who has never established auditory "coupling" with the ongoingness of the world is not depressed by the absence of this coupling as the adult is by the loss of it. Nor has the child developed through training and experience any urgent aesthetic needs of an auditory nature. And once communication has been established, whether by visual reading, speechreading, the manual alphabet, or the language of signs, the deaf child is able to formulate successfully in nonauditory terms the structure for his thoughts and for his moral code.

Practical Suggestions

Hearing loss presents obvious problems at the language level even for an adult. Unless the hearing loss is very mild, situations involving spoken language as a means of communication are difficult and remain difficult. *The first step toward surmounting the difficulty is to admit it frankly and realistically.* Much of the tension of social situations is eased for the deafened as well as for others if the impairment is regarded as factually and objectively as the need for glasses. Society accepts glasses for impaired vision and will accept with equal readiness the wearing of a hearing aid and also the need for face-to-face conversation to facilitate speechreading by those whose impairment is too severe for a hearing aid.

A few simple suggestions will help those with hearing loss to master practical situations which must be met. The complexity of even such a simple transaction as buying a railroad ticket may be great. Here the experience of those who have most successfully surmounted such difficulties has taught them to study the situation, to anticipate the difficulties which may arise, and to attempt by so doing to avoid confusion. If you wish to buy a railroad ticket from Columbus to Cincinnati, for example, you should if possible consult a timetable in which the three alternate routes are listed before asking for your ticket. You will then be familiar with the names of railroad lines and train schedules so that you can more easily recognize the words used in answer to your questions. Such advance knowledge makes it possible for you to ask pertinent questions and reduces the chance of your getting on the wrong train. A hearing aid in this situation is valuable, not only as an amplifier but also, if visible, as a sign and reminder impairment. It relieves the wearer from the need of frequently mentioning his handicap and signifies to strangers that his difficulty in the situation depends on a physical and not on an intellectual defect.

When a conversation is primarily the exchange of experiences with friends, no bluff at all should be attempted. The handicap should be frankly admitted so that the strain of keeping up with the conversation may be eased. An effort should be made, however, to participate whenever possible and an attitude of dependence should be avoided. Here, as in the simple transaction of buying a ticket, a careful analysis of social patterns will provide a useful repertoire of anticipations which will facilitate in advance the adjustment to the inevitable difficulties of a social situation.

Social situations are not infinitely variable. There are not more patterns to learn than exist, for example, on a checker board. A mastery of social amenities is helpful and can be acquired without inducing a feeling of submission or dependency. Viewed realistically, the anticipation of the demands of a situation can become a competitive game.

Many who are deaf believe it important to be able to hear in order to make new friends. If the deaf who hold this belief would distinguish between friendship and casual acquaintance, they would realize that although friendship is undeniably carried on through the senses, it does not follow that the loss or impairment of only one of them destroys, makes impossible, or even lessens the depth of such a relation. The deaf man is in no way handicapped in the exchange of warm and affectionate experiences if he has developed the requisite deep sensibilities.

There are many situations in which none of us need or use our hearing. In such instances, where communication is unnecessary, the practical if not the emotional problems of the hearing and of the hard-of-hearing or deafened person are almost the same. For instance, all of us must face the problem of occupying leisure hours. For the hearing and for the deaf alike, idle times passes slowly, but occupied time passes quickly. The only difference in the problem for the two is that the hard-of-hearing or deafened person is more apt to fill his leisure hours with self-pity than with the chitchat of casual companions by which others may attempt to cover up a poor capacity for solitude.

Recreation should find a central place in the life of those suffering from hearing loss. They should habitually fill their leisure hours with some creative activity or avocation. If they do, they will soon realize that each person has his own individual and unique pattern of life and that it is worth while to find some definite interests and objectives as an outlet for this individuality. Since activity in a chosen field invariably leads to a relationship with others who share the same interests, those with hearing loss should make a careful survey of their interests and capabilities and discover the mechanical, artistic, or creative sphere in which they can express themselves. Those with mechanical ability can profitably spend their spare time repairing radios, electrical appliances, or watches. They can learn to refinish and upholster furniture or to rebuild antiques. An interest in furniture might lead eventually to cabinetmaking. A frequent approach to the artistic field is through model making. Models of airplanes, ships, houses, or trains may be made for personal pleasure alone or, if the individual develops sufficient skill, for the commercial market. Those with an interest in botany, biology, or medicine can apply their knowledge making models for classroom study. In the creative sphere, painting, writing, and modeling or sculpturing offer natural outlets. The amount of talent possessed is not important. If the individual is interested in one of these forms of creative work, he should try it as a means of personal expression and for the pleasure it brings. By identifying himself with a group interested in the same avocation, he may in part compensate for being unable to feel himself an intimate part of as large a social group as he could before hearing loss narrowed his conversational circle.

The experience of one man who developed a successful business from spare-time activity illustrates the professional possibilities of many avocations. Having time on his hands, he began by helping his mother, who was secretary of a large club, address the notices that she had to send out to its members. Friends of hers learned of his assistance and gave him letters to address for organizations with which they were connected. Requests for his aid increased. Today he runs a mailing and letter service that employs two assistants.

Interest in the problems of deafness, and assisting those who are similarly afflicted, is a common and very effective and useful form of social activity for the hard of hearing, provided that it does not turn into a form of mutual self-pity. Even better, if it can be achieved, is participation in more general social interests that do not depend on the handicap and do not make life and thoughts revolve about and continually emphasize it. More effort and skill may be required, but the most successful adjustment is the one that overrides and submerges the handicap in normal activity centering outside one's self.

FEELINGS OF SUSPICION

There is an additional reason why it is psychologically healthful for the deaf to make a decided effort to center their interests and activities outside themselves. There is in many persons with normal hearing a tendency to feel that conversation interrupted upon their entrance into a room must have been about them or that half-heard remarks were critical and unfriendly. *Deafness accentuates this tendency and may make an oversensitive person unduly suspicious of hostility in those around him.* A word of explanation and warning is needed about such so-called *paranoid* reactions. Since the term "paranoid" is often used, perhaps erroneously, to characterize this hypersensitivity of the deaf, a simple explanation of the term is needed.

Not all persons can accept criticism without being hurt. It is possible for a friend to criticize your suit without implying any criticism of you. We all have a tendency, however, to interpret any criticism of something that is "mine" as a criticism of "me." If the tendency is strong, the person is described as sensitive. It is easy to imagine a person so sensitive that he is suspicious and anticipates that others are being critical of him. When the suspicion, reflecting a basic insecurity, is developed to this point, we speak of "paranoid reactions."

The tendency toward paranoid reactions exists to some degree in nearly all of us, but it is generally kept under control. Since control is lessened when a person is depressed, sensitiveness and suspicion are more easily aroused. *Deafness seems to be a powerful stimulus to any latent paranoid trend in the personality,* possibly because of the invariable association between depression and deafness.

We frequently observe that deaf people often think that conversations which they cannot hear are about them. They may often go so far as to think that derogatory remarks are being directed toward them in tones too low for them to hear. This is a typical "paranoid trend." Deafness alone, however, or even the insecurity that deafness may bring, is not enough to produce a paranoid trend. The person who becomes suspicious has a life pattern of placing his own insecurity in center stage and is preoccupied with the fear that others may see the lack which he feels. *A person secure in his own emotional life will develop no paranoid trends even when deafened.* The frequency of such paranoid trends shows, however, how many persons feel insure in their social relations. Deafness may not be the fundamental cause of the trends, but it waters the seeds and encourages them to grow.

The conquest of this morbid symptom reduces to the problem of attaining a mature point of view that is centered outside one's self. If one has developed a genuine interest in other people and in outside activities, statements not heard will be interpreted as objective statements of fact, not as remarks about one's self.

THE OBJECTIVE ATTITUDE

The explanation of the psychology of hearing given in this chapter and the effect of impairment at the different levels have been realistically presented. There is no disguising the fact that anyone who becomes deaf or hard of hearing experiences an almost catastrophic loss when he must adjust himself to a completely or partially silent world. Only after he has faced this fact honestly and objectively can he determine the extent to which compensation is possible. An objective attitude furnishes the only sound basis upon which to build a readjustment.

Psychologically speaking, no permanent adjustment is possible until the individual realizes that the cause of his depressive state lies in the loss of the primitive function and until he faces the practical difficulties imposed by the loss at the two higher levels. Since depression and the feeling of deadness are the most destructive psychological effects of hearing impairment, it is fortunate that *the major step in recovering from these emotional states lies in a clear understanding of their cause.*

The suggestions made to facilitate mastery of the practical difficulties are by no means exhaustive. Each individual will work out his own, in accordance with the demands of his particular environment and his own personality and abilities.

The man with severe hearing loss will save himself much pain if he will realize that, although the difficulties imposed by deafness are now receiving recognition, he must not expect the general public to understand the problems of adjustment that are involved. Although this indifference is cruel, it does require him to develop a usefully independent and objective attitude toward his handicap.

Suggested Readings

CANFIELD, N. *Hearing: A Handbook for Laymen.* New York: Doubleday & Company, 1959.
An otologist talks to hard-of-hearing laymen.
MEYERSON, L. "Somatopsychological Significance of Impaired Hearing," in *Adjustment to Physical Handicap and Illness: A Survey of the Social Psychology of Physique and Disability,* R. G. Barker, ed. New York: Social Science Research Council, 1953, Chap. 5.

PART 6

SOCIAL AND ECONOMIC PROBLEMS

19

THE VETERANS ADMINISTRATION AUDIOLOGY PROGRAM

Bernard M. Anderman, Ed.D.

History

The Veterans Administration is one of the heirs of the legacy of the World War II military audiology program. During that war, military centers, furnishing what was then termed "aural rehabilitation services," were established at Deshon (Pennsylvania), Borden (Oklahoma), and Hoff Army General (California) Hospitals, for the Army and at the United States Naval Hospital in Philadelphia for the Navy. The military programs met the requirements of their times in most commendable fashion and treated an estimated 15,000 servicemen for hearing impairment. Today, approximately 56,000 veterans of World War II have service-connected hearing impairments or diseases of the ear. The Veterans Administration program was established to assist them, and the estimated 24,000 additional veterans who served during other periods, through audiological examination, treatment, and guidance.

Under Veterans Administration policy, outpatient beneficiaries may receive hearing aids and training when the disability is service-connected and when there is a need for them. For hospitalized patients, there must be a medically established need in the case of a service-connected condition, as well as in certain categories of adjunct or auxiliary treatment when the hearing condition is not service-connected.

The overwhelming majority of veterans who are furnished hearing aids and training are those whose condition is service-connected, and they are treated on an outpatient basis. A service-connected impair-

477

ment is one which was incurred or aggravated in line of duty in the active military, naval, or air service. For purposes of outpatient medical services, any impairment of a veteran of the Spanish-American War is considered to be service-connected.

Facilities providing adequate audiological services were rare in the years immediately following World War II. Most veterans eligible for hearing aids were referred directly to dealers after medical examination but without intervening audiological evaluation. However, with the growth of audiology, increasing numbers of clinics, both governmental and private, were established throughout the country.

The first Veterans Administration Audiology Clinic was established in the New York City Regional Office in 1946. A large unit, it was designed to meet the needs of the huge veteran population in southern New England and metropolitan New York. Other clinics were subsequently established in a number of large population areas. Eleven are presently in operation, each serving the needs of neighboring localities as well as the one in which it is located. A list of the clinics and their locations is given at the end of this chapter. To provide needed audiological assistance for eligible veterans who lived at a distance from these centers, contracts were established with qualified university, hospital, and community clinics. As a consequence, more and more of the hearing aid selection for veterans has been carried out in clinics.

Present Status

The Veterans Administration audiology program has many facets. It provides direct services to eligible veterans, including auditory assessment and rehabilitation, and it carries on research, training, and consultation of considerable scope.

REHABILITATION

The philosophy underlying the Veterans Administration rehabilitation effort is one which was originally developed in World War II military practice. At its core is a unified, integrated program involving the extensive use of educational techniques and personal counseling as well as the selection of hearing aids.

No single standard or model rehabilitation program has been provided by the Veterans Administration for its audiology clinics. Individual approaches have been developed in varying patterns to suit local needs and conditions. Then, too, many veterans are served by the network of clinics that provide services under contracts.

A basic activity both in the Veterans Administration's own and in

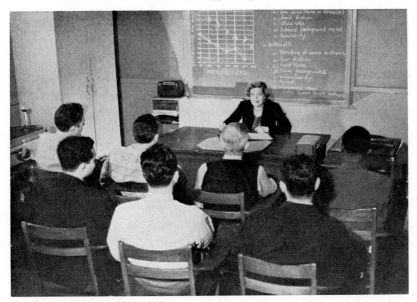

Fig. 19-1. One of the first steps in rehabilitation is to give accurate information about the nature of hearing impairment. (*Veterans Administration.*)

its contract clinics is the evaluation of hearing aids for eligible veterans. Testing is done under controlled conditions to determine whether or not the veteran is likely to benefit by wearing a hearing aid. Acoustic features of the instrument (described in Chapter 10) and audiological assessment of the veterans are considered in relation to his less tangible social, economic, and psychological needs. When the issuance of a hearing aid is indicated, selection is made from among a representative group of instruments which have been placed in the clinic stock. An important feature of the selection procedure is that the veteran receives the actual hearing aid used in the trial process. This provides the veteran with an instrument that has been found to suit his particular needs, and one whose limitations for the veteran, where present, have been ascertained. Thus the necessary adjustments can be made during his training.

The New York Regional Office Audiology Clinic is a good example of the application of the principles underlying the Veterans Administration Program of Rehabilitation. The veteran is given a course of instruction that is planned to restore his efficiency in communication as completely as possible. He is taught speechreading and speech conservation and is given auditory training and speech correction. The veteran is helped to understand the nature and extent of his impairment and is informed about the general problems related to loss of hearing. Psychological and social work assistance are offered when needed.

At the New York Regional Office Audiology Clinic group teaching has proved to be the most effective. The size of the class is limited so that attention may be given to individual needs while the benefits of group instruction and interaction are realized. The teachers have always strived to employ dynamic and meaningful teaching materials, geared to the level of the adult veteran. There is a choice of either a four-week program consisting of twenty half-days, or a shorter program of three days' duration. Approximately 5400 veterans have participated in this form of training in the New York Regional Office Audiology Clinic, with slightly more than one half electing to attend the four-week sessions. The success of this program has, in part, been related to careful and sympathetic counseling of the veteran. The counseling has been carried out not only in the audiology clinic but also in the office of the prosthetic specialist in the Veterans Administration. The latter is himself a physically disabled veteran who has a background of special training and who relates effectively to handicapped veterans requiring a hearing aid.

A somewhat modified rehabilitation program has been in effect in the audiology clinic in the Los Angeles Regional Office of the Veterans Administration. There the extended program consists of ten half-days and the limited program runs for three half-days. Again, the goal is to improve the skills of communication while helping the veteran to attain a realistic estimate of his handicap due to hearing loss and of his progress in overcoming it. Frequently, special problems create the need for a special program of individual instruction, but group work is more typical. A social worker and a psychologist participate actively in the program. In common with the experience of the New York Regional Office, the office in Los Angeles has found that many veterans who have completed the program return later for further training. In Los Angeles, where the program developed more recently than that in New York, almost 500 veterans have attended, most of them for the extended course.

Numerous elderly veterans, particularly those who served in the Spanish-American War, have been referred to Veterans Administration Audiology Clinics. Clinicians who have assisted these patients are astonished by the large percentage who have been benefited. Unexpectedly large numbers of older veterans have learned to use hearing aids successfully, while many have participated enthusiastically in training programs. This experience runs counter to the notion that there is little that can be done for the amelioration of hearing loss in elderly persons.

It is now recognized that the immediate costs for rehabilitation are ultimately more than recovered in economic gains to the individual and to society. For example, a veteran who was experiencing job problems in his home city enrolled in the training program in Los Angeles. Before leaving he applied for a position in Los Angeles with a company that was known to be favorably inclined to the hard of hearing. The veteran was offered and accepted a job; he has since won several awards for outstanding sales ability. There have been many similar reports of benefits following the furnishing of a hearing aid, rehabilitation training, and counseling.

The military and veterans' programs are considered to have had a subtle yet important influence on public acceptance of hearing aids. Before World War II, hearing aids were not often seen in public and were especially shunned by young adults with hearing loss. A shift in attitude occurred when thousands of men in military service were furnished hearing aids before discharge during the final period of the war, and when, following its termination, additional thousands qualified for receipt of hearing aids as eligible veterans. It is likely that the example set by these groups encouraged the more general use of hearing aids. Perhaps, too, the attitudes of employers and the general public were favorably affected by veterans with impaired hearing who sought to overcome their handicap. Today, in Veterans Administration Audiology Clinics, one rarely encounters any reluctance to be seen wearing a hearing aid, a reluctance which was often strong among young veterans immediately after World War II.

ASSESSMENT OF SOCIAL EFFICIENCY

Veterans Administration Audiology Clinics play a significant role in examining hearing function in claims for disability compensation. Immediately following World War II, these examinations were conducted in the various outpatient medical clinics, utilizing the traditional spoken-voice, distance-fraction tests.

Aware of the weaknesses in measuring hearing loss by the spoken-voice method, the Veterans Administration revised its procedures for evaluating hearing impairment. In 1952 it turned to a rating schedule based on pure tone and speech audiometry. The veteran generally went to the outpatient clinic nearest his home, where the examination was carried out. Although this procedure was demonstrably superior to the one previously employed, it too showed several weaknesses: poor acoustic conditions in many of the clinics, insufficient experience and training of some technicians, and limitations of the available audiometric equipment.

In 1955 came a fuller recognition of the fact that accurate assessment of auditory function was not a simple matter. A system was developed that took advantage of the growth which had occurred in the field of audiology. Within the Veterans Administration and available on a contract basis throughout most of the country were clinics with highly trained personnel and excellent equipment. An effort was made to take advantage of such facilities wherever possible.

The Veterans Administration, using selected audiology clinics, then instituted a program of re-examining veterans who had been receiving compensation for a service-connected hearing impairment. These audiology clinics, either under contract or as part of the Veterans Administration, were required to possess hearing evaluation equipment meeting specified technical standards. Further, a uniform minimum level of training and experience was established for all participating clinicians.

For purposes of compensation, a minimum battery of tests was established for examinations related to evaluation of hearing impairment. This presently includes air- and bone-conduction audiometry, electrodermal audiometry at one or more frequencies, speech reception threshold, and speech intelligibility tests, for each ear. When these tests give results which are equivocal, additional tests must be performed. These include the Stenger and the Doerfler-Stewart tests and tests based on the principle of delayed speech. These tests are described in Chapters 7 and 8. Consultants continually monitor the test findings, the status of equipment, and the performance of personnel. This testing program has since been extended to the evaluation of veterans who present new claims for loss of hearing.

The audiological re-examination program has been important in many ways. It has provided the Veterans Administration with a significant advance in procedures for determination of hearing impairment and, because of its insistence on minimum standards for personnel and equipment, the Veterans Administration has helped in the development of competent clinics in the few areas where they were not previously available.

THE PROBLEM OF NONORGANIC DEAFNESS

One of the most interesting aspects of the Veterans Administration audiology program is its concern with the problem of functional or psychogenic deafness. (The Veterans Administration uses the broad term "nonorganic," which includes "functional" and psychogenic deafness.) Psychogenic deafness and the other forms of central dysacusis are described in Chapter 4. It is noted there that the incidence of psychogenic deafness in the general population seems to be very small. In all probability this is partly due to the failure to employ appropriate procedures routinely, since the detection of psychogenic deafness requires both an awareness of the problem and a willingness to use the necessary techniques, even though the tests may be more elaborate than those for threshold audiometry.

Nonorganic deafness has been observed quite frequently in Veterans Administration Audiology Clinics. Its difference from organic hearing loss is often a subtle one. For this reason, the decision to have examinations for rating purposes conducted in audiology clinics has proved wise because it has encouraged audiological evaluations of a most exacting nature. Were they to be done in a cursory manner, nonorganic deafness might not be recognized and the possibilities of award of compensation and issue of a hearing aid might very well lead veterans to accept easily the idea that they have an organic impairment when actually they do not. This is especially likely when one reflects on the nature of nonorganic or "functional" hearing loss. Typically, it appears in conjunction with a mild organic impairment.

Electrodermal audiometry is particularly useful in the audiological test battery, principally because it may suggest that the impairment is not organic. Other tests which have been successfully employed for this purpose in addition to the minimum battery of pure-tone audiometry, speech audiometry, and electrodermal pure-tone audiometry, are Stenger, shifting-voice, electrodermal speech audiometry, Doerfler-Stewart, delayed sidetone, and determination of the difference limen for intensity—all tests described in Chapters 7 and 8. Psychological and psychiatric procedures have also proved helpful in evaluation.

Nonorganic deafness has long been a poorly understood and rarely discussed phenomenon outside the military and veterans' sphere. Partly because of the use of contract clinics for Veterans Administration examinations, there has developed a much more widespread knowledge and appreciation of the condition. The awareness of what it is and that it exists in the civilian population, including children, is increasing.

INTERDEPARTMENTAL RELATIONS

Veterans Administration Audiology Clinics have had the advantages of good physical plants as well as versatile and modern equipment. Quite naturally, therefore, they have worked closely with the Departments of Otolaryngology, Neurology, Psychology, Psychiatry, and related specialties. As the evaluation of auditory function has become more complex and revealing, the possible professional contribution of the clinical audiologist has grown. Such associations have been fostered in research and training also.

RESEARCH

Audiological research in the Veterans Administration has a strong orientation to clinical needs. Research activities help create a stimulating professional environment which in turn results in improved treatment of patients. Audiology clinics have shared in the general growth of research throughout the Veterans Administration's Department of Medicine and Surgery. Research projects typically develop secondarily to regular clinical duties. In some situations, however, the primary activity is research. The study of hearing aids, nonorganic deafness, and hearing problems related to aging are among the research interests.

TRAINING

Veterans Administration Audiology Clinics have encountered difficulties in securing the services of qualified personnel, largely because of the national shortage. Various types of training programs designed to stimulate interest and improve competence in audiology have been established in order to alleviate this situation. To college students who have completed their senior year and who have majored in speech and hearing science the Veterans Administration offers an opportunity to participate in a program which serves as an introduction to the field of audiology. This training program is offered during the summer months and includes study at five Veterans Administration Audiology Clinics. At higher levels there are training programs which allow students to work part-time in Veterans Administration clinics while they attend neighboring universities to study for advanced degrees. Many audiologists presently employed in the Veterans Administration are former students in these training programs. Other former trainees who may be employed in its contract clinics also assist the Veterans Administration. The remainder have gone on to help meet the ever-increasing demand for audiological services throughout the nation.

CONSULTANTS

A large government program must always recognize the danger of stagnation. Consultants provide an excellent antidote to such a possibility. The Veterans Administration audiology program is presently receiving the consultation services of outstanding specialists in the fields of otology and audiology, who act as advisers and monitors of the program.

One group of consultants is composed of thirteen otologists, who evaluate the work done in the various clinics and whose opinions and advice are solicited on important policy matters. Another consists of eight audiologists, who, in addition to their roles in supervision and recommendation, also participate directly in the conduct of the program.

HEARING AID PROCUREMENT

Since World War II, the Veterans Administration has been furnishing hearing aids to large numbers of eligible veterans. Its Department of Medicine and Surgery quite naturally is keenly interested in the quality of commercially available hearing aids and, as it does with other prosthetic and sensory-aid devices, it actively supports research and other programs aimed at fostering improvements.

As we have said, the Veterans Administration prefers to furnish the veteran with the actual instrument which is selected in the hearing aid evaluation. A complicating factor in the whole procedure is the large number of manufacturers, each of whom is likely to have a variety of models which are subject to periodic change. The decision as to which instruments to stock in the audiology clinics is thus a difficult one. It would be undesirable for the stock to lag significantly behind current models, yet too-frequent addition of new but very different models could result in a continually increasing inventory of out-of-date hearing aids. Furthermore, not every change necessarily represents an improvement over the existing models.

For a number of years the Veterans Administration procured its hearing aids on the basis of negotiated contracts with the various manufacturers. Many companies were represented and, as a result, the variety of models in stock was so extensive that it created administrative problems in the clinics without compensating professional advantages.

In 1956 the hearing aid procurement policy was changed. One goal was to reduce to a smaller and more manageable level the number of different models that the individual clinics were required to stock. In addition, and insofar as possible, it was hoped to achieve lowered costs while obtaining hearing aids of the highest quality.

A special consultant group was organized to assist in the management of this new program. The plan is to evaluate the performance characteristics of hearing aids submitted to the Veterans Administration for proposed inclusion in its clinic stock. Competitive bids are then invited from the manufacturers whose instruments score highest in the performance tests. Final procurement thus rests on a relation between performance scores and bid prices, or cost-per-point-of-quality.

The cooperation of the National Bureau of Standards has been enlisted for the actual measurement of the performance characteristics. The bureau tests the various models of hearing aids for a number of acoustic features and submits the results to the Veterans Administration. The Veterans Administration then subjects the data to statistical and comparative analyses which in turn lead to a solicitation to bid.

The Veterans Administration has retained the right to eliminate from consideration any instruments which it regards as clinically unacceptable. In addition, each manufacturer desiring to participate in the program must have been actively engaged in the business of manufacturing hearing aids for a period of not less than three years. Furthermore, because hearing aids must occasionally be procured through local commercial dealers rather than from the factory, each manufacturer must have established dealers or distributors in most of the major cities of the United States. The plan has never contemplated the development of formal specifications. Instead, emphasis is placed on actual comparative performance of the instruments, in the hope of stimulating research and benefiting from continuing design improvements in the hearing aid industry. To meet unusual needs which may arise, the Veterans Administration has also reserved the right to procure hearing aids having special characteristics that may not be included in the basic program.

The manufacturers are, of course, free to decide which of their models to submit for evaluation. A maximum number of models per manufacturer has been established, however. The manufacturers are given a description of the tests which will be made. It is their responsibility to decide which tone settings, adjustments, and battery voltages they wish to specify for a particular model. They are advised to select those settings that will yield a frequency response curve that is close to a 5 db per octave rise. Three randomly selected samples of each hearing aid model are then given the entire series of tests.

The tests for evaluation include measurements of maximum power output, of frequency response, of gain, of battery drain, of nonlinear distortion, and of signal-to-noise ratio. (These various characteristics and the importance of each have been described in Chapters 10 and 11.) The models are then classified, on the basis of gain and maximum power output, into three categories: mild, moderate, and strong. The results from the other measurements of the three samples of each model are then averaged to yield a performance score for that model on each test item. The raw scores representing the various physical measures are then weighted according to a ranking that has been assigned to their relative importance. This ranking and the consequent weighting of the scores is based on the advice of the special consultants, and every effort is made to ensure that they also reflect the needs and the experience of the audiologists in the various Veterans Administration clinics.

The cost of each model to the Veterans Administration is divided by the quality-point score of that model. The cost-per-point-of-quality establishes a ranking for the various models in each of the three categories of mild, moderate, and strong. The clinical needs of the Veterans Administration are being successfully met by procuring a selected number of instruments for each of these three categories.

It should be clearly recognized that this description is intended to furnish a general outline of the Veterans Administration goals and policies in this field. It has not been a complete analysis of the program for procurement of hearing aids. Further, there is a continuing review of objectives and evaluation of results. Important changes and minor modifications have been introduced annually.

The Veterans Administration intends that its hearing aid test program should assist in reducing the number of different models that must be stocked in its clinics. It further seeks to provide a means for competitive bidding while still assuring the acquisition of hearing aids which have high performance ratings. The physical features evaluated are those which the Veterans Administration considers to be important in a large procurement program. The cost factor is related to quantity purchasing. The hearing aids are ultimately selected on the basis of a series of factors which are most meaningful to the Veterans Administration, but the Veterans Administration has never suggested that the results of this program be used to guide other governmental or private agencies, or individuals, in their choice of hearing aids.

Prospects

The demands for audiological services in the Veterans Administration will continue to be heavy for many years to come. Present plans contemplate the establishment of several additional Veterans Administration Audiology Clinics in the future in order to provide complete geographical representation in accordance with changing population patterns. The ultimate goal is a group of approximately fifteen Veterans Administration clinics which, together with approximately thirty-five contract clinics, will make it possible for the nation's eligible veterans to obtain any necessary audiological assistance within a reasonable distance from their homes.

Outpatient medical clinics are being consolidated into large hospital settings. Audiological treatment, research, and training activities should prosper in such an environment. We believe that while serving the veterans the Veterans Administration program will greatly enrich the field of audiology.

Appendix: Veterans Administration Audiology Clinics

CALIFORNIA
VA Regional Office, Los Angeles
VA Hospital, San Francisco
DISTRICT OF COLUMBIA
Veterans Benefits Office, Washington
FLORIDA
VA Regional Office, St. Petersburg
GEORGIA
VA Regional Office, Atlanta
ILLINOIS
VA (West Side) Hospital, Chicago
LOUISIANA
VA Hospital, New Orleans
MASSACHUSETTS
VA Outpatient Clinic, Boston
MISSOURI
VA Regional Office, Kansas City
NEW YORK
VA Regional Office, New York City
TEXAS
VA Hospital, Dallas

Suggested Readings

MOE
✳ BERGMAN, M. "The Audiology Clinic," *Acta Oto-Laryngologica*, 1950, Supp. 89, 1–107.
This is a description of the Audiology Clinic in the Veterans Administration Regional Office, New York.

20

ORGANIZATIONS AND AGENCIES FOR THE AURALLY HANDICAPPED

Betty C. Wright
(Revised by Ada Morgan Hill
and S. R. Silverman, Ph.D.)

If you are deaf or hard of hearing, you owe a debt to the pioneers who realized that your social, economic, and educational status could be improved through organizations. Organizations for the aurally handicapped vary in purpose and scope, but they are similar in that their accomplishments have benefited you directly or indirectly and have focused attention on your problems. You may be one of the 190,000 deaf in the United States without sense of hearing from birth or early childhood; or you may belong to the larger company of the hard of hearing (9,500,000 estimated),[1] who have some useful hearing. Many of you should supplement it by a hearing aid or speechreading or both; but whatever your degree of hearing loss and however it came about, one or more of the following organizations are working for you.

THE CONVENTION OF AMERICAN INSTRUCTORS OF THE DEAF

The Convention of American Instructors of the Deaf (formerly the Convention of American Instructors of the Deaf and Dumb) held

---

[1] This figure, representing our best guess, is from the November, 1958, issue of the *National Hearing Aid Journal*. A "panel" for gathering the information consisted of 100 manufacturers of hearing aids, component parts, accessories, or supplies, as well as some advertising agencies who had been handling hearing aid accounts. The *Journal* also indicates that the estimate agrees well with government statistics. Although criteria of hearing impairment are not given, it is obvious that it is of practical importance for commercial organizations to estimate their potential market as accurately as possible.

489

its first meeting in New York City in 1850. Membership is limited to those engaged in teaching the deaf. The Convention does not stand committed to any particular method or system of teaching the deaf; its general object is the "promotion of the education of the deaf on the broadest, most advanced and practical lines." Through its organization it seeks harmony of all persons instructing the deaf in America and provides for general and local meetings where different points of view can be aired. It has been said that its influence penetrates the classroom and extends into every portion of the field of activity by and for the deaf. The program of its recent annual meeting included sections on language, speechreading, secondary education, vocational training, multiple handicaps, auditory training, preschool and kindergarten, research, health and physical education, social studies, visual education, as well as sections for deaf teachers, day school teachers, and principals and supervising teachers.

The Convention is one of the few educational organizations in the United States that has been in continuous existence and activity for more than a century. Among its valuable contributions have been the reports of its meetings, held biannually, which have contained addresses on almost every aspect of deafness. The *Proceedings* of the Convention of American Instructors of the Deaf have been published for many years by the United States Government Printing Office. Its official organ is the *American Annals of the Deaf*.

THE CONFERENCE OF EXECUTIVES OF AMERICAN SCHOOLS FOR THE DEAF

The Conference, formed in 1868, was an informal organization until its incorporation seventy years later. Its membership is limited to the administrative heads of schools for the deaf. Associate members include assistant superintendents or principals of large institutions. The object of the Conference is "to promote the management and operation of schools for the deaf along the broadest and most efficient lines and to further and promote the general welfare of the deaf." Through its meetings and discussions it has emphasized the importance of vocational training. It has also assisted in standardizing the requirements for the special training of teachers of the deaf and has outlined a course of study for teacher-training classes. It has charge of the certification of teachers of the deaf. The Conference has promoted legislation beneficial to the deaf and has created public understanding of their problems. Perhaps its most noteworthy contribution is the publication of the *American Annals of the Deaf*, which contains its proceedings. The *Annals*, edited at Gallaudet College, Washington 2, D.C., is the oldest journal in America dealing with the education of the deaf. Its first issue appeared on October 1, 1847. It has published all types of material on the deaf and is the official organ of both the Convention and the Conference. It is widely read by educators of the deaf, and its contents yield valuable research material and directories.

THE NATIONAL ASSOCIATION OF THE DEAF

Seventy-nine years ago, in 1880, the National Deaf-Mute Convention, now the National Association of the Deaf (NAD), held its first meeting. In 1890 a constitution was adopted and purposes were stated: "Mutual assistance and encouragement in bettering their standing in society at large, and the enjoyment of social pleasure attendant upon the periodical reunion of a widely scattered class of people."

To carry out these purposes, the NAD has striven quite successfully to eliminate unjust liability, compensation, and traffic laws. It has worked to remove barriers against the deaf in civil service and in other employment. At its triennial meetings, conducted in the language of signs and the manual alphabet, the NAD has gone on record, through formal resolutions, as standing in favor of the preservation of the language of signs. It has advocated that a strong campaign be undertaken to educate the public toward a better understanding of "the true place of the language of signs in the lives of the deaf as a means of facile communication for which no practical substitute has yet been devised."

The deaf as a class are proud and independent and do not wish to be considered recipients of charity. The self-respecting deaf are the first to denounce peddling or panhandling by irresponsible deaf persons. The National Association of the Deaf believes that there is no necessity for an educated deaf person to beg because of his deafness. It has been proved that in some cases hearing people have feigned deafness in order to arouse sympathy, and these people rightly deserve the scorn of the self-respecting deaf. The Association has announced that "stringent laws should be enacted, making it a penal offense to ask pecuniary aid on account of deafness or on pretense of being 'deaf and dumb.'"

The National Association appointed a committee to study the matter of workmen's compensation and employers' liability insurance, and the committee found that no state had any law that would bar the deaf man from working for any company. In the opinion of the committee, the employers who did not want to hire deaf men took refuge in saying that the insurance laws prohibited the hiring of the deaf or they accepted the arbitrary decisions of their insurance companies. It was felt that perhaps the deaf workmen in some portions of the country had in some way created prejudice on the part of some employers and that other employers did not know the true abilities of the deaf.

The National Association has encouraged homes for the aged and infirm deaf, maintained by organizations for the deaf. Homes are located in several states, including California, Georgia, Illinois, Indiana, Massachusetts, New York, Ohio, and Pennsylvania, and in Montreal, Canada.

In 1923 the NAD established a Traffic Bureau to assist deaf automobile drivers who had been discriminated against because of their deafness. It has cooperated with other organizations and agencies in gathering facts showing that the deaf are safe drivers. It has worked for special employment agencies for the deaf and has emphasized the necessity of compulsory-education laws for deaf children.

In March, 1946, a cooperative relationship between the Office of Vocational Rehabilitation, the Federal Security Agency, and the NAD was worked out. The National Association and the Office of Vocational Rehabilitation outlined the services available through both agencies. The National Association agreed to encourage its affiliated state associations of the deaf to establish working relationships with the state rehabilitation agencies and to acquaint their membership with the available vocational rehabilitation services. It also agreed to extend to the state rehabilitation agencies the services of interpreters of the manual alphabet and the language of signs. The agreement provided for joint studies and projects as well as for the preparation and distribution of literature and information on the rehabilitation of the deaf.

In recent years, the NAD has been reorganizing itself and at its 1957 convention in St. Louis it adopted new bylaws. The preamble states the aims and purposes of the Association: "The National Association of the Deaf shall be the focal point of the activities of all cooperating state and provincial associations of the deaf in promoting the welfare of the deaf in educational measures, in employment, in legislation, and in any other field pertaining to or affecting the deaf of America in their pursuit of economic security, social equality, and all their just rights and privileges as citizens." It further states that the NAD shall cooperate with its member associations of the deaf and give assistance when requested and that the NAD shall be in fact a federation of cooperating associations of the deaf, and shall also render assistance when possible to individual deaf persons and local groups of deaf persons.

The past few years have been characterized by greatly increased activity. An official publication, *The Silent Worker,* has been published monthly, and a national headquarters has been established. Opportunities for deaf workers have increased, particularly through contacts with the United States Civil Service Commission and the United States Bureau of Employment Security. Large federal grants have been obtained to help in an Occupational Survey of the Deaf, which is now in progress, and a training institute for vocational and social workers with the deaf was held in New York in the fall of 1957. The National Association continues to maintain vigilance to prevent discriminatory legislation and misleading propaganda. In the future, conventions will be held in alternate years.

Further information concerning the publications issued by the NAD and the plans for the future are obtainable from the Secretary, Mr. Robert M. Greenmun, School for the Deaf, St. Augustine, Florida.

THE NATIONAL FRATERNAL SOCIETY OF THE DEAF

The story of the National Fraternal Society of the Deaf (formerly the Fraternal Society of the Deaf) is a story of initiative, resourcefulness, mutual protection, and sound business. The Society was organized in Flint, Michigan, in 1901 by some young deaf men just out of school who rebelled against the classification of the deaf, by fraternal orders and by insurance companies, as "undesirable members or risks." And they realized that even if some deaf men became members of lodges, they would feel left out because of their deafness and loss of speech and their inability to take part fully in the ceremonies and ritual.

These men combined their need for adequate insurance (to cover sickness, accident, and death) with their need for social life (where all were on the same plane as far as communication was concerned). They formed the nonsectarian National Fraternal Society of the Deaf.

Membership in the Fraternal Society is open to deaf men and women of all creeds and stations in life; however, not all of them are eligible for membership. Members must be between the ages of eighteen and fifty-five and have "good bodily and mental health and industrious habits." In addition to its sickness, accident, and death benefits, the Society is pledged to give moral, financial, and material aid to its members in time of need. Among other benefits, the Society can provide safe and reliable car insurance for the deaf automobile driver, with public-liability and property-damage coverage. It encourages each member to feel that his interests are the interests of his fellow members. There is a strong feeling of good fellowship, and its members enjoy parties, balls, picnics, lectures, and the like, from time to time. Its meetings are conducted in the language of signs. *The Frat* is its official publication.

The Society operates under the supervision of the Insurance Department of the state of Illinois and is licensed in thirty-eight states and in the Dominion of Canada. Local units or divisions are maintained in all the principal cities of the United States and in the provinces of Ontario and Quebec. There are 10,500 members enrolled in the Society, and, during its existence, life insurance has been written on the lives of more than 17,000 deaf men and women. Additional information about the National Fraternal Society for the Deaf may be obtained from its home office: 6701 West North Avenue, Oak Park, Illinois. Its executive secretary is L. S. Cherry.

THE ALEXANDER GRAHAM BELL ASSOCIATION FOR THE DEAF, INC., AND THE VOLTA BUREAU

The history of this Association (formerly the American Association to Promote the Teaching of Speech to the Deaf, also the Volta Speech Association for the Deaf), which has served the deaf and the hard of hearing since it was incorporated in 1890, is interwoven with the life of a man whose genius has benefited all mankind, a man whose knowledge of speech and of the fundamentals of sound has opened up new worlds for the deaf, the hard of hearing, and those with normal hearing. Alexander Graham Bell was a great friend to the deaf and hard of hearing, and his influence on the development of the teaching of speech and speechreading is incalculable. Bell is even more widely known as the inventor of the telephone; and, as was pointed out in Chapter 10, the modern electric hearing aid is a development from the telephone. Today, an inestimable number of persons who would otherwise have been left out of things have been virtually restored to normal living with the aid of an electric hearing device.

Alexander Graham Bell, born in Scotland, came by his interest in speech naturally. His grandfather was an authority on speech. His father, Alexander Melville Bell, was acknowledged as the leading phonetician of his day and perfected a system of symbols known as "visible speech," [2] by which any sound made in speaking could be exactly expressed in writing. These symbols were originally intended to be used as a method of universal language instruction. The symbols described in Chapter 16 are good for training the ear and were the forerunners of the present International Phonetic Alphabet.

The Bell family moved to Canada in 1870. When Alexander Melville Bell was invited to give a course in the use of his Visible Speech Symbols to a group of teachers in Boston, he replied that he was too busy to come but that his son, Alexander Graham Bell, knew as much about the symbols as he did and would be available. Young Bell was only twenty-three years old when he went to Boston. His work there (quite apart from his electrical inventions) was the beginning of a

[2] Not to be confused with the Visible Speech machine mentioned in Chapter 14.

movement which was to spread over America and result in strong differences of opinion as to whether the deaf child should be taught by speech or by a manual method. Although Bell knew that deaf children could be taught how to speak, it was not until he became convinced of the practical value of speechreading that he became enthusiastic over its possibilities. Thousands of deaf people today who speech-read and speak owe their skill to the pioneering efforts of this genius with unusual mental gifts and a winning personality.

Perhaps in some people's minds the name "Volta Bureau" means a place where electricity is generated. The name owes its origin to three extraordinary men: Alessandro Volta, Napoleon Bonaparte, and Alexander Graham Bell. Fred DeLand has told this interesting story in his *Story of Lip Reading:*

> In 1800, Volta, an Italian scientist who had been experimenting with a chemical generator of electricity, described his battery at a meeting of the National Institute in Paris. Napoleon, who was a member of the Institute, was present. He grasped the value of the invention, and immediately proposed that France should award Volta a gold medal and a gift of 6000 francs. He also established a permanent fund from which a sum of money, known as the "Volta Prize" should be conferred upon those who made important contributions to the new science of electricity. In 1880, this prize which now amounted to 50,000 francs, was bestowed upon Alexander Graham Bell for the invention of the electric speaking telephone. He determined to invest this money in such a way that it would promote scientific research and at the same time would remain a permanent fund. This he accomplished in a characteristic fashion by using part of the Volta Fund to further the improvement of phonograph records, the patent rights to which, when sold, brought him $200,000. June 27, 1887, he turned over to his father, Alexander Melville Bell, $100,000 to be held in trust and used "for the purpose of founding and maintaining a Bureau for the increase and diffusion of knowledge relating to the deaf." [3]

Three years later (1890) Bell, not being eligible for membership in the Convention of American Instructors of the Deaf because he was not employed as a teacher of the deaf, organized the American Association to Promote the Teaching of Speech to the Deaf. In 1908, the Volta Fund, which Bell had created in 1887, was placed in the charge of the Association. All the activities of the Volta Bureau and of the Association have been carried on in the Volta Bureau Building since 1894. Helen Keller turned the first sod to break ground for the construction of this building.

[3] F. DeLand, *The Story of Lip-Reading* (Washington, D.C.: The Volta Bureau, 1931).

Membership in the Association has always been open to anyone interested in having children taught speech and speechreading. Alexander Graham Bell realized the importance of opening the membership to parents of deaf children, educators, scientists, physicians, philanthropists, and the general public. Soon hard-of-hearing adults began to seek membership, and today, after sixty-seven years, many Association members are hard of hearing.

Parents of deaf children have found the Association a wise counselor and a never-failing friend. Through personal correspondence and through literature prepared by experts, thousands of bewildered parents have learned what to do for their deaf children. They have also been told what they should not do if they desired their children to develop into well-adjusted adults, able to converse intelligibly and to speechread. In 1957 the Association provided for an expanded national program, in the interest of deaf children, by organizing a Parents' Section for individuals and establishing a membership classification whereby parent groups may become affiliated with the Association.

Teachers of the deaf have received inspiration and practical help through the Association's professional meetings, publications, and staff services; other teachers have found challenging new positions through services rendered by the Association. Hard-of-hearing adults the world over have left the influence of the Association's work in their behalf. The Association established the first standards for certification of teachers of the deaf, and later turned its function in the field of certification over to another professional group. Through its various committees it has consistently worked for the betterment of the deaf child, the hard-of-hearing child, and hard-of-hearing adults. It is constantly working toward the ideal of its founder: speech for all deaf children. The results of its efforts are encouraging. In every school for the deaf (private, residential, denominational, and day schools) provision is now made for the teaching of speech.

Since the Volta Bureau is owned by the Association, its work can rightfully be regarded as a part of the Association's work. The Volta Bureau contains the largest collection of books on the deaf and deafness in America, perhaps the largest in the world. Research workers from various foreign lands have used the facilities of its library, where there are books in fourteen languages. Priceless manuscripts, as well as rare editions of books and pamphlets, are carefully preserved. The research worker can find reports of schools for the deaf that will give him a step-by-step knowledge of the evolution of the teaching of speech and of speechreading. During World War II the facilities of the Volta Bureau were used freely by members of the Armed Forces.

The first magazine published by the Association was the *Association Review*. In 1910, the name was changed to the *Volta Review*. The *Volta Review* has published thousands of articles dealing with speech-reading, the teaching of speech, hearing aids, auditory training, problems of parents of deaf children, and methods of teaching deaf children and hard-of-hearing adults, as well as stories of individuals who have overcome the handicap of impaired hearing, and informative articles dealing with various phases of work with the acoustically handicapped. The *Volta Review* for many years also served as the official organ of the American Hearing Society. Later, the Volta Bureau published the *Auditory Outlook* for the American Hearing Society, until April, 1933, when the Society decided to issue its own publication, *Hearing News*.

A fine service rendered by the Association and the Volta Bureau was the assistance given to the present American Hearing Society. It provided quarters for the Society in the Volta Bureau Building and publicized the work of the Society in the *Volta Review*. Through its policy of "Help thy brother's boat across, and lo! thy own hath reached the shore," the Association is now stronger and is serving more people than ever before.

Further information about the Alexander Graham Bell Association for the Deaf may be obtained by writing to Mrs. Jeanette N. Johnson, the present executive secretary, at 1537 35th Street, N.W., Washington 7, D.C.

THE AMERICAN HEARING SOCIETY

This national organization has changed its name several times. It was first the American Association for the Hard of Hearing, then the American Federation of Organizations for the Hard of Hearing, then the American Society for the Hard of Hearing, and, since 1946, the American Hearing Society, but it has not changed its three major purposes: the prevention of deafness, the conservation of hearing, and the rehabilitation of the hard of hearing.

The story of the American Hearing Society is one of vision, courage, and the will to attempt an organized attack on the social, educational, and economic problems of hard-of-hearing children and adults. As described above, a great deal had already been done for the deaf before the Society was formed, and the organization owes much to the early pioneers, especially to Alexander Graham Bell and the Volta Bureau. But, while the problems of the deaf and of a limited number of the hard of hearing were receiving concerted attention, there was a vast group of acoustically handicapped persons who were isolated even in the midst of their families and friends, standing on the outskirts of social life, neither deaf nor normally hearing. They were misunderstood, discriminated against, and neglected.

Schools of speechreading for heard-of-hearing adults began to be established, usually by teachers who were themselves hard of hearing and wanted to show others how life could be worth living again by learning to speechread. One of these teachers was Edward Bartlett Nitchie of New York. Some of his well-to-do pupils provided scholarships for those who could not afford to pay for instruction. One of his less fortunate pupils could not find employment and one day told Mr. Nitchie that he would commit suicide if he continued to be unsuccessful. He was never seen again. Out of that pupil's great mental stress and tragedy grew the American Hearing Society. The pupils in Nitchie's school formed the Nitchie School Alumni Association, which later became the Nitchie Service League. The members of the League began to realize that they were doing true social pioneering—pioneering in which its workers themselves turned the searchlight on their own problems, worked out readjustments, and helped each other. This was a unique type of social work. As the Nitchie Service League grew in strength and influence, its leaders (and particularly Nitchie) decided that a name should be chosen to indicate that there was no connection with any one school or individual. And so the name "New York League for the Hard of Hearing" was given to the first organization for the hard of hearing in America.

By 1919 there were local organizations for the hard of hearing in Boston, Chicago, Cleveland, Los Angeles, Newark, Philadelphia, Toledo, and San Francisco. All of these organizations had received much help and guidance from the New York League. In that year Dr. Wendell C. Phillips, prominent otologist of New York, united the scattered groups into a national organization. Under his leadership representatives of existing organizations for the hard of hearing formed what is now the American Hearing Society. The program of the Society is "to serve as an information center on problems of defective hearing; to improve the educational, economic, and social conditions among both adults and children whose hearing is impaired; and to stimulate scientific efforts in the prevention of deafness and the conservation of hearing."

Fifty-one persons, most of them hard of hearing, attended the first conference of the new Society, which was held in Boston in 1921 in conjunction with a meeting of the Otological Section of the American Medical Association. Years later, one delegate, in reporting on that first meeting said, "How could we, an obscure little organization, with only one hundred direct members and with only nine local organizations, influence the handling of children scattered through the schools of the United States like needles in a haystack? The task seemed insurmountable. Nevertheless, we know today that when that meeting closed, the hard of hearing child had found his best and most convincing friend—the American Hearing Society."

From 1919 to 1923 the business of the American Hearing Society was carried on entirely by volunteers. In March, 1923, headquarters were moved from New York to Washington, where, for over three years, its office quarters were provided by the Volta Bureau. The Society then maintained its own offices in the Volta Bureau Building until 1948. Headquarters are now located at 919 18th Street, N.W., Washington 6, D.C.

In 1924 the first Committee on Hard-of-Hearing Children surveyed the opportunities for the education of hard-of-hearing children in public schools. It found that prior to 1916 practically all hard-of-hearing children were sent to special schools for the deaf or were untaught because no provision was made for them elsewhere.

The Committee appealed to the Bell Telephone Laboratories for an instrument that could test the hearing of large numbers of children. As a result, the group audiometer was developed.

Another report of the Committee, in 1925, became the nucleus of the Society's Conservation of Hearing Program. The program calls for medical prevention of deafness through hearing tests; otolaryngological examinations and treatment; use of hearing aids when indicated; instruction in speechreading and auditory training in regular schools for the children who need it; special classes for children who are severely hard of hearing; special training in speech when necessary; and, finally, vocational guidance for the hard of hearing. From time to time the Society has made available free hearing aids for children and elderly persons from special funds contributed to it.

Hearing News, a bimonthly periodical, is the official publication of the American Hearing Society and is sent to all members of the Society. It carries organization news and articles on developments in the treatment of hearing loss, selection of hearing aids, and aural rehabilitation. Speechreading, speech correction, and auditory training are all covered, and advice as to employment and the choice of vocations is featured. The magazine advertises hearing aids and accessories.

The American Hearing Society also distributes at nominal cost pamphlets dealing with hard-of-hearing children, hearing clinics, tests of hearing, and related subjects. In 1955 it published *A Guide for Self-Study of Hearing Programs* which is widely used in setting up community hearing services and in evaluating and expanding existing programs.

The Society's Committee on Legislation distributed informative

material designed to influence various states to adopt measures benefiting hard-of-hearing children.

Field workers of the Society have visited almost every state and
some of the provinces of Canada, giving advice to groups of hard-of-
hearing people, talking before civic groups, pointing out to school
officials the needs of hard-of-hearing children, and making contacts
with social workers and with physicians. At first the field workers
carried with them large trunks of electrical equipment. Group hearing
aids were set up, and with these the people who were interested in
forming a local hearing society could hear what was going on. The
American Hearing Society organized local chapters in many large
cities and in a number of those chapters group hearing aids were available. Today these aids have been supplanted by public-address
systems.

During World War II the Society cooperated with the Office of
Civilian Defense, the Red Cross, and interested government agencies
in programs related to the hard of hearing.

In 1956 the American Hearing Society changed the name "chapters" to "member organizations," which are divided into two groups:
member agencies and member affiliates (the former offering a well-
rounded community service by a professional staff, and the latter
operating on a volunteer basis). Of these organizations, forty-nine
are supported by local Community Chests or United Funds. These
organizations aim to alleviate the social isolation of individual hard-of-
hearing men and women and to help them in their adjustment to many
problems. Sympathetic understanding helps to make easier their contacts with the normally hearing world. The member organizations
have been termed "hope filling stations," for they give their members
hope and enable them to take their rightful places in the world of
normally hearing people.

The local groups also serve as information centers. Social agencies,
physicians, school officials, and the general public turn to these organizations for information on various problems affecting the acoustically handicapped. Speechreading practice classes and social activities are provided. In some of the larger member agencies there are
also employment bureaus, evaluations of hearing aids, speech therapy,
and auditory training. Some groups offer guidance to parents of hard-
of-hearing children. There are clubs for current events, bowling,
nature study, sewing, photography, dramatics, and bridge. The organizations for the hard of hearing not only help those who are in
need of guidance and training but lift the morale of all who work for
their purposes. A feeling of fellowship and mutual helpfulness prevails,

combined with the ideal of helping all in the community with a hearing handicap.

A hearing workshop, cosponsored by the American Hearing Society and the Office of Vocational Rehabilitation, United States Department of Health, Education, and Welfare, was held in Washington, D.C., in 1954. Theme of the workshop was "Community Attack on the Hearing Problems of Adults." This program brought together experts on hearing problems from all over the United States, and the deliberations and conclusions were published in the *Proceedings*, which can be obtained from the American Hearing Society.

In 1956 the American Hearing Society published *A Syllabus on Special Problems of the Deaf and the Hard of Hearing for Orientation Institutes*, prepared under a grant from the Office of Vocational Rehabilitation. Copies are available from the Society.

Through another grant from the Office of Vocational Rehabilitation, under Public Law 565, the American Hearing Society is working on a special rehabilitation project to assemble data, requirements, methods, and procedures to aid communities wishing to establish or expand facilities for rehabilitation of persons with hearing and/or speech defects. Information about the American Hearing Society may be obtained from Crayton Walker, its executive director, 919 18th Street, N.W., Washington 6, D.C.

THE AMERICAN SPEECH AND HEARING ASSOCIATION

The American Speech and Hearing Association is a professional and learned association. Begun in 1925 as the American Academy of Speech Correction, the organization became the American Society for the Study of Disorders of Speech in 1927, and the American Speech Correction Association in 1934. It assumed its present name in 1947. Annual conventions are held regularly. The bylaws state: "The purposes of this organization shall be to encourage basic scientific study of the processes of individual human speech and hearing, promote investigation of speech and hearing disorders, and foster improvement of therapeutic procedures with such disorders; to stimulate exchange of information among persons thus engaged, and to disseminate such information." The Association has set up certain requirements, criteria, and standards for certification and carries on a program of clinical certification for members. It maintains a Placement Registry Service for all members seeking employment or change of employment. The Association has been chosen by United Cerebral Palsy for the distribution of substantial scholarship funds. The Association carries on a program of public relations to interpret the profession of speech and hearing therapy to the public, to related professional groups, and to prospective professional workers. Its official publications are *The Journal of Speech and Hearing Disorders* and *The Journal of Speech and Hearing Research,* which are published quarterly.

The code of ethics of the Association has become an influential standard for professional conduct, and its annual directory is a valuable source of information about speech and hearing workers and their qualifications. The Office of Vocational Rehabilitation has contributed support to the establishment of a national office for the Association and has sponsored a conference arranged by the Association on research needs in speech and hearing. The Executive Secretary is Dr. Kenneth O. Johnson, 1001 Connecticut Avenue, N.W., Washington 6, D.C.

MEDICAL GROUPS

The American Academy of Ophthalmology and Otolaryngology is the chief American organization of certified otolaryngologists. Through its Committee on the Conservation of Hearing it sponsors public information and research activities about hearing and deafness. It publishes manuals for its own members and for related groups, and in general makes known the attitudes of the profession of otolaryngology on such questions as standards for audiometers and medicolegal principles for the evaluation of hearing loss. With the cooperation of the manufacturers of audiometers and certain independent laboratories the Academy has recently instituted a program for testing audiometers to determine whether they meet mutually agreed standards published by the American Standards Association. The Secretary of the Committee on Conservation of Hearing is Dr. Dean M. Lierle, State University of Iowa, Iowa City.

A significant and active group under the Committee on the Conservation of Hearing is the Subcommittee on Noise. Its purposes are to disseminate information through publication, conferences, and lectures about the effects of noise on man and to conduct research to add to our knowledge of this problem. These purposes are achieved through a well-equipped research center, enlarged to its present (1959) scope in 1954. The research center has recently become affiliated with the University of Southern California. The director is Dr. Aram Glorig, 327 South Alvarado, Los Angeles 57, California.

Another important group under the aegis of the Committee on Conservation of Hearing is the Subcommittee on Hearing in Children. The specific aims of this committee are to develop the most efficient case-finding methods and to use these methods in estimating the magnitude of the problems in the country; to study state laws and review current practices and facilities for children with hearing handicaps; to develop methods and standards for medical and surgical rehabilitation of children; and ultimately to use Subcommittee findings in assisting professional workers to improve and expand programs related to hearing loss. The full-time executive director is Dr. Eldon L. Eagles, whose offices are at the Graduate School of Public Health, University of Pittsburgh, Pittsburgh, Pennsylvania.

The American Otological Society is the senior society of American and Canadian otologists. The Society publishes transactions of its annual meetings and finances a research bureau whose chief interest is the investigation of otosclerosis. The secretary of the Society (1958) is Dr. Lawrence Boies, University of Minnesota, Minneapolis, Minnesota.

GOVERNMENT AGENCIES

In addition to these organized groups, agencies of the government have also been active in the field of hearing and deafness.

The Armed Forces–National Research Council Committee on Hearing and Bio-Acoustics (CHABA) was organized originally (through a contract between the Department of Defense and the Central Institute for the Deaf) to furnish expert consulting services to the Armed Forces related to hearing and bio-acoustics. Among the problems on which CHABA has been consulted are methods of audiometry, the conservation of hearing in the Armed Forces, problems arising from noise in the neighborhood of military airports, and interference by noise with communication and with the performance of military duties. The executive secretary of CHABA, Dr. Milton Whitcomb, can be reached through the National Academy of Sciences, 2101 Constitution Avenue, Washington, D.C.

The Department of Health, Education, and Welfare has become active in hearing and deafness in order to carry out the increasing interest of Congress in matters of health and rehabilitation. Through its National Institute on Neurological Diseases and Blindness the National Institutes of Health furnish funds for basic and applied research and for training purposes. The training aims to increase the quality as well as the number of investigators and teachers who are committed to work on problems of deafness. The Office of Vocational Rehabilitation, as we have seen, is interested in promoting and in upgrading the employability of the deaf and hard of hearing through grants for research, for rehabilitation, and for the training of professional personnel. It has sponsored valuable conferences and has encouraged participation by the deaf and hard of hearing themselves. The Office of Education gathers statistics about handicapped children and promotes studies about them. Among recent significant activities are studies of the competencies needed for teachers of the deaf and the hard of hearing. Acoustically handicapped children are also of interest to the Children's Bureau. The Department of Health, Education, and Welfare may be reached at Washington, D.C.

The extensive work of the Veterans Administration in auditory rehabilitation has been described in Chapter 19.

Other organizations whose activities touch on problems of hearing and deafness are the following:

The Acoustical Society of America
The American Federation for the Physically Handicapped
The American Public Health Association
The Council for Exceptional Children
The National Rehabilitation Association
The National Society for Crippled Children and Adults

The list of organized groups and agencies is formidable and impressive, and it suggests that we may be encouraged by the outlook for the deaf and hard of hearing in the years ahead.

Suggested Readings

KURTZ, R. H. *Social Work Yearbook.* New York: National Association of Social Workers, 1957.
A valuable reference book with brief descriptions of the aims, purposes, and activities of national organizations.

SILVERMAN, S. R. "The Hearing Handicapped: Their Education and Rehabilitation," *Postgraduate Medicine,* 23: 321–330 (1958).
One of a series on physical medicine and rehabilitation that cites the factors responsible for increased interest in hearing impairment and the organizations active in the field.

Nearly all of the organizations that we have described publish periodicals regularly. For information about them we suggest direct correspondence.

21

EMPLOYMENT FOR THE HARD OF HEARING

Ada Morgan Hill

The employment problems of the hard of hearing are legion. Until the beginning of World War II, when the shortage of manpower became acute, many employees with impaired hearing had been the first to lose their jobs whenever a reduction in personnel was necessary. Prior to the war, the number of hard-of-hearing persons who were unemployed had grown to alarming proportions, and it became increasingly evident that vocational counseling, had it been given these people, might have helped some of them to retain their employment. Many hard-of-hearing workers had been placed in jobs where their lack of hearing was definitely a handicap. Either they had decided on their lifework without giving due consideration to their loss of hearing, or they had received no vocational guidance and were placed, more or less by chance, in occupations where they could not succeed.

Many pitfalls could have been avoided, and disappointments over failure lessened, if vocational guidance had been sought and heeded. Once a hard-of-hearing person is trained and placed in employment for which his training has fitted him, his morale is greatly lowered if he finds he cannot continue in his chosen field of endeavor. He usually blames his lack of hearing, entirely unaware of the fact that had he been properly advised in the first place about his own limitations and the requirements of that type of work, he could almost certainly have avoided the calamity. The effect of unemployment on the morale of persons who are hard of hearing seems to be unusually severe, and often it is difficult for them to pull themselves out of an apathetic attitude and seek another kind of work.

TESTS AND GUIDANCE

In most states there are public agencies which give aptitude tests and advice concerning vocations to the normal and the handicapped alike. State rehabilitation services have been of inestimable help in advising many hard-of-hearing persons regarding their vocational problems. Their counselors and supervisors have cooperated with the American Hearing Society and its member agencies in offering understanding help, guidance, and training to the hearing handicapped and in placing them in profitable occupations.

In some communities, testing and guidance programs are offered by private and public schools, colleges, and universities on a fee basis, although these institutions do not undertake to find jobs for the unemployed. These tests help to uncover such capabilities as mechanical comprehension, manual dexterity, artistic, literary, and clerical aptitudes, speed, memory, and general intelligence. With this information, counselors are better able to advise as to what occupations are best suited to a client's particular talents and abilities. Tests of this sort frequently disclose latent abilities that had not been fully realized or even suspected by the person. Many local hearing societies are equipped to offer guidance in vocational and employment problems, as a community service to the hearing handicapped.

THE COUNSELOR

The number of counselors giving vocational guidance to the hard of hearing has grown considerably during the last few years, but not everyone is qualified to undertake this sort of work. Not only must a good counselor have at his or her fingertips a wealth of information concerning job analyses and working conditions in various types of work, the special abilities that make for success in each line, and the physical demands or hazards that make them unsuited for those with this particular physical handicap; he must also understand the prognosis of the condition which causes the defect. Above all, the counselor must have a keen understanding of human nature and of the psychological effects of deafness if he is to deal successfully with the hard of hearing. He must see both sides of the problem, that of the employer and that of the employee. He must be able to recognize that just because some hard-of-hearing persons are emotionally unstable, it does not follow that all persons with a hearing loss are likewise unstable. He must think of each client as an individual with his own particular combination of abilities and disabilities, and not merely as a member of a group with the special handicap of hearing loss.

CONSULTATION WITH THE COUNSELOR

From the point of view of the counselor, the ideal way to give vocational guidance is through a series of personal interviews. The personal contact enables the counselor better to evaluate the abilities and personality of the client and to gain his confidence. In a face-to-face talk the counselor can determine many points for himself which might remain uncertain if he were forced to depend only on the client's opinion of himself or even on opinions given by associates, relatives, or employers. The client should give the counselor full and frank information regarding his education, his training, his occupational experience (if any), and his aptitudes, abilities, or special interest in (or dislike for) various types of work. He should also discuss his hobbies with the counselor because often the experience gained in working on a hobby is valuable and leads to a job with a good salary. An example is the photographic enthusiast who has a dark room and the necessary equipment to develop and enlarge all his own pictures. He could easily capitalize on that hobby. The counselor might also find the same potentialities for the man who had spent all his free time (and money!) in his cabinetmaking shop, or for the woman who possessed unusual ability in crafts or in the culinary arts. Such hobbies (and many others) can be turned into profitable employment.

The counselor requires reliable medical information as to the nature of the hearing loss and its prognosis and, quite as important, the general state of the client's health and the presence or absence of any other physical handicaps. Obviously, the difficulty in communication by speech is not as severe for the hard of hearing as it is for the deaf. The counselor endeavors to appraise the client's assets, such as good health, initiative, judgment, conscientiousness, reliability, education, special training, and so on. The skillful counselor is always on the alert to discover hidden abilities and capacities that may have been unsuspected by the client himself. Neither counselor nor client should allow the loss of hearing to obscure the abilities and assets. Most persons with physical handicaps have far more ability than disability. On the other hand, it is the duty of the counselor to advise his client against trying to enter a profession that is known to be overcrowded, or to train for any kind of work that is likely to be beyond his reach mentally and physically. If the client has more than one disability, both must be taken into consideration. This is particularly true of the double handicap of poor vision and poor hearing because the combination is more handicapping than either one alone.

There is no need for a list of occupations in which the hard of hearing are employed because such a list would contain practically all types of work. They are engaged in medicine, nursing, teaching, salesmanship, creative art work, social work, engineering, scientific research, photography, and innumerable other vocations. Many of them are following successfully occupations that would at first sight seem to be closed to the hard of hearing or at least to be extremely difficult for them. In general, however, there are certain types of skilled work that seem especially well suited for those hard-of-hearing persons who do not want to have daily contacts with the general public. These occupations include, among others, library work with its cataloguing, indexing, filing, and arranging of books; work in a stockroom with its marking, sorting, listing, and bundle-wrapping; and many of the various branches of bookkeeping and accounting. There are semiskilled and unskilled jobs in every community which can be filled satisfactorily by persons with a hearing loss. The choice of a vocation should never be made simply on the basis of a hearing loss, nor should the loss and its complications be ignored. This is especially true in the selection of an occupation for young persons with progressive deafness. On the other hand, there are favorable factors that are fully as important, such as education, temperament, and native ability. The total assets and liabilities should be considered in every case.

EDUCATION AND SOCIAL ADJUSTMENT

Education and training are necessary for success in any kind of work and the hard of hearing are no exceptions to this rule. The hard of hearing who become deaf after they have acquired a good education or substantial experience have just that much advantage over those whose deafness was so severe in childhood that they were retarded in their schooling. A first and most obvious bit of vocational advice, which cannot be given too early, is hardly "vocational" at all. It is that the hard-of-hearing youngster should obtain all the education that his abilities indicate and that, in addition, he or she should adopt a sound mental attitude toward the hearing loss, learn to speech-read and to use a hearing aid, aim to keep his voice and speech as nearly normal as possible, and above all develop or keep a pleasing personality. *Personality more often than the state of a man's hearing is the deciding factor in keeping or losing a job.* Frequently a bad voice and faulty speech are more of a handicap than loss of hearing. Auditory training and speech therapy will do much to improve a voice that is not pleasing. The value of speechreading and of a good hearing aid can hardly be overemphasized.

Like any other intelligent young men and women, young adults who are hard-of-hearing, should capitalize on their abilities and minimize their disabilities. Intelligence tests and aptitude tests can show whether anyone possesses superior ability, and if he does, regardless of the state of his hearing, he has a right to expect to be given work where his ability and training can be utilized, provided that he has successfully overcome his hearing loss. He should never expect, however, to be shown special favors because of his hearing loss or to use his disability in any way as an excuse for unusual demands on his employer or associates. He must be prepared to make himself just a little more skilled at his job than are his fellow workers, to work harmoniously with others, and to adapt his methods to the routine of his position.

SELECTIVE PLACEMENT

We can better understand some of the earlier reports that were not so favorable to the hard of hearing in industry if we recall that before the problems of the hard of hearing were so widely discussed and so generally known, many employees with hearing losses were placed in occupations which they could not and did not fill successfully. When the causes of their failure were listed, the impairment of hearing was almost invariably placed at the top of the list, although it may have been only one of several contributing factors. Lack of proper general education or of specific training for a particular job was often overlooked, as well as the possibility that the hard-of-hearing man may have been a disturbing element among his co-workers. We now recognize that more men leave their jobs because of personality factors than because of lack of skill. In the more recent surveys all of these factors are recognized and reasonably evaluated.

The need for selective placement of the physically handicapped in industry is generally recognized today. With proper analysis of the prospective employee and the job, square pegs are not so often put into round holes. Selective placement is receiving more and more attention from industry and government alike, to the benefit of both employer and employee.

In recent years a routine physical examination and screening have been included more and more frequently as a part of selective-placement programs. Sometimes these examinations have been abused, and discrimination against the hard of hearing has been evident. For example, instances are on record of an examining physician's refusing to allow a hard-of-hearing applicant to wear his hearing aid during the physical examination, although not demanding that he remove his eyeglasses. It is hoped, however, that the examination is now done intelligently to assist in placing the right employees in the right job and not as a screen to keep the physically handicapped out of jobs they can perform.

THE HARD OF HEARING IN UNFAVORABLE SURROUNDINGS

In connection with the selective placement of the hard of hearing there has long been an impression that noisy places of employment are suitable for them. This impression probably arises from the fact that for years such places were recommended for the deaf, and there are still many persons today who fail to differentiate between the deaf and the hard of hearing. Moreover, few people realize that many of the hard of hearing are just as sensitive to *loud* noise as are those with normal hearing. Some hard of hearing, in fact, are abnormally annoyed or disturbed by loud sounds. Sensory-neural hearing loss, it will be recalled, may destroy a man's ability to hear faint sounds but still leave him normally sensitive to loud noises, which are likely to be both startling and annoying. For such a man it is not only ridiculous but harmful to recommend employment in noisy surroundings. The man with a conductive hearing loss, however, is partly protected against the noise and, in consequence, has a distinct advantage over his normal companion in noisy surroundings. If he ordinarily wears a hearing aid, he only needs to turn down its volume control or turn it off altogether.

It is obvious that no blanket rule can be laid down concerning the fitness of the hard of hearing for work in noisy situations. We do not recommend noisy surroundings as desirable for anyone, but as long as we have such surroundings, the hard of hearing who are automatically protected by their very disability may well take advantage of the situation. On the other hand, the hard-of-hearing man who tires quickly and becomes careless and irritable under the strain of trying to distinguish voices from noise should not be placed in noisy surroundings. Any alert examining physician should be able to recognize the difference between the two types of hearing loss and not be misled by unsound generalizations. Here again, the temperament of the client is quite as important as his hearing loss in determining whether or not he is fit to work in noisy surroundings.

The whole question of the effects of industrial noise on man is being studied by the Subcommittee on Noise of the American Academy of Ophthalmology and Otolaryngology, which has published some excellent pamphlets on the subject, notably its *Guide for Conservation of Hearing in Noise.*

In addition to noise, there are other surroundings which may affect hard-of-hearing persons unfavorably, such as dusty and damp places, and locations where there are sudden changes of temperature, but it is certainly true that not all hard-of-hearing persons are unduly affected by any of these situations.

INDUSTRIAL INSURANCE

Some employers have refused to hire physically handicapped workers on the grounds that their insurance rates would be increased as a result. On the other hand, the Association of Casualty and Surety Executives has stated: "The physical defects of such workers are not considered in the formulas for determining the initial rate for insurance, and no higher rate is charged because of employment of physically disabled persons." In spite of this, some cases have been reported to the American Hearing Society where hard-of-hearing persons were told they could not be given employment because the insurance rates for the positions to which they were seeking appointment would be raised. It was not always the employer himself who was trying to hide behind insurance rates. The examining physician was sometimes to blame. In one particular instance, a placement agent advised the American Hearing Society that the employer in a certain factory was willing and ready to hire a hard-of-hearing person, but stated that the examining physician would not pass the worker for fear that if an accident occurred, he, the physician, would be blamed. Such practices are unfair to physically handicapped persons and defeat the very purposes of the law. A workmen's compensation insurance policy makes no provision for the physical condition of the workers an insured employer may hire, and his insurance rates are not increased if he does employ a disabled person. Workmen's compensation premium rates are based upon hazards inherent in the industry and the experience record in the payment of benefits for work injuries sustained over specified periods of time.

It is true that insurance costs do rise or fall with the frequency and severity of an employer's accidents. Accidents may occur because the employer has failed to place and safeguard his employees properly, whether they are physically handicapped or able-bodied. This condition only emphasizes more than ever the great necessity for selective placement.

SENIOR WORKERS

Today the problem of employment for the older age group is perplexing management and labor as never before. Discrimination against the worker forty-five to sixty-five years of age and older must diminish and more of these persons must be retained in their jobs or transferred to work that is more compatible with their abilities. The problems of the older worker have become a community responsibility, and the federal government is giving the whole matter serious study. Conferences on the aging are being held to determine and fix the responsibilities for the welfare of this group.

Many older persons are unhappy in enforced retirement, or they find their pensions inadequate to meet living costs. When hearing loss is added to old age, as it frequently is, the person finds himself with a double handicap. As life expectancy increases, the number of people sixty-five years and older who need vocational guidance continues to grow. The vocational counselor should be skilled in techniques of counseling the elderly as well as the young. He will need the help of all the disciplines at his command, for these older persons must be helped into productive and fruitful occupations. Their experiences and techniques are of untold value to the world; society has need for all that her citizens can contribute to her welfare.

SUCCESS OF THE HARD OF HEARING IN INDUSTRY

The hard of hearing are part, and an important part, of a larger group of physically handicapped employees numbering approximately seven million men and women. Many surveys have been made among employees to determine the performance of physically handicapped workers as compared with those who are able-bodied. A recent report from The President's Committee on Employment of the Physically Handicapped stated:

> The records show that the handicapped are *adaptable*. They adjust quickly and satisfactorily to the conditions of the job. They're *productive*. In job performance they often surpass the production records of other employees. They're *careful*. Safety records of the handicapped are as good as those of other workers. They're *regular*. Handicapped have job attendance records that equal those of other workers doing the same type of work. They're *reliable*. The handicapped are not "job-hoppers." Finally, they're *capable*. They do any kind of work where their impairments are not handicaps—and do it as well as those who are unimpaired.

The favorable reports of the government commissions concerning the performance of physically handicapped workers in general should be quite as inspiring to the deaf and the hard of hearing as the familiar examples of geniuses, such as Ludwig van Beethoven, Sir Joshua Reynolds, and Thomas Edison, to name a few, who have made history in spite of the handicap of their hearing losses.

THE ECONOMIC AND PSYCHOLOGICAL VALUE OF REHABILITATION

The economic value of employing hard-of-hearing workers is perfectly obvious. Each man employed means one less on the charity rolls, one more self-supporting citizen, and another taxpayer added to the list. The Vocational Rehabilitation Services have published statistics which show that the earnings of men and women who have been rehabilitated are many times the amount spent for their rehabilitation. But, in addition to the economic benefits, the psychological value of the hard-of-hearing person who has been given suitable and continual employment is beyond tabulation. Every individual has certain basic psychological needs. Every man and woman likes to have a sense of achievement, a sense of personal worth, and a sense of contributing to the joys of others. Hearing loss is only a part of a man's make-up, and he should not, because of this handicap, be denied the rights and opportunities to which he is entitled.

Suggested Readings

BLUETT, CHARLES G., coordinator. *Handbook of Information for the Hard of Hearing.* Sponsored by the California State Departments of Public Health and Education. Sacramento: 1947.

———, and ADA M. HILL. *An Employment Survey,* conducted by the American Hearing Society. Washington, D.C.: 1946.

BORDEN, EDWARD S. *Psychological Counseling.* New York: Appleton-Century-Crofts, Inc., 1955.

GARRET, JAMES F., ed. *Psychological Aspects of Disability.* Rehabilitation Service Series No. 210. Office of Vocational Rehabilitation, United State Department of Health, Education, and Welfare. Washington, D.C.

HAMILTON, KENNETH W. *Counseling the Handicapped.* New York: The Ronald Press Company, 1950.

HARVEY, VERNE. A Guide to the Placement of the Physically Handicapped. Washington, D.C.: Government Printing Office, Pt. I, *Aircraft Positions,* 1952; Pt. II, *Ordnance and Ordnance Stores Positions,* 1953; Pt. III, *Shipbuilding Positions,* 1953; Pt. IV, *Positions in Five Technical Agencies,* 1955.

HEINER, MARIE HAYS. *Hearing Is Believing.* Cleveland: The World Publishing Company, 1949.

MURPHY, GRACE E. BARSTOW. *Your Deafness Is Not You.* New York: Harper & Brothers, 1954.

Number of Disabled Persons in Need of Vocational Rehabilitation. Rehabilitation Service Series No. 274. Office of Vocational Rehabilitation, United States Department of Health, Education, and Welfare. Washington, D.C.: 1954.

Orientation Training for Vocational Rehabilitation Counselors. Betty C. Wright, comp. Washington, D.C.: American Hearing Society, 1956.
A syllabus on special problems of the deaf and the hard of hearing for orientation institutes.

Rehabilitation Counselor Training: Eighth Annual Workshop on Guidance, Training and Placement. Report of Proceedings. Rehabilitation Service Series No. 331. Office of Vocational Rehabilitation, United States Department of Health, Education, and Welfare. Washington, D.C., Pt. I.

Report to the President of the Federal Council on Aging. Department of Health, Education, and Welfare. Washington, D.C.: 1957.

SILVERMAN, S. R. "The Hearing Handicapped: Their Education and Rehabilitation," *Postgraduate Medicine,* 23: 321–329 (1958).

TYLER, LEONA E. *The Work of the Counselor.* New York: Appleton-Century-Crofts, Inc., 1953.

Vocational Rehabilitation Counselor: Health Careers Guidebook. New York: The National Health Council, 1955, pp. 142–143.

Workshops for the Disabled. Rehabilitation Service Series No. 371. Office of Vocational Rehabilitation, United States Department of Health, Education, and Welfare. Washington, D.C.: 1956.

22

VOCATIONAL GUIDANCE
FOR THE DEAF

Boyce R. Williams, LL.D.

This chapter will discuss the common vocational guidance resources for deaf people in the United States. Also, it will give special attention to desirable practices in counseling and in psychological diagnosis. Counseling and psychological evaluation, two of the most critical tools in the vocational guidance process, are frequently misused with deaf people. The chapter will review recent data on rehabilitants and the results of vocational guidance in some jobs at which deaf people work, and it will examine important employment principles specific to deaf workers in industry. Finally, it will make some suggestions on the employability of deaf people that we believe will be helpful to audiologists and those in relevant fields.

Definitions

For the purposes of this discussion three definitions are necessary. The first is for vocational guidance, the second is for the deaf, and the third is for the vocational guidance team.

WHAT IS VOCATIONAL GUIDANCE?

According to an accurate, popular definition, "vocational guidance is the process of assisting individuals to understand their capabilities and interests, to choose a suitable occupation, and to prepare for, enter, and make successful progress in it."

Definitions of vocational guidance suggest that all people can do many jobs very well. They have not encouraged the concept of a one best job for the individual. Moreover, they recognize that people grow, that change is healthy, that it is natural for people to look for more challenging, attractive, or appropriate employment. Accordingly,

515

vocational guidance is a continuing process rather than a one-time undertaking.

WHO ARE THE DEAF?

There are many opinions among specialists from various fields regarding proper definition of the deaf. Educational circumstances in different communities, variations in individual response to equivalent hearing losses, different family backgrounds, a clearly recognizable core of wishful thinking, different ages at onset of loss are a few of the many variables. They produce the exceptions that weaken definitions. In another chapter this matter is fully covered. Here only the essentials will be stated.

The common denominators of our group are their ages at onset and the severity of their hearing losses, and their needs for special education. In other words, they lost their hearing early enough and the amount of loss was severe enough to require special education. They should have had at least part of their educational experience in a public or private residential school for the deaf, a day school or class for the deaf, or a nursery school for the deaf. Our group includes those who missed the special education pattern despite meeting the criteria of age-at-onset and severity. Most of them should not have missed it. They tax our vocational guidance resources to the utmost.

All of the group have severe problems of communication. They communicate principally through their eyes rather than ears. Many speak too poorly to be understood at all or they may be understood only by an experienced teacher of the deaf. Many with reasonably acceptable speech are insecure in its use except with family and friends. The written language of many is full of errors and bizarre expressions. Many with poor expressive spoken or written language are excellent speechreaders. Many with excellent ability in speech and writing are poor speechreaders. Most communicate very fluently by manual methods. They prefer sign language and finger spelling among themselves and in interrelationships with other people whenever this talent is available. In fact, they are likely to gravitate to vocational guidance resources where such methods of communication are used.

These are the deaf. They are a small group. We estimate that they numbered roughly about 188,000 in 1953.[1] There are probably 200,000 now. Moreover, the fact that they are spread relatively thinly throughout the country complicates all problems of providing them with useful services, including vocational guidance.

[1] "Estimates of the Number of Deaf and Partially Deaf in the U.S.," Division of Program Statistics and Special Studies, Office of Vocational Rehabilitation, United States Department of Health, Education, and Welfare, December 10, 1954.

THE TEAM

The common concept of the team is a group that interacts to achieve a common objective. Workers in many fields are daily involved in teamwork around conference table, in the clinic, or in the rehabilitation center. However, when such people and their clients are relatively few, as is true of the deaf, we must adopt more practical patterns of teamwork if we are to avoid self-defeating limitations.

Time, distance, and the relatively small number of clients preclude much if any simultaneous coming together of the relevant experts. The essential teamwork lies in joint acceptance of a common goal or responsibility, in free and full exchange of thinking and information, in respect for the contribution of each discipline, in courage to call for change or to reject proposals, in prompt and wholehearted response to calls for action.

In some places such a team concept serves the deaf effectively although seldom if ever is there a group meeting. Telephone calls, correspondence, verbal messages passed along by the client, or case folder memoranda—all are common tools by which the team coordinator marshals, evaluates, and integrates a flow of valuable information and opinion. The coordinator or primary manager is not always the same team member. He may be a teacher, principal, school counselor, audiologist, vocational rehabilitation counselor, physician, placement specialist, social worker, or psychologist. He is whichever worker presses the action. Team efficiency rests upon his skill in stimulating the best contributions from each team member and helping the individual to interpret them effectively.

What We Have

Resources available to help deaf people choose, prepare for, enter upon, and progress in suitable occupations include special schools for the deaf, state vocational rehabilitation agencies, state employment services, and professional and voluntary workers. A persisting sense of sparseness in vocational guidance for the deaf is due partly to time and distance factors associated with the spread of both the resources and deaf people. It is due also to inadequate teamwork. Ideally these resources complement each other in identifying and meeting the needs of each deaf person. In day-to-day operations, this goal is frequently not attained because the responsibilities, techniques, and practices of teamwork are only now gaining acceptance among the various team members.

The three public programs are the main framework of vocational guidance services for the deaf. However, it should be noted that four states have important additional public services that contribute extensively: the Minnesota Services for the Deaf in the Department of Public Welfare, the North Carolina Labor Bureau in the Department of Labor, the Michigan Division for the Deaf and the Deafened in the Employment Security Commission, and the Wisconsin Service Bureau in the State Association of the Deaf. Each has a rich and varied program that encourages great personal assistance to deaf people who have need of it.

Professional and voluntary sources provide information useful in vocational guidance of the deaf. The National Association of the Deaf and its constituent state associations are one constellation of sources of help. The National Fraternal Society of the Deaf and its divisions which exist in many metropolitan areas are another. Social clubs for the deaf found in urban settings are a third. Contributions to the team are increasing from almost four hundred speech and hearing clinics throughout the country as well as other professional workers.

SCHOOLS FOR THE DEAF

The main pillar of the vocational guidance structure is the school for the deaf. *The American Annals of the Deaf* [2] lists 71 public residential schools for the deaf, 10 day schools, 206 day classes, 16 denominational and private residential schools, 45 denominational and private day classes, and 11 schools and classes for the multiple handicapped deaf. These 359 centers of information about the deaf are all useful in vocational guidance work.

The large schools, with their impressive array of shops, are likely to have well-developed vocational programs and may on their own initiative assume the coordinating function in the vocational guidance activity. The common practice is for the student from ten to twelve years and upward to rotate by semesters through all shops, which may number more than a half-dozen units. He may be exposed to even more teachers, and many more vocational subjects. During these three or more school years he has a wide range of experience in manipulating basic materials, such as wood, glass, metal, mortar, finishes, plastics. He aims at acquiring good work habits and the attitudes that are critical for job success. In his later school years, he concentrates on one or several vocational subjects, developing a core of specific knowledge and manual skills plus further strength in habits and attitudes.

For many deaf persons, the choice of an occupation and actual preparation may begin in this period of shop concentration. For all, these years of shop specialization have real significance for whatever

[2] *American Annals of the Deaf*, 103: 120 (1958).

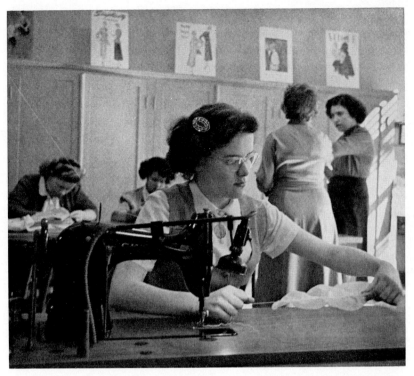

Fig. 22-1. Deaf girls learn to operate power machines used in the garment industry. (*Lexington School for the Deaf.*)

occupational choice and preparation is eventually undertaken. The guidance process bridges the period from school to postschool life. Choice of occupation and preparation for it may very well originate or even be completed during school days.

The school serves important functions in addition to providing fundamentals of shopwork. It may well coordinate the team and provide significant information regarding each deaf person for the benefit of the vocational rehabilitation counselor, the placement specialist, the other team members, and the deaf person himself.

The increasing number of guidance workers in the larger schools for the deaf is encouraging. They logically spend a fair share of their time on student vocational interests. As many as eighteen residential schools for the deaf now have trained guidance workers (twelve full-time, six part-time), and more would be employed if they were available. In several states, schools and vocational rehabilitation agencies are combining forces to recruit and maintain specially trained vocational rehabilitation counselors for the deaf.

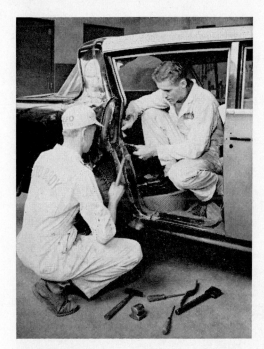

Fig. 22-2. Deaf boys learn to repair automobile bodies. (*New Jersey School for the Deaf.*)

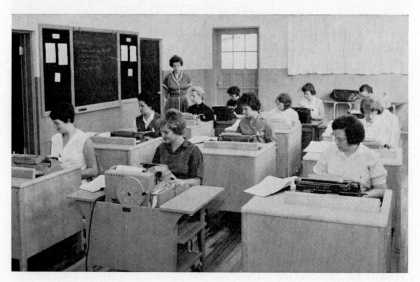

Fig. 22-3. Deaf girls learn to operate business machines. (*New Jersey School for the Deaf.*)

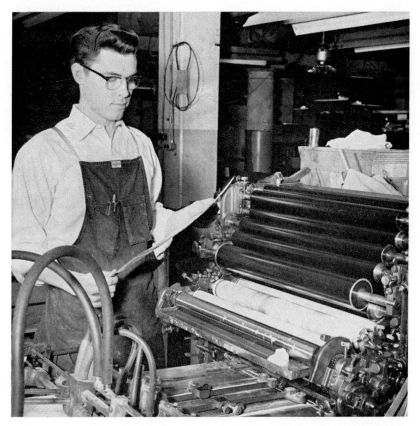

Fig. 22-4. A deaf printer checks proofs. (*Commercial Letter Service, Inc., St. Louis.*)

Information about the quality and depth of vocational guidance work in the special schools may indicate the direction of growth. It appears that the following six functions of vocational guidance would be appropriate for schools for the deaf: imparting occupational information; collecting and coordinating personal history data; psychological testing and evaluation; counseling; coordinating community services; and following up on the job.

VOCATIONAL REHABILITATION AGENCIES

Each of the fifty states, the District of Columbia, Guam, Puerto Rico, and the Virgin Islands has a vocational rehabilitation program that serves eligible deaf clients. The number of deaf clients "closed" as rehabilitated by the states in four recent years increased from 851 in 1954 to 1494 in 1957. All of the 1957 deaf clients were employed at closure, 92 per cent as earners, and the balance as farm or family workers. Eighty-four per cent were unemployed when they applied. Group earnings rose from an estimated rate of $335,800 before rehabilitation to an estimated $3,337,100 after. Clearly, the vocational rehabilitation program makes an important contribution to deaf people and to society.

The determination of a deaf person's eligibility and the actual extension of services are functions of the state vocational rehabilitation agencies. The three universal criteria of eligibility are the presence of a physical or mental impairment; the existence of a substantial handicap to employment from the impairment; and reasonable expectation that vocational rehabilitation services may render the individual fit to engage in a remunerative occupation. Each state agency has a minimal age level at which a person can be accepted for services, generally sixteen years or the age at which employment is legal. Moreover, each state agency has its own residence requirement, ranging from intention to reside to as long as one year in actual residence.

Rehabilitation services are provided in accordance with a plan worked out by the client and his rehabilitation counselor, assisted by the vocational guidance team:

1. Thorough physical, mental, and aural examinations
2. Necessary medical, surgical, psychiatric, and hospital services
3. Hearing aids, speechreading, speech correction, and auditory training, if necessary
4. Individual counseling and guidance, including attention to problems of personal adjustment as they influence employment
5. Training for jobs—in schools, on the job, by correspondence, or by tutor
6. Maintenance and transportation during rehabilitation, if necessary
7. Necessary tools, equipment, and licenses
8. Placement in the right job
9. Follow-up to make sure that the rehabilitated workers and the jobs are properly matched

The fifty-four general state rehabilitation agencies have more than 1800 counseling and placement workers in over 525 offices throughout the country. By experience and training they are highly skilled in techniques of vocational guidance. They are especially effective when another team member has skills to communicate and to coordinate the thinking of team and client. Of course, their effectiveness is increased to the extent that they have had experience in serving deaf clients.

STATE EMPLOYMENT SERVICES

The significant member of the vocational guidance team is the state employment service, because of its specific objectives for the handicapped and its many outlets for a wide variety of services. Its aims are

1. Equal opportunity for employment and equal pay in competition with other applicants
2. Employment at highest skills suitable to physical capacities and other occupational qualifications
3. Satisfactory adjustment to chosen occupation and work situation
4. Employment that will not aggravate physical impairments nor endanger other employees

These important aims are implemented through the 1787 local employment offices in all the states and territories. Each office has a worker who gives special attention to handicapped job seekers.

The specialized services that the state employment services offer handicapped persons include

1. Selective placement, requiring
   a. Appraisal of the individual's assets, with special emphasis on the recognition of the impairment and the evaluation of physical capacity.
   b. Analysis of job requirements, with special emphasis on physical demands and working conditions.
   c. Selective matching in which the physical capacities and other qualifications of the handicapped applicant are matched with the physical and other requirements of the job.
2. Employment counseling, where the handicapped applicant is in need of assistance in formulating a plan to reach a vocational goal or adjustment in a job consistent with his disability.
3. Evaluation of need for services of other agencies to improve physical capacities or otherwise enhance employability.
4. Individualized job development when no job order is available which is consistent with the individual's physical capacities and other qualifications.
5. Preparation of the applicant and employer for the interview so that the factor of the handicap is seen in proper perspective.
6. Recommendations concerning job modifications to meet the applicant's physical capacities.
7. Follow-up to ensure that the applicant, with his disability, can perform the job safely and efficiently, and is making a satisfactory adjustment to it.

All of these services assist the individual to meet his need for employment suitable to his physical capacities and other qualifications.

The staff is skilled in applying the principles of selective placement and their knowledge of the current job market, and their experience in intricate employer-employee adjustments are rich resources for the deaf.

Special Knowledges Needed

The effectiveness of vocational guidance for the deaf rests considerably upon the availability of special knowledges and skills in certain areas of the work, specifically the evaluative and counseling activities.

COUNSELING STANDARDS

Counseling work with the deaf, as with any other severely handicapped group, must be carried on by one who is an expert counselor and who has had experience with deaf people. He must be able to weigh the significance of evaluative tools and conclusions, and also the desirability of job objectives. Finally, he must be able to communicate freely with all types of deaf clients. Public agencies are anxious to reduce their inadequacies in these respects. For example, the Office of Vocational Rehabilitation supports well-attended training programs for counselors, placement officers, and related workers for the deaf at Gallaudet College in Washington in addition to short courses elsewhere.

A free flow of thinking between counselor and counselee is the principal ingredient for the joint decisions of successful guidance work and for the supportive counseling so many clients need. Experienced guidance workers for people with hearing impairment are very sensitive to this critical factor of communication. A group of them made the following recommendations regarding standards for counseling clients with impaired hearing:

Counseling the hard of hearing.

1. A desk model hearing aid, described in Chapter 10, should be used for interviewing hard-of-hearing clients. A normal speech volume and range should be employed, with consonants and vowels articulated slowly and clearly and directly to the client, repeating when necessary, eliminating all slurring and mouthing, and keeping the lips unobstructed.

2. Interviews, especially the first one, should be conducted in quiet surroundings, preferably a private room, with the client's better ear not more than two yards from the counselor and with the client's back to the brightest light.

3. Writing should be resorted to when amplification is not suitable and when the client does not speech-read sufficiently well for free and easy exchange of thought.

4. The client should be interviewed alone, unless the presence of a close associate is essential to the establishment of rapport.

Counseling the deaf.

1. Skill in the use of the sign language and the manual alphabet.

2. Writing may be resorted to when the client has language patterns that permit free and easy exchange of thought by this medium.

3. Speechreading is a desirable medium for those who understand normal conversation by this means.

4. Whenever applicable, the standards followed with the hard of hearing should be used with the deaf.

PSYCHOLOGICAL TESTING AND EVALUATION

Although exploration of individual potentials, interests, and achievements by objective tests is a well-established procedure in guidance, there is no other aspect of guidance work with the deaf in which there are so many well-intentioned transgressions. Misdirection of deaf persons' job prospects and consequently their whole lives on the basis of improper evaluation is most serious. These improprieties frequently consist of wrong administration, wrong tests, and wrong interpretations. They suggest that full use should be made of psychological tests as a corrective action.

Myerson cites a typical example and effectively points up the continuing, pressing need for proper and complete interpretation of test findings.[3] In doing so, he brings out also the wide range of special knowledges to which the counselor must be alert if he is to do an adequate job with the deaf.

> . . . the counselor feels blocked and frustrated by the difficulties in communication. When speech is poor in quality and limited in quantity and when lip reading seems faltering and uncertain, there is a strong tendency . . . to consider the client stupid and push him off into some unskilled occupation. Even when . . . the deaf client is bright, the counselor often doesn't understand the situation and doesn't know what to do. . . . recently . . . a young deaf boy . . . from _____ School, whose score on the verbal portion of the Wechsler Adult Intelligence Scale was very low but whose I.Q. on the performance portion was 135 . . . . Since the boy's behavior was sharp and alert, the counselor knew enough to disregard the verbal I.Q. as a measure of intelligence, but he didn't know how to interpret the performance portion. "How is it that such a bright boy never learned to speak and to lip-read?" Further, the counselor didn't know what to

[3] Lee Meyerson, Department of Psychology, University of Houston, in a personal communication, January 28, 1958.

do. Apparently neither he nor his supervisor . . . thought of Gallaudet, no one knew anything about the army of deaf workers in _____, and no one ever heard of _____ [a nearby authority on the deaf]. At last report they were thinking of placing this boy as janitor's apprentice!

A committee of the First Institute for Special Workers for the Aural Disabled gave concentrated attention to the needs of the state vocational rehabilitation agencies in meeting the urgent problems in psychological evaluation. Their conclusions and recommendations are useful to all workers serving the deaf.

> Psychological tests are not a counseling short-cut but rather a supplement. They should be interpreted only in the light of adequate case data. Evaluations of difficult deaf cases should be undertaken by qualified psychologists. Guidance workers for the deaf have a special responsibility to increase the number of qualified psychologists to extend their experience and capacities in serving deaf clients.
>
> After arbitrarily dividing deaf clients into non-reading and reading groups, the committee concluded that few tests, largely performance, could be used with the former while many more were suitable for the latter. It emphasized the need for clear understanding of directions before testing, using sign language or amplification, as necessary.
>
> The committee cautioned that its dozen guides for psychological testing of the deaf and the severely hard of hearing are just guides, not formulas.
>
> 1. Scores on verbal tests may be depressed for persons with language habits arising from early onset or long-standing hearing loss. Careful interpretation is indicated.
>
> 2. The later the age at onset, the less are verbal test scores apt to be affected.
>
> 3. Verbal test scores of deaf people are more safely considered as minimal levels of abilities rather than upper limits.
>
> 4. When deafness results from injury to the nervous system, for example, test results should be evaluated primarily in terms of the more basic condition and secondarily in terms of deafness.
>
> 5. Sub-test scores of different mental abilities rather than the single-score I.Q. should be emphasized in case study.
>
> 6. Both total test scores and separate test items should be studied for richer, more accurate interpretation of test and other case data.
>
> 7. Individual testing is preferable for the deaf.
>
> 8. Special precautions should be taken to assure that good rapport prevails between examiner and deaf client. Free exchange of thinking by any means and preconditioning of both tester and testee are important.

9. The reasons for any gaps in a deaf testee's formal education should be used in interpreting scores.

10. The impact of emotional stresses, idleness, and isolation upon test scores must be related to the underlying conditions for interpretation and prognosis.

11. Overemphasis on deafness itself may obscure other major factors in the case study, such as poor attitudes, parental domination, physical or mental illness.

12. Qualitative observation of the deaf testee may reveal personality traits such as confidence and persistence that permit better interpretation of test performance.[4]

The Deaf at Work

The performance of deaf people in competitive employment is the main test of our vocational guidance efforts. And surely we can feel increasing satisfaction over the progress which indicates that in a normal labor market, the fully employable deaf are fully employed; moreover, there is some evidence that more of them are working at higher-grade jobs than was formerly true.

Our best evidence shows that the deaf have proved to be good employees. World War II increased their opportunities that were severely restricted during and even before the depression of the thirties. They made a splendid record during the war and they apparently have held their gains since then. Reported unemployment seems to reflect community circumstances and individual inadequacies rather than deafness itself.

DEAF REHABILITANTS

The large numbers of deaf people who are rehabilitated each year is a useful source of information about the jobs deaf people hold. Interesting comparisons are shown in the table.

The appreciable percentage differences between all rehabilitants and the deaf in the professional, managerial, sales, and protective service categories seem to point at the communication problem, for these groups include many types of employment in which speech and hearing are very important. Some readers may be surprised at the comparatively minor differences in clerical lines, for most of us are accustomed to think of clerical workers as being involved in telephoning, dictation, and similar tasks requiring hearing. Students of deaf society explain the

[4] R. M. Phillips, Chairman, S. G. DiMichael, Consultant, Committee on Psychological Services to the Deaf and the Severely Hard of Hearing, Reports of the Committees of the First Institute for Special Workers for the Aural Disabled, Federal Security Agency, Office of Vocational Rehabilitation, June, 1950, pp. 10–18.

Deaf Rehabilitants Compared to All Rehabilitants by Major Occupational Group at Closure, Fiscal Years 1956 and 1957

Major occupational group at closure	1956				1957			
	All Rehabilitants		Deaf		All Rehabilitants		Deaf	
	No.	%	No.	%	No.	%	No.	%
Total	65,640	100.0	1,278	100.0	70,940	100.0	1,494	100.0
Professional	3,279	5.0	38	3.0	3,270	4.6	35	2.3
Semiprofessional	1,584	2.4	21	1.6	1,693	2.4	35	2.3
Managerial	1,740	2.7	2	0.2	1,727	2.4	7	0.5
Clerical	9,773	14.9	180	14.1	10,342	14.6	244	16.3
Sales	3,010	4.6	9	0.7	3,255	4.6	23	1.5
Service,								
Domestic	3,300	5.0	54	4.2	3,854	5.4	44	2.9
Personal	4,680	7.2	89	7.0	5,349	7.6	79	5.3
Protective	874	1.3	1	0.1	1,072	1.5	15	1.0
Building	2,263	3.4	35	2.7	2,635	3.7	46	3.1
total:	11,117	16.9	179	14.0	12,910	18.2	184	12.3
Agricultural	5,614	8.6	42	3.3	6,022	8.5	47	3.1
Skilled	8,094	12.3	259	20.3	8,201	11.6	285	19.1
Semiskilled	9,781	14.9	332	26.0	10,480	14.8	366	24.7
Unskilled	4,413	6.7	141	11.0	4,771	6.7	165	11.0
Family workers	1,404	2.1	21	1.6	1,499	2.1	20	1.3
Housewives	5,823	8.9	54	4.2	6,767	9.5	83	5.6
Not reported	8	—			3	—		

Source: Reports of Division of Program Statistics and Special Services, Office of Vocational Rehabilitation.

differences in the agricultural classification with the information that rural life is too dull for many deaf people who, being gregarious like most of us, prefer urban areas where mutual-interest groups with easy communication abound. The sharp differences in the skilled and semi-skilled categories seem to bring out the great values in the excellent shop training most schools for the deaf feature. Finally, one wonders if the larger percentage of deaf persons in unskilled work is an indi-cator partly of the need for training facilities for deaf adults whose educational experience have been inadequate and partly of the need for better vocational guidance.

Specific jobs in which deaf rehabilitants were closed in several major occupational groups are also interesting.

Such lists of jobs should be regarded only as suggestive. We must be aware that our samples are limited only to people who have pre-sented themselves for rehabilitation. Some deaf people, already suc-cessful, are not likely to seek guidance services, and others who are

Some Jobs in Which Deaf Rehabilitants Were Closed Frequently in 1954, 1955, 1956, and 1957

Major Occupational Group and Specific Job	1954	1955	1956	1957
Professional				
Teachers	19	13	20	13
Accountants	6	7	3	1
Semiprofessional				
Draftsmen	9	11	12	20
Laboratory technicians	1	11	3	6
Clerical				
Office machine operators	28	27	49	91
Typists and clerks	49	69	96	120
Personal service				
Kitchen workers	15	21	32	33
Barbers, beauticians	11	12	25	13
Skilled				
Dressmakers, etc.	16	19	20	21
Printers, etc.	59	56	91	85
Mechanics, auto	14	10	12	18
Semiskilled				
Food products	8	8	18	11
Textile products	42	53	69	46
Printing, etc.	12	11	25	18
Laundering, cleaning, etc.	29	23	36	40
Packing, etc.	6	16	11	10
Unskilled				
Food products	6	12	13	16
Packing	9	16	11	12

less successful may not have the initiative and the intelligence to seek them. Care should be taken that our statistics do not lead to stereotyped thinking. B. M. Schowe of Firestone Tire and Rubber Company, Akron, Ohio, succinctly brought this into focus with a well-illustrated poster bearing this legend: "Range of Employability—The creative self-expression of the deaf, individually and collectively, is often stifled through unwarranted restriction to a narrow range of employment opportunities. At the Firestone Tire and Rubber Company in Akron, Ohio, deaf men and women are successfully employed at all levels of skill and training from common labor to Senior Research Chemist."

PLACEMENT GUIDE LINES

In another of his important contributions, Mr. Schowe identifies simple basic principles to observe with deaf workers and an effective orientation pattern for them.[5] He emphasizes that employers should *show* job processes and safety principles, rather than talk about them. He cautions that some deaf workers may be very sensitive to noise; that generally only one deaf worker should be hired at first; that deaf workers should usually be integrated with hearing workers, not segregated; and that some guidance from an older, friendly employee until he is a part of the shop team is desirable when a deaf employee is a novelty. To these fundamental observations the counselor or placement specialist will add that some deaf people should not work in high or dark places or wherever a fine sense of balance is essential, since they may have serious problems of equilibrium.

BETTER JOBS

Steadily increasing emphasis by business and government on employment of physically handicapped workers in recent years arises in large part from the very practical reasons of filling manpower needs and of making taxpayers out of tax consumers. Circumstances are most favorable for deaf people to prove their mettle. More and more employers are coming to understand that after a brief orientation period most jobs require little communication and that properly trained and placed deaf workers are very resourceful in compensating.

We have, however, scarcely begun. Jobs that do not begin to tap a person's capacities are a major continuing problem in the vocational guidance of deaf persons. There is need for understanding that properly motivated, trained deaf people bring to their jobs skills and powers of compensation that reduce the communication difficulties to small significance. All disciplines that serve the deaf share the responsibility for creating understanding.

Suggested Readings

GLEASON, CLYDE W. "State Employment Service Program of Service to the Handicapped," Division of Counseling, Selective Placement and Testing, United States Employment Service, Bureau of Employment Security, Department of Labor. Washington, D.C.: 1957.

HOAG, RALPH L. "Cooperative Relationships between Public Residential Schools for the Deaf and State Rehabilitation Agencies," Staff Development Aids No. 5. Office of Vocational Rehabilitation, Department of Health, Education, and Welfare. Washington, D.C.: 1948.

LUNDE, ANDERS S., and STANLEY K. BIGMAN. "Occupational Conditions Among the Deaf."
A report on a national survey conducted by Gallaudet College and the National Association of the Deaf, September 1, 1959.

[5] B. M. Schowe, "Guide Lines for the Employment of Deaf Workers," *Employment Security Review*, December, 1951, pp. 30–31.

"Opportunities for the Deaf and the Hard of Hearing," Office of Vocational Rehabilitation, Federal Security Agency. Washington, D.C.: 1949, pp. 1–2.

"The Performance of Physically Impaired Workers in Manufacturing Industries," Bulletin No. 923. Bureau of Labor Statistics, United States Department of Labor. Washington, D.C.: 1948, pp. 74–83.

SEAL, A. G., Chairman, B. R. WILLIAMS, Consultant, Committee on Standards for Special Casework and Counseling Procedures for the Deaf and the Severely Hard of Hearing. *Reports* of the Committees of the First Institute for Special Workers for the Aural Disabled, Federal Security Agency, Office of Vocational Rehabilitation, Department of Health, Education, and Welfare. Washington, D.C.: June, 1950, p. 19.

WILLIAMS, BOYCE R. "The Guidance Program in a School for the Deaf," *Report* of the Proceedings of the Thirty-sixth Meeting of the Convention of American Instructors of the Deaf. Washington, D.C.: Government Printing Office, 1954, pp. 190–196.

————. "Occupational Placement of the Deaf—Past, Present, and Future," *Report* of the Proceedings of the Thirty-eighth Meeting of the Convention of American Instructors of the Deaf, Knoxville, Tennessee, 1958, pp. 32–35.

APPENDIX

GLOSSARY

INDEXES

APPENDIX

In this appendix are presented nine different collections of words or sentences that are widely used as tests of hearing. Several of the word and sentence lists are also useful for auditory training and as test material in the selection of hearing aids.

The principles of the tests that employ these words and sentences are explained in Chapter 7, and their use in the selection of hearing aids is discussed in Chapter 11. It is pointed out in Chapter 7, for example, that a "discrimination score" obtained with the PB monosyllabic word lists has a totally different meaning from a "hearing level for speech" measured with the two-syllable word lists. The principles of the different types of test will not be discussed again, but a brief statement introduces each set of lists, telling something of their properties, how and where they were constructed, and their general fields of usefulness.

Some of the shorter lists are given in full; others are represented only by samples, but by more generous samples than could properly be included in the text. The lists are given primarily for the benefit of readers who may wish to use them personally or professionally. It must be remembered, however, that word lists or sentences alone do not make a test of hearing. The loudness and clarity with which they are spoken and the acoustic conditions of the test are equally important. These lists are only the materials. As explained in Chapter 7, they must be correctly and intelligently used.

1. Spondaic Words (CID)

Auditory tests W-1 and W-2 were developed at Central Institute for the Deaf as modifications of Auditory Test No. 9 of the Psycho-Acoustic Laboratory of Harvard University. The test material is a list of thirty-six words, each composed of two syllables that are equally stressed (spondees). The words were chosen for familiarity and also

535

for equal intelligibility when spoken at the same intensity as measured by the VU meter. Six different scramblings of the thirty-six words have been recorded.

Tests W-1 and W-2 are particularly suited to measuring the threshold hearing level for speech. In Test W-1 all of the spondaic words are recorded at the same intensity. The carrier phrase is recorded at a level 10 db higher. A 1000 cps calibration tone is also recorded at this level. In W-2 the intensity of the words descends systematically by 3 db for each successive group of three words. With this form of test it is only necessary to count the number of words repeated correctly. Each word correct lowers the threshold level by 1 db.

Phonographic recordings of these tests, either 78 or 33⅓ rpm, may be purchased from the Technisonic Studios, Inc., 1201 South Brentwood Blvd., Richmond Heights 17, Missouri. These tests are described in an article entitled "C.I.D. Auditory Tests W-1 and W-2," by R. W. Benson, H. Davis, C. E. Harrison, I. J. Hirsh, E. G. Reynolds, and S. R. Silverman, in *Journal of the Acoustical Society of America,* 23: 719 (1951), and, in more detail, "Development of Materials for Speech Audiometry," by I. J. Hirsh, H. Davis, S. R. Silverman, E. G. Reynolds, E. Eldert, and R. W. Benson in *Journal of Speech and Hearing Disorders,* 17: 321–337 (1952). (These tests were developed under contracts with the Office of Naval Research and the Veterans Administration.)

SPONDAIC WORDS OF AUDITORY TESTS W-1 AND W-2

1. airplane	10. eardrum	19. iceberg	28. railroad
2. armchair	11. farewell	20. inkwell	29. schoolboy
3. baseball	12. grandson	21. mousetrap	30. sidewalk
4. birthday	13. greyhound	22. mushroom	31. stairway
5. cowboy	14. hardware	23. northwest	32. sunset
6. daybreak	15. headlight	24. oatmeal	33. toothbrush
7. doormat	16. horseshoe	25. padlock	34. whitewash
8. drawbridge	17. hotdog	26. pancake	35. woodwork
9. duckpond	18. hothouse	27. playground	36. workshop

2. PB (Phonetically Balanced) Word Lists

First in this section are presented four of the fifty-word phonetically balanced word lists prepared by the Psycho-Acoustic Laboratory. All twenty of the fifty-word lists are given in the article by J. P. Egan entitled "Articulation Testing Methods" in *The Laryngoscope,* 58: 955–991 (1948). Each list consists of fifty common English monosyllables arranged in alphabetical order. For articulation testing, the words should be arranged in different random order for each presentation. The special merits of these lists and the uses to which they may be put are described in Chapter 7. The words range in difficulty from quite intelligible to rather difficult. The lists given here are among those recorded at Central Institute for the Deaf with Rush Hughes as the talker.

PB-50—LIST 5

1. add	11. feed	21. love	31. rind	41. thud
2. bake	12. flap	22. mast	32. rode	42. trade
3. bathe	13. good	23. nose	33. roe	43. true
4. beck	14. Greek	24. odds	34. scare	44. tug
5. black	15. grudge	25. owls	35. shine	45. vase
6. bronze	16. high	26. pass	36. shove	46. watch
7. cheat	17. hill	27. pipe	37. shy	47. wink
8. choose	18. inch	28. puff	38. sick	48. wrath
9. curse	19. kid	29. punt	39. solve	49. yawn
10. drive	20. lend	30. rear	40. thick	50. zone

PB-50—LIST 6

1. as	11. deep	21. gap	31. ode	41. scan
2. badge	12. eat	22. grope	32. plug	42. shank
3. beg	13. eyes	23. hitch	33. prime	43. slouch
4. best	14. fall	24. hull	34. pun	44. sup
5. chart	15. fee	25. jag	35. pus	45. thigh
6. cloth	16. flick	26. kept	36. raise	46. thus
7. clothes	17. flop	27. leg	37. ray	47. tongue
8. cob	18. forge	28. mash	38. reap	48. wait
9. crib	19. fowl	29. match	39. rooms	49. wasp
10. dad	20. gage	30. nigh	40. rough	50. wife

PB-50—LIST 7

1. act	11. dope	21. jug	31. quiz	41. siege
2. aim	12. dose	22. knit	32. raid	42. sin
3. am	13. dwarf	23. meet	33. range	43. sledge
4. but	14. fake	24. mud	34. rash	44. sniff
5. by	15. fling	25. nine	35. rich	45. south
6. chop	16. fort	26. off	36. roar	46. though
7. coast	17. gasp	27. pent	37. sag	47. whip
8. comes	18. grade	28. pig	38. scout	48. wire
9. cook	19. gun	29. plod	39. shaft	49. woe
10. cut	20. him	30. pounce	40. shave	50. woo

PB-50—LIST 8

1. ask	11. cod	21. forth	31. lick	41. rot
2. bid	12. crack	22. freak	32. look	42. shack
3. bind	13. day	23. frock	33. night	43. slide
4. bolt	14. deuce	24. front	34. pint	44. spice
5. bored	15. dumb	25. guess	35. queen	45. this
6. calf	16. each	26. horse	36. rest	46. thread
7. catch	17. ease	27. hum	37. rhyme	47. till
8. chant	18. fad	28. jell	38. rod	48. us
9. chew	19. flip	29. kill	39. roll	49. wig
10. clod	20. food	30. left	40. rope	50. yeast

CID Auditory Test W-22 is a set of recordings of phonetically balanced word lists that represent a more restricted and simpler vocabulary than the original Psycho-Acoustic Laboratory lists. The talker is Ira Hirsh. These recordings are considerably more intelligible than the Rush Hughes version. Test W-22 is described in detail, including the criteria for phonetic balance, in the article entitled "Development of Materials for Speech Audiometry" cited in Chapter 7.

Both CID Auditory Test W-22 and the Rush Hughes version of the PB-50 test can be obtained from Technisonic Studios, 1201 South Brentwood Blvd., Richmond Heights 17, Missouri.

W-22 WORD LISTS

PB-50—LIST 1

1. ace	12. deaf	21. it	31. owl	41. toe
2. ache	13. earn	22. jam	32. poor	42. true
3. an	(urn)	23. knees	33. ran	43. twins
4. as	14. east	24. law	34. see (sea)	44. yard
5. bathe	15. felt	25. low	35. she	45. up
6. bells	16. give	26. me	36. skin	46. us
7. carve	17. high	27. mew	37. stove	47. wet
8. chew	18. him	28. none	38. them	48. what
9. could	19. hunt	(nun)	39. there	49. wire
10. dad	20. isle	29. not (knot)	(their)	50. you
11. day	(aisle)	30. or (oar)	40. thing	(ewe)

PB-50—LIST 2

1. ail (ale)	5. by (buy)	10. does	15. flat	20. ice
2. air (heir)	6. cap	11. dumb	16. gave	21. ill
3. and	7. cars	12. ease	17. ham	22. jaw
4. bin	8. chest	13. eat	18. hit	23. key
(been)	9. die (dye)	14. else	19. hurt	24. knee

PB-50—LIST 2 (*continued*)

25. live	30. odd	36. send	42. then	47. well
(verb)	31. off	37. show	43. thin	48. with
26. move	32. one	38. smart	44. too	49. yore
27. new	(won)	39. star	(two, to)	(your)
(knew)	33. own	40. tare	45. tree	50. young
28. now	34. pew	(tear)	46. way	
29. oak	35. rooms	41. that	(weigh)	

PB-50—LIST 3

1. add (ad)	11. done	21. is	31. out	42. though
2. aim	(dun)	22. jar	32. owes	43. three
3. are	12. dull	23. king	33. pie	44. tie
4. ate (eight)	13. ears	24. knit	34. raw	45. use
5. bill	14. end	25. lie (lye)	35. say	(yews)
6. book	15. farm	26. may	36. shove	46. we
7. camp	16. glove	27. nest	37. smooth	47. west
8. chair	17. hand	28. no	38. start	48. when
9. cute	18. have	(know)	39. tan	49. wool
10. do	19. he	29. oil	40. ten	50. year
	20. if	30. on	41. this	

PB-50—LIST 4

1. aid	11. clothes	21. his	31. ought	40. they
2. all (awl)	12. cook	22. in (inn)	(aught)	41. through
3. am	13. darn	23. jump	32. our	42. tin
4. arm	14. dolls	24. leave	(hour)	43. toy
5. art	15. dust	25. men	33. pale (pail)	44. where
6. at	16. ear	26. my	34. save	45. who
7. bee (be)	17. eyes	27. near	35. shoe	46. why
8. bread	(ayes)	28. net	36. so (sew)	47. will
(bred)	18. few	29. nuts	37. stiff	48. wood
9. can	19. go	30. of	38. tea (tee)	(would)
10. chin	20. hang		39. than	49. yes
				50. yet

3. The R Lists

The two following word lists are useful when a limited number of different words are required for abbreviated articulation tests. The words were selected so that they resemble one another as much as possible and at the same time sample the various sounds of speech. The fifteen vowels and diphthongs are represented by six words each. An effort was made to distribute all the different consonant sounds among these ninety words. The remaining ten words of each hundred are used to sample some of the compound consonants. The lists are intended to be used in the same way and for the same general purposes as the PB lists. They should be well adapted for use in the selection of hearing aids, as described in Chapters 10 and 11.

R LIST 1

1. aisle	21. dame	41. jack	61. rack	81. still
2. barb	22. done	42. jam	62. ram	82. tale
3. barge	23. dub	43. law	63. ring	83. tame
4. bark	24. feed	44. lawn	64. rip	84. toil
5. baste	25. feet	45. lisle	65. rub	85. ton
6. bead	26. file	46. live	66. run	86. trill
7. beet	27. five	47. loon	67. sale	87. tub
8. beige	28. foil	48. loop	68. same	88. vouch
9. boil	29. fume	49. mess	69. shod	89. vow
10. choke	30. fuse	50. met	70. shop	90. whack
11. chore	31. get	51. neat	71. should	91. wham
12. cod	32. good	52. need	72. shrill	92. woe
13. coil	33. guess	53. oil	73. sing	93. woke
14. coon	34. hews	54. ouch	74. sip	94. would
15. coop	35. hive	55. paw	75. skill	95. yaw
16. cop	36. hod	56. pawn	76. soil	96. yawn
17. couch	37. hood	57. pews	77. soon	97. yes
18. could	38. hop	58. poke	78. soot	98. yet
19. cow	39. how	59. pour	79. soup	99. zing
20. dale	40. huge	60. pure	80. spill	100. zip

R LIST 2

1. ball	21. dial	41. hen	61. peep	81. tap
2. bar	22. dig	42. huff	62. peeve	82. them
3. bob	23. dine	43. hush	63. phase	83. then
4. bong	24. ditch	44. jar	64. pull	84. title
5. book	25. doubt	45. job	65. put	85. tine
6. boot	26. dowel	46. joy	66. raid	86. tong
7. booth	27. drain	47. joys	67. raze	87. toot
8. bout	28. em	48. kirk	68. rich	88. tooth
9. bowel	29. en	49. leap	69. rig	89. tout
10. boy	30. fade	50. leave	70. ream	90. towel
11. boys	31. far	51. made	71. roe	91. toy
12. brain	32. foam	52. maize	72. root	92. toys
13. bull	33. fob	53. mew	73. rough	93. weave
14. crane	34. foe	54. muff	74. rush	94. weep
15. cue	35. foot	55. mush	75. ruth	95. while
16. curb	36. full	56. mute	76. sack	96. whine
17. curd	37. gall	57. new	77. sap	97. wig
18. curse	38. gong	58. newt	78. slain	98. witch
19. curt	39. grain	59. oh	79. tack	99. yak
20. cute	40. hem	60. ohm	80. tall	100. yap

4. Multiple-Choice Word Lists

A multiple-choice word-intelligibility test has been developed by Professor John W. Black of Ohio State University in collaboration with the United States Naval School of Aviation Medicine. It has been used extensively in tests of talkers speaking under various conditions of interest to military aviation. The talker is given a list of words to read. The listeners mark prepared blanks on which each word read by the talker appears as one of four rather similar possible choices. Twenty-four of these lists are published in the *Journal of Speech and Hearing Disorders*, 22: 213–235 (1957). The first of these lists is given here as a sample. The word in each group actually read by the talker is italicized.

groove	modern	*vice*
drew	moderate	fight
crew	modesty	mice
grew	*modest*	bite
say	forbade	*chink*
stay	*pervade*	kink
stayed	surveyed	check
spade	survey	chin
stung	drunk	*intent*
stun	*grunt*	intend
sun	brunt	content
stunned	runt	intense
quench	busy	wade
went	physics	waves
whence	*physic*	*wave*
when	visit	way
pass	clearly	*fine*
past	weary	find
cast	quarry	sign
task	*query*	kind
popular	nurse	*get*
poplar	first	gap
hopper	birth	guess
opera	*burst*	guest
immense	named	only
commence	*name*	woman
emit	main	pullman
cement	knave	*omen*

latter	*last*	swain
ladder	lash	*slain*
lattice	laugh	flame
rabbit	glass	plain
crash	gold	pail
crab	bowl	poor
craft	cold	*polo*
crack	*bold*	palace

5. *The Larsen Sound-Discrimination Lists*

The following lists were prepared by Miss Laila Larsen for use in auditory training at Deshon General Hospital. They are likely to be useful also in tests for the selection of hearing aids. One word of each pair is read by the tester and the subject checks the word he thinks he hears. Of course, in this test, as in all articulation tests, the loudness with which the words are spoken must be standardized.

SOUND-DISCRIMINATION TEST AND DRILL SHEET

1. f and ch		2. p and b		3. m and l		4. sh and f	
fin	chin	pin	bin	mine	line	show	foe
few	chew	pie	buy	mast	last	shore	four
filed	child	pole	bowl	moan	loan	shade	fade
calf	catch	cap	cab	name	nail	cash	calf
four	chore	rope	robe	home	hole	leash	leaf

5. f and k		6. b and m		7. n and v		8. d and n	
fit	kit	bill	mill	nice	vice	dot	not
four	core	boast	most	nurse	verse	die	nigh
find	kind	bake	make	nine	vine	deed	need
cliff	click	robe	roam	loans	loaves	ode	own
laugh	lack	tab	tam	lean	leave	did	din

9. k and g		10. m and v		11. t and th		12. p and f	
coal	goal	mice	vice	tie	thigh	pour	four
came	game	ham	have	tin	thin	pile	file
coat	goat	glum	glove	trill	thrill	par	far
luck	lug	mine	vine	mit	myth	cap	calf
rack	rug	mile	vile	pat	path	cup	cuff

13. v and z

live	lies
have	has
rave	raise
view	zoo
wives	wise

14. l and v

lane	vane
lie	vie
lace	vase
lull	love
rail	rave

15. l and z

lip	zip
loan	zone
lisle	lies
dole	doze
male	maze

16. v and f

five	fife
vase	face
leave	leaf
view	few
loaves	loafs
vine	fine

17. l and n

lame	name
light	night
loan	known
dial	dine
pail	pain
rail	rain

18. b and d

bid	did
big	dig
buy	die
rob	rod
bell	dell
robe	road

19. s and sh

lease	leash
sew	show
sign	shine
sip	ship
save	shave
lass	lash

20. f and b

fun	bun
fig	big
fan	ban
cuff	cub
calf	cab
graph	grab

21. k and t

kick	tick
kite	tight
code	toad
shirk	shirt
park	part
kin	tin

22. m and n

mine	nine
mew	knew
time	tine
dime	dine
dumb	done
loam	lone

23. b and v

bet	vet
bow	vow
bile	vile
bigger	vigor
robe	rove
boat	vote

24. th and v

than	van
thy	vie
that	vat
thine	vine
loathes	loaves

25. f and t

four	tore
fall	tall
fan	tan
fill	till
free	tree
fry	try

26. k and p

pike	pipe
car	par
core	pore
coke	poke
cock	cop
crock	crop
cry	pry
coal	pole

27. d and g

door	gore
dot	got
doe	go
date	gate
drove	grove
bud	bug
dye	guy
dad	gag

28. s and z

ice	eyes
seal	zeal
sip	zip
loose	lose
bus	buzz
lice	lies
juice	Jews
fuss	fuzz

29. t and p

tore	pore
tine	pine
tail	pail
cat	cap
cut	cup
tar	par
toll	pole
coat	cope

30. f and s

fine	sign
fur	sir
four	soar
flat	slat
cuff	cuss
knife	nice
lift	list
loft	lost

31. th and s

theme	seam
thin	sin
thumb	sum
truth	truce
path	pass
myth	miss
thing	sing
thank	sank

32. ch and sh

chop	shop
chip	ship
chair	share
chew	shoe
watch	wash
catch	cash
which	wish
cheap	sheep

33. th and f		34. Word endings		
thin	fin	store	stored	stores
thirst	first	close	closes	closed
three	free	will	wills	willed
Thor	for	start	starts	started
thought	fought	cough	coughs	coughed
throw	fro	cap	caps	capped
thrill	frill	try	tries	tried
		fee	fees	feed

6. Question-Answer Type of Sentence Lists

The following sentences are the basis of Auditory Test No. 12, prepared by the Psycho-Acoustic Laboratory. The questions are relatively simple and can be answered by a single word. This feature makes them useful when a written test for use in group testing is desired. If only one subject is being tested, he may be allowed to repeat the entire sentence. This procedure allows him to concentrate more fully on his listening.

These sentences have been recorded phonographically in groups of four at successively lower intensities. In this form the test is useful for obtaining a *threshold* for speech. The threshold level determined by this test is normally about 4 db above the threshold measured by the spondaic two-syllable words. This test, together with Test No. 9 (spondaic words), is described in detail in the article entitled "The Development of Recorded Auditory Tests for Measuring Hearing Loss for Speech," by C. V. Hudgins, J. E. Hawkins, J. E. Karlin, and S. S. Stevens, and published in *The Laryngoscope*, 47: 57–89 (1947).

Recordings of Auditory Test No. 12 can be obtained from Technisonic Studios, Inc., 1201 South Brentwood Blvd., Richmond Heights 17, Missouri.

LIST 1

Level	Answer	Question
0 db	B	1. What letter comes between A and C?
	Yes	2. Do flies have wings?
	Monday	3. What day comes after Sunday?
−6 db	3 or 4	4. How many colors are there in the American Flag?
	11	5. What number comes after 10?
	Hammer	6. What tool do you drive nails with?
−12 db	7	7. What number comes between 6 and 8?
	Yes	8. Are moths dangerous to clothing?

Level	Answer	Question
	February	9. What month comes after January?
−18 db	5	10. How many pennies are there in a nickel?
	No	11. Is there a lot of water in the desert?
	Weak	12. What is the opposite of strong?
−24 db	9	13. What number comes before 10?
	Bullets	14. Does a gun shoot flowers or bullets?
	Old	15. What is the opposite of new?
−30 db	France	16. In what country is Paris?
	No	17. Do you climb mountains in a sailboat?
	X	18. What letter comes after W?
−36 db	Tuesday	19. What day comes after Monday?
	Light	20. What is the opposite of dark?
	12	21. What number comes after 11?

LIST 5

Level	Answer	Question
0 db	Night	1. Which is darker, night or day?
	Pen	2. Do you write with a chair or a pen?
	E	3. What letter comes after D?
	Long, tall	4. What is the opposite of short?
−4 db	Red	5. What is the color of blood?
	24	6. How many hours are there in a day?
	Pacific	7. What is the ocean west of the United States?
	Thursday	8. What day comes after Wednesday?
−8 db	Tongue	9. What does a cat lick with?
	Cord, string	10. What do you tie a package with?
	Fish	11. Does a cat eat fish or straw?
	N	12. What is the first letter in "never"?
−12 db	Bottom	13. What is the opposite of top?
	Hay	14. Does a cow eat hay or stones?
	Sour	15. Is a lemon sour or salty?
	20	16. What number comes between 19 and 21?
−16 db	Ugly, homely	17. What is the opposite of pretty?
	White	18. What color is a Ping-pong ball?
	13	19. What number comes between 12 and 14?
	Pacific	20. In what ocean is Pearl Harbor?
−20 db	Thursday	21. What day comes before Friday?
	Glass	22. What are windows made of?

Level	Answer	Question
	Sun	23. What shines in the sky in the daytime?
	White	24. Is a polar bear white or green?
−24 db	6	25. What number comes between 5 and 7?
	2	26. How many legs does a man have?
	60	27. How many seconds in a minute?
	No	28. Do fish swim in trees?

7. S-1 Type of Sentence Test

These lists of sentences were prepared at the Psycho-Acoustic Laboratory for testing sentence intelligibility. The listener writes down or repeats each sentence. Scoring is based only on the five italicized words in each sentence. One point is scored for each word heard correctly. In each sentence the five key words consist of four monosyllables and one dissyllable. The vocabulary is fairly simple; nevertheless, the sentences tend to hold the attention of the listener. The lists are useful for practice in listening as well as for the elaborate articulation testing for which they were designed.

LIST 1

1. The *birch canoe slid* on the *smooth planks.*
2. *Glue* the *sheet* to the *dark blue background.*
3. *It's easy* to *tell* the *depth* of a *well.*
4. These *days* a *chicken leg* is a *rare dish.*
5. *Rice* is *often served* in *round bowls.*
6. *John* is *just* a *dope of long standing.*
7. The *juice* of *lemons makes fine punch.*
8. The *chest* was *thrown beside* the *parked truck.*
9. The *hogs* were *fed chopped corn* and *garbage.*
10. A *cry* in the *night chills my marrow.*
11. *Blow high* or *low* but *follow* the *notes.*
12. *Four hours* of *steady work faced* us.
13. A *large size* in *stockings* is *hard* to *sell.*
14. *Many* are *taught* to *breathe through* the *nose.*
15. *Ten days leave is coming up.*
16. The *Frenchman* was *shot when* the *sun rose.*
17. A *rod* is *used* to *catch pink salmon.*
18. He *smoked* a *pipe until* it *burned* his *tongue.*
19. The *light flashed* the *message* to the *eyes* of the *watchers.*
20. The *source* of the *huge river* is the *clear spring.*

LIST 2

1. *Death marks* the *end of our efforts.*
2. The *gift of speech* was *denied* the *poor child.*

3. *Never kill a snake* with your *bare hands.*
4. *Kick* the *ball straight* and *follow through.*
5. *Help* the *woman get back* to her *feet.*
6. *Put* a *dot* on the *i* and *sharpen* the *point.*
7. The *hum* of *bees made Jim sleepy.*
8. A *pint* of *tea helps* to *pass* the *evening.*
9. *Smoky fires lack flame* and *heat.*
10. The *soft cushion broke* the *man's fall.*
11. *While* he *spoke,* the *others took* their *leave.*
12. The *core* of the *apple housed a green worm.*
13. The *salt breeze came across* from the *sea.*
14. The *girl* at the *booth sold fifty bonds.*
15. The *purple pup gnawed a hole* in the *sock.*
16. The *fish twisted* and *turned* on the *bent hook.*
17. A *lot* of *fat slows* a *mile racer.*
18. *Press* the *pants* and *sew a button* on the *vest.*
19. The *swan dive* was *far short* of *perfect.*
20. *James tried* his *best* to *gain ground.*

8. The BTL Sentences

The Bell Telephone Laboratories sentences, of which the following lists are samples, were for many years a standard tool for testing hearing and for testing the performance of instruments, such as telephone and radio. The original collection contains forty-nine lists of fifty sentences each. The questions are longer and more difficult in vocabulary than the Psycho-Acoustic Laboratory sentences, and for this reason they are not so satisfactory for routine clinical use. The scoring is a little less certain; and for many listeners, the difficulty may be in understanding or remembering rather than in correct hearing.

INTELLIGIBILITY LIST 3

1. What is meant by "A stitch in time saves nine"?
2. What is the first letter of your last name?
3. Why is there a spring in a window shade roller?
4. What is meant by the expression "during rush hours"?
5. How many judges make up the Supreme Court?
6. Why is it necessary to build foundations for houses?
7. Name the tool with which a burglar opens a window.
8. Of what benefit was the Red Cross to soldiers during the war?
9. What man is called the "Father of his country"?
10. What instrument do we use to drive nails into wood?
11. How many miles do you travel daily?
12. Three inches is what part of one foot?
13. Name a large steamer that sails from this port.
14. What substance is employed for the manufacture of lead pencils?

15. Name some furniture made from pine.
16. What is used at home parties for dance music?
17. Why does oil float on the surface of water?
18. What flowers float on the top of the water?
19. What harm is done by waves at sea?
20. What do we mean when we say that the storm has abated?
21. How does a man differ from other animals?
22. Mention a winter sport of Canada.
23. Why is it desirable to paint an iron fence?
24. Where does a sailor spend most of his time?
25. What is the principal beauty of Niagara Falls?
26. Of what advantage is a hooked beak to a parrot?
27. Of what assistance to the duck is its webbed feet?
28. How many of your grandparents are living at present?
29. Why do people wear low shoes in summer?
30. Describe the appearance of a falling star.
31. Make a list of articles made of wool.
32. Why do we use more coal in winter than in summer?
33. Why is it dangerous to fall from a great height?
34. Name an organization for the benefit of the soldiers.
35. What is the color of the suit worn by policemen?
36. Why are electric lights covered by frosted shades?
37. When are roof gardens more comfortable than theaters?
38. What can be done to avoid teeth decaying?
39. In what way will prohibition benefit drunkards?
40. Name an animal that lives on vegetation.
41. For what purpose are life buoys placed in the water?
42. How many hours sleep did you have last night?
43. Name a large hotel in New York City.
44. What time of the year are parsnips planted?
45. What is the purpose of putting knobs on doors?
46. What city gets notoriety for baked beans?
47. Name a state belonging to New England.
48. What kind of shoe polish do you use?
49. Mention some important part of a lamp.
50. Why do men carry matches in their pockets?

9. Everyday Speech (CID)

A set of sentences has been prepared at Central Institute for the Deaf to represent "everyday American speech." The specifications for such a sample were laid down by a Working Group (chairman, Dr. Grant Fairbanks) of the Armed Forces–National Research Council Committee on Hearing and Bio-Acoustics. Some of the more important characteristics are as follows:

1. The vocabulary is appropriate to adults.

2. The words appear with high frequency in one or more of the well-known word counts of the English language.
3. Proper names and proper nouns are not used.
4. Common nonslang idioms and contractions are used freely.
5. Phonetic loading and "tongue-twisting" are avoided.
6. Redundancy is high.
7. The level of abstraction is low.
8. Grammatical structure varies freely.
9. Sentence length varies in the following proportion:

Two to four words	1
Five to nine words	2
Ten to twelve words	1

10. Sentence forms are in the following proportion:

Declarative	6	Imperative	2
Rising interrogative	1	Falling interrogative	1

The sentences have been recorded but have not yet (1959) been released for general use until the properties of the speech sample have been thoroughly studied. Ten talkers were employed, five male and five female. None were trained speakers. Much effort was devoted to obtaining natural, spontaneous, everyday inflection, tempo, and emphasis, with a realistic range of individual variation.

No "test" has ben developed from this material. It represents a sample of American speech of high face validity against which more specific tests of intelligibility or of "correct hearing" may be validated. In scoring the "correctness of hearing" of the new speech material, a system based on the correct repetition of fifty key words in each list of ten sentences has proved satisfactory.

The actual sentences, with the key words italicized, are as follows:

LIST A

1. *Walking's my favorite exercise.*
2. *Here's* a *nice quiet place* to *rest.*
3. *Our janitor sweeps* the *floors every night.*
4. It *would* be *much easier if everyone* would *help.*
5. *Good morning.*
6. *Open* your *window before* you *go* to *bed!*
7. *Do* you *think* that *she should stay out* so *late?*
8. *How do* you *feel* about *changing* the *time when we begin work?*
9. *Here we go.*
10. *Move out* of the *way!*

LIST B

1. The *water's too cold* for *swimming.*
2. *Why should I get* up *so early* in the *morning?*

3. *Here* are *your shoes.*
4. *It's raining.*
5. *Where are* you *going?*
6. *Come here when* I *call you!*
7. *Don't try* to *get out of it this time!*
8. *Should we let little children go* to the *movies* by *themselves?*
9. *There isn't enough paint* to *finish* the *room.*
10. *Do* you *want* an *egg* for *breakfast?*

LIST C

1. *Everybody* should *brush* his *teeth* after *meals.*
2. *Everything's* all *right.*
3. *Don't use up all* the *paper* when you *write your letter.*
4. *That's right.*
5. *People ought* to *see* a *doctor once* a *year.*
6. *Those windows* are *so dirty* I *can't* see *anything outside.*
7. *Pass* the *bread* and *butter please!*
8. *Don't forget* to *pay* your *bill before* the *first* of the *month.*
9. *Don't let* the *dog out* of the *house!*
10. *There's* a *good ballgame* this *afternoon.*

LIST D

1. *It's time* to *go.*
2. *If* you *don't want these old magazines, throw* them *out.*
3. *Do* you *want* to *wash up?*
4. *It's* a *real dark night so watch your driving.*
5. *I'll carry* the *package* for *you.*
6. *Did you forget* to *shut off* the *water?*
7. *Fishing* in a *mountain stream* is my *idea* of a *good time.*
8. *Fathers spend* more *time* with their *children than* they *used* to.
9. *Be careful not* to *break your glasses!*
10. *I'm sorry.*

LIST E

1. *You can catch* the *bus across* the *street.*
2. *Call her* on the *phone and tell her* the *news.*
3. *I'll catch up* with *you later.*
4. *I'll think* it *over.*
5. *I don't want* to *go* to the *movies tonight.*
6. *If your tooth hurts that much* you *ought* to *see* a *dentist.*
7. *Put that cookie back* in the *box!*
8. *Stop fooling around!*
9. *Time's up.*
10. *How* do you *spell your name?*

LIST F

1. *Music always cheers* me *up.*

2. My *brother's in town* for a *short while* on *business*.
3. *We live* a *few miles* from the *main road*.
4. *This suit needs* to *go* to the *cleaners*.
5. *They ate enough green apples* to *make* them *sick for* a *week*.
6. *Where* have *you been all this* time?
7. *Have* you been *working hard lately?*
8. There's *not enough room* in the *kitchen* for a *new table*.
9. *Where is he?*
10. *Look out!*

LIST G

1. I'll *see you right after lunch*.
2. *See you later*.
3. *White shoes* are *awful* to *keep clean*.
4. *Stand there* and *don't move until I tell you!*
5. *There's* a *big piece* of *cake left over* from *dinner*.
6. *Wait* for *me at* the *corner in front* of the *drugstore*.
7. *It's no trouble at all*.
8. *Hurry up!*
9. The *morning paper didn't say anything* about *rain this afternoon* or *tonight*.
10. The *phone call's for you*.

LIST H

1. *Believe me!*
2. *Let's get* a *cup* of *coffee*.
3. *Let's get out* of *here before it's too late*.
4. I *hate driving at night*.
5. *There was water* in the *cellar after that heavy* rain *yesterday*.
6. *She'll only* be *gone* a *few minutes*.
7. *How do you know?*
8. *Children like candy*.
9. *If* we *don't get rain soon*, *we'll have no grass*.
10. *They're not listed* in the *new phone book*.

LIST I

1. *Where can I find* a *place* to *park?*
2. *I like those big red apples* we *always get* in the *fall*.
3. *You'll get fat eating candy*.
4. The *show's over*.
5. *Why don't* they *paint their walls* some *other color?*
6. *What's new?*
7. *What are* you *hiding under* your *coat?*
8. *How come I should always* be the *one to go first?*
9. *I'll* take *sugar* and *cream* in my *coffee*.
10. *Wait just* a *minute!*

LIST J

1. *Breakfast is ready.*
2. *I don't know what's wrong with the car, but it won't start.*
3. *It sure takes a sharp knife to cut this meat.*
4. *I haven't read a newspaper since we bought a television set.*
5. *Weeds are spoiling the yard.*
6. *Call me a little later!*
7. *Do you have change for a five-dollar bill?*
8. *How are you?*
9. *I'd like some ice cream with my pie.*
10. *I don't think I'll have any dessert.*

A BRIEF GLOSSARY
OF AUDITORY TERMS

Several terms or usages employed in this book, particularly in Chapters 4, 5, 6, 7, 8, 9, and 16, are relatively new but are believed to be clarifications of or improvements over certain older usages. The following definitions (in logical rather than alphabetical order) form a self-consistent system and are in agreement with current American Standard Acoustical Terminology and, to the best of our ability, with relevant authoritative statements by the American Academy of Ophthalmology and Otolaryngology and the American Medical Association.

Hearing impairment. This is the most general term for malfunction of the auditory mechanism. It does not distinguish either the anatomical area primarily involved (central vs. peripheral), or the functional nature of the impairment (sensitivity, frequency range, discrimination, sense of loudness or of pitch, recognition of meaning, and the like). In a medicolegal context "hearing impairment" implies a severity sufficient to "affect personal efficiency in the activities of daily living," specifically in respect to communication. (The term "disability of hearing" is sometimes misused for "impairment of hearing." This is confusing in the medicolegal context because there "disability" has the added connotation that the impairment reduces a person's ability to engage in gainful activity. Impairment is only a contributing factor to disability.)

Normal hearing. "Normal" hearing refers to the hearing of a group of individuals of both sexes whose ears, on otological inspection, show no indications of present or past otological disease or anatomical deviation that might interfere with acoustic transmission, who have no history of past otological disease or abnormality, who are between the ages of adolescence and old age (approximately fifteen to sixty-five years), who have no hearing complaints, and who understand and cooperate in the tests of hearing that may be applied. Many psycho-acoustic relations have been established for such individuals, including threshold of sensitivity as a function of frequency, discrimination of loudness, of pitch, of words, and the like, as well as the relation of subjective loudness to physical intensity, and so on. For all quantitative tests of hearing such a group of normal individuals shows a range of performance. The performance of the group is usually expressed as the mean or the median accompanied by some measure of the dispersion (scatter), such as the standard deviation.

Normal threshold of hearing. The threshold of sensitivity for a group of normal-hearing individuals as defined above is a function among other things of the frequency of the test tone and of the age and the motivation of the subject. With respect to age, the hearing of adult subjects between approximately eighteen and thirty is usually found to be most sensitive and is chosen as the reference. The threshold is usually defined as the intensity of the tone which elicits responses on 50 per cent of the trials. The manner of listening (open acoustic field or under an earphone) and the place and method of measuring the sound pressure level must be defined. There are thus many different values for the normal threshold of hearing.

Reference level for audiometry or "audiometric zero." An arbitrary choice has been approved and published by the American Standards Association of a set of sound pressure levels, generated by certain types of earphone used for audiometry and measured in a standard acoustic coupler, to be used as the zero for the intensity scale of audiometers. This set of values was chosen to represent as well as possible the thresholds of hearing of normal young adults in the United States, as measured under the conditions of the United States Public Health Survey of 1936. The British Standard Audiometric Zero, based on other and more recent measurements, is on the average about 10 db more sensitive (lower sound pressure levels) than the American Standard. There is at present (1959) no International Standard for Audiometric Zero.

Hearing loss. This term has acquired three distinct meanings:

1. The symptom or condition of impaired hearing, particularly impairment of the sensitivity of hearing as tested by either pure tones or speech. For this meaning the terms "hearing loss" and "hypoacusis" are employed in this book.

2. The ratio, expressed in decibels, of the threshold of hearing of an ear at a specified freqency to a standard audiometric threshold. For this meaning the new term "hearing-threshold level" or "hearing level" is employed. This term should always be used instead of "hearing loss" when a numerical value in decibels is given. The set of standard

reference levels employed (American, British, or other) must be specified.

3. A change for the worse in an individual's threshold of hearing. This meaning carries the connotation of disease, injury, or deterioration, as in the common phrase "to suffer a hearing loss." To avoid these connotations the term threshold shift is often employed. It is helpful to specify whether the threshold shift is *temporary* or *persistent*. The consistent use of the distinctive terms "hypoacusis," "hearing level," and "threshold shift" is particularly helpful and desirable in medico-legal contexts.

Audiogram (threshold audiogram). An audiogram is a graph that shows hearing level as a function of frequency.

Hearing level for speech. Hearing level for speech (formerly hearing loss for speech) is the difference in decibels between the speech levels at which the average normal ear and a particular ear reach the same intelligibility, often arbitrarily set at 50 per cent. (There is no American Reference Standard for speech. Each speech test must be calibrated individually. For estimating the hearing level for speech in order to evaluate an impairment of hearing the Committee on Conservation of Hearing recommends the average hearing level for the three pure tones 500, 1000, and 2000 cps.)

Deafness (Anacusis). Deafness is the traditional term for a severe or complete impairment of hearing. For adults it should only be used if the hearing level for speech, estimated as recommended above, is 82 db (American Standard) or worse. This implies a hearing loss sufficient to make auditory communication difficult or impossible without amplification. For children the cutoff level is often set as low as 60 db for educational purposes, as explained in Chapter 16. "Deafness" usually implies that the abnormality is peripheral and is primarily a loss of auditory sensitivity.

Dysacusis. Any impairment of hearing that is not primarily a loss of auditory sensitivity is called dysacusis. The cause of dysacusis may be a malfunction or injury of either the central nervous system, the auditory nerve, or the sense organ. Dysacusis is not relieved, like hypoacusis, by simple amplification of speech, and therefore is not measured in decibels.

Among the many types of dysacusis are

Discrimination loss for words, syllables, or phonemes.

Reduced intelligibility for sentences.

Auditory agnosia or *central auditory imperception*. This condition is explained in Chapter 4. It is also called "sensory aphasia," "receptive aphasia," "auditory aphasia," or "word deafness."

Phonemic regression. This is the symptom, found in elderly folk, of loss of the ability to comprehend all of the words in a sentence, or even single words, spoken at normal tempo, in spite of relatively good sensitivity for pure tones or slow speech.

Recruitment. The recruitment of loudness (Fowler) is an abnormally rapid increase in subjective loudness as a function of sound pressure level.

Binaural diplacusis. In this condition a single pure tone, presented alternately to the right and left ears, is judged to have a different pitch in each ear.

Monaural diplacusis. In this condition a single pure tone, presented monaurally, is heard as a group of tones, a noise, or both.

Aphasia. Loss or impairment of the capacity to use words as symbols of ideas. The predominant defect may affect the ability to speak (*motor aphasia* or *expressive aphasia*) or the failure may be a lack of comprehension of the spoken word (*sensory aphasia* or *receptive aphasia*), or both. Receptive aphasia may be visual (*alexia*) as well as auditory.

Combined hearing impairment. This term implies the combination of hypoacusis (a peripheral reduction of sensitivity) with a central dysacusis. This term is not applied to a combination of conductive and sensory-neural hearing loss (mixed hearing loss).

Air conduction. Air conduction is the process by which sound is conducted to the inner ear through the air in the outer ear canal as part of the pathway.

Bone conduction. Bone conduction is the process by which sound is conducted to the inner ear through the cranial bones. (There is no American Reference Standard for hearing by bone conduction. Manufacturers try to approximate "normal" in their calibration of bone-conduction vibrators.)

Air-bone gap. The difference in decibels between the hearing levels for a particular frequency as determined by air conduction and by bone conduction.

Conductive hearing loss. A hearing impairment due to interference with the acoustic transmission of sound to the sense organ, usually in the outer or middle ear. (In pure conductive hearing loss, the hearing threshold levels measured by bone conduction are usually near normal and the air-bone gaps are large.)

Sensory-neural hearing loss. A hearing impairment due to abnormality of the sense organ, the auditory nerve, or both. Some or all hearing levels by bone conduction are abnormal, but the air-bone gaps are small or absent. (The old terminology was "nerve deafness," "perceptive hearing loss," and the like.)

Mixed hearing loss. A combination of conductive with sensory-neural hearing loss. This term is restricted by custom to peripheral hearing losses.

NAME INDEX

Agricola, R., 407
Albrite, J. P., 254
Aristotle, 405
Arnoldi, J. L. F., 407

Bárány, R., 152
Barry, K. E., 446
Beasley, W., 254
Bede, 407
Beethoven, L. v., 512
Békésy, G. v., 58, 75, 202
Bell, A. G., 409, 432, 494
Bell, A. M., 409, 432, 495
Black, J. W., 541
Boies, L., 503
Bonaparte, N., 495
Bonet, J. P., 407
Braidwood family, 409
Bulwer, J., 407
Bunch, C. C., 102

Cardano, G., 407
Clerc, L., 409, 419
Cox, J. R. Jr., 40, 267, 309

Dalgarno, G., 407
DeLand, F., 495

Eagles, E. L., 503
Edison, T., 512
de l'Épée, C. M., 408, 419
Ernaud, 407
Ewing, A. W. G., 422
Ewing, I., 422

Fairbanks, G., 548
Fitzgerald, E., 446

Fletcher, H., 181, 187
Fuller, S., 409

Gallaudet, E. M., 409
Gallaudet, T. H., 409, 419
Glorig, A., 107, 502
Goldstein, M. A., 409
Greenberger, D., 447
Greenmun, R. M., 493
Groht, M., 447

Heider, F. K. and G. M., 445
Heinicke, S., 408
Hirsh, I. J., 538
Holder, W., 407
Holmgren, G., 153
Hudgins, C. V., 429
Hughes, R., 537

Itard, J. M. G., 415

Jenkins, G. J., 152
Jeremiah, 406
John, Bishop of York, 407
Johnson, J. N., 497
Johnson, K. O., 502

Keller, H., 495
Kessel, 152

Larsen, L., 542
Lasius, O., 407
Lempert, J., 153
Lierle, D. M., 502

McGinnis, M., 448

559

SUBJECT INDEX